Panels

Phil Michal Thomas

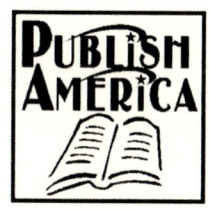

PublishAmerica
Baltimore

© 2004 by Phil Michal Thomas.
All rights reserved. No part of this book may be reproduced, stored in a retrieval system or transmitted in any form or by any means without the prior written permission of the publishers, except by a reviewer who may quote brief passages in a review to be printed in a newspaper, magazine or journal.

First printing

ISBN: 1-4137-3741-2
PUBLISHED BY PUBLISHAMERICA, LLLP
www.publishamerica.com
Baltimore

Printed in the United States of America

To those that continue to live within our hearts. Their lives are not forgotten.

There are many people that I owe my gratitude. Not only those individuals that shared their thoughts with me but also the countless numbers of friends, colleagues, associates, writers that supported me along the way. I would like to thank Susan Ford Wiltshire and Brenda Barnes. These two women were able to read an extremely raw draft and yet realize the real lives amidst the errors. To fine gifted writers such as Martha W. Hickman and the entire Nashville Writers Group for their much indebted support and experiences shared. To Pat Floyd, Nancy Crutcher, Ed Hendricks, Al Byrce, Bill Barnes, Bob Coleman, Lynda Lewis, Mattielyn Williams, Kathy Mathea, and the entire congregation of Edgehill United Methodist Church that believed in the Jesus story that reminded us that we are indeed a child of God as well as a wonder of God. To Dwayne Jenkins and the Brothers United Nashville Chapter for their tireless efforts to educate the African Americans of the risk of AIDS. To Dr. Stephen Raffanti, Dr. Lisa Brumble, Dr. Wendy Mangialardi, and Dr. Roy Sanders for never giving up on their patients when the patients themselves have given up on their will to live. To Comprehensive Care Clinic, Nashville Cares, Mental Health Cooperative, PFLAG-Nashville, Vanderbilt University Hospital and AID Atlanta for their dedication. To Robert Conley for his immeasurable support and encouragement especially for enduring countless midnight hours of hearing the typing sounds of the revisions in progress. To my family for their support especially my twin sister Phyllis and my grandmother, a real Duchess.

To finish my appreciation, I thank God.

I thought on the way to the Medieval Renaissance Festival would be a good time to tell her. It was on a hot Saturday afternoon in May that Cleo, her darling daughter, my godchild, Theresa, and I decided to escape from our stale world of routine life and go to a land of make believe. The radio blared in the background as Theresa perched herself forward between our seats. She was full of energy. An occasional bump in the road only made her laugh louder.

"So, Michal, where exactly am I driving us?" Cleo asked. "Where is this Medieval Renaissance Festival being held?"

"According to the directions, stay on this road until you come to the end of the road," I said. "It's near Triune."

"Where in the world is Triune?"

"Somewhere down this road. Just drive until it ends, I guess."

"The story of my life…always going to the end of the road or is it the end of the rope…I can't remember." She laughed.

"Whatever…just drive," I cut back at Cleo. She was so damn perky that it was getting on my nerves. I wanted to be serious. I wanted to talk to her.

"Mama, are we going to see a real castle with a real king?" .

"The castle may be real but I really don't think the king will be real…who knows, maybe it will have a queen."

"That's all we need are some more fake queens," I moaned.

"Lord knows you have had your fair share of queens."

"Uncle Michal, do you know a real live queen?" Her eyes beamed from innocence. I loved this dear child but I wished that she wasn't here with us today. I wished that I had Cleo all to myself. I was ready to talk. I so desperately wanted her to know.

" Not really…your mama was just talking nonsense."

"Oh, uncle Michal, I wish you and mama got married…then I will have you as my daddy!"

"Yeah, Michal, you should marry me and make me an honest woman."

Cleo smirked as she glanced across at me. "Imagine the expression on your parents' faces as we drive up for the holidays! I can see it now, a new version of 'Guess Who's Coming to Dinner.' It would be a hoot!"

"Whatever!" I paused.

"Uncle Michal, you never told if you knew a real queen!"

"No, sweetheart, I don't know any queens."

"Oh, Michal, don't be so modest…I'm sure you have fallen to the floor on your knees a few times and knighted."

"Whatever, anyway, Theresa, don't listen to your mom; the sun is making her crazy."

Cleo looked over at us and smiled. Theresa leaned over and hugged me from behind. I could smell the fragrance of her hair as she laid her head against my cheek. Her tiny hands folded over my head. She kissed the side of my face.

"There it is! There it is! I can see it! The castle…mama, there it is. But, mama, I don't see the draw bridge…and where's the water?"

"Baby, this is an American castle and the water isn't needed. But, isn't it lovely? Look at the beautiful gardens. "

"Well, I'm impressed already and I haven't even set foot inside."

"I can just see us living here. We would be so far away from the madness of the world. Finding peace and quiet. Michal, I might even let you have your own tower."

"I hate to burst your bubble, honey, but did you notice how close this mighty fortress is to the interstate?"

"What! How dare the peasants destroy my land with their shoddy wagons! I will have their heads! Command my soldiers to return my land back to me." Cleo laughed.

We toured through the massive stone building. The first room was the kitchen. Quite small and simple. A burning fireplace reflected across the cobble stone floor. Hanging overhead arches made me bend low to avoid hitting my head. Modern appliances were installed and appeared working. The path continued and my heart continued to race.

We climbed a narrow staircase to ascend to another level. An aged gent with a kilt and a Scottish accent was seated behind a long wooden table. Displayed were various pieces of armor as well as a Scottish coat of arms. We continued.

The higher we climbed, the narrower the stairwell became; my anxiety increased. Suddenly, we found ourselves in an open area that crossed over to the other side, which was locked.

"Just look! Look at this marvelous landscape. Beautiful stone sculptures and cozy benches around the flowers. Michal, honey, isn't this to die for!" Cleo was beside herself. "I would love to wake up around here and see this."

"Mama, why is glass missing from some of the windows?"

"It makes it easy to climb into and save the dame in distress," I said.

"I think they were called 'damsels' and not dames." Cleo lowered her eyes at me. "Honey, we will have to ask them why they don't have window panes, okay...You know, Michal, the only thing I would change is to make the rooms wider. I simply have to keep my antiques...the high ceilings are marvelous for the paintings. With the right lighted sconces and some track lighting, child, we got a winner."

"Theresa, be careful, your mama may be buying you both a castle."

"Good, then I can be a little princess. I can have my slaves do things for me."

"Honey, they are called hired help and not slaves," Cleo whispered.

"Is there really any difference?" I moaned.

"You'll be alright in the morning...Now, you guys, let's get ready and go see the human chess match." Cleo dashed away.

Theresa skipped along the road in total awe of the people dressed in period clothing. She was wide eyed with anticipation. Cleo and I tried to keep pace with her. Maybe Cleo was trying but somehow I felt myself slowing down. I didn't want to talk in front of the child.

Moments later, we sat on a row of wooden bleachers that semi-circled a grassy lot. People flocked to find any available seats before the match began. The sun was beating down on us. Cleo was busy applying sun block on both Theresa and herself. She dabbed the tip of my nose. There was no slight of a breeze in the air.

Inside the semi-circle were people dressed in various period clothing. Some carried swords. They were divided into social classes, one being of nobility while the other was the gypsy peasant. We sat on the side of the peasants. We cheered when they were victorious over the nobility and booed the nobility when they proved victorious over us. The grass was painted to create a rather large chessboard. Each participant stood in a square on opposite sides. Suddenly we had to stand as the King and his court arrived and was seated. The game began.

Glancing around me, I noticed people laughing and talking. Everyone appeared to be having fun, except for me. My heart was not really into the game. The sun became hotter as it began to beat across the back of my neck. I needed to talk to someone. I needed to talk to Cleo. I just had to tell her.

I watched as one of the peasant players fought against his adversary of nobility yielding a sword while he stood with only a book in his hands. He smirked rather confidently that he was prepared to battle because he had the book on sword fighting. He fenced while he read. He pranced about the ground with much glee. Nonetheless, his choice of weapons proved no match for his foe. Instead of tears, the crowd reacted in laughter while we booed the challenger.

As ludicrous as this may sound, I began to wonder if I was fighting my own battle in this same fashion. Instead of using a book, I was using silence. Was that using common sense, I wondered. I took a deep breath and turned to Cleo. This was the time.

"Have you heard the one about the guy that went to see his doctor about his health?"

"No, but is this a joke?" Cleo appeared puzzled and somewhat annoyed at my distraction.

"Well, maybe, anyway, there he was, sitting on the examination table staring out a window when his doctor enters. Before he could say anything, the doctor proceeds to tell him that he had just tested positive."

Cleo looked straight into my eyes. Her eyes appeared cold and stoned. I looked away from her glaring eyes. Now, I wished she was watching the chess match.

"What's the punch line to this morbid chatter?" Out of the corner of my eye, I could see that she was still watching me. I tried to ignore her staring. Finally, she turned back to the game. "Michal, what are you trying to say?"

"I really don't know…I'm still trying to find out myself."

"Mama, isn't this fun! And look, nobody's getting hurt for real."

"Yeah, honey, no one is being hurt…again." Cleo glanced over at me.

That conversation took place many years ago. I was such a liar and a coward. I tried to convince myself that I didn't tell her because I didn't want to hurt her anymore. She had already suffered from the hell of living through all the other deaths. Maybe I will tell her later, maybe. Maybe I'm wishing like hell that it was indeed a bad joke or even a bad dream and I will soon wake up. Maybe!

My name is Michal Cameron and I'm thirty-eight years old. Reared in St.

PANELS

Louis but formally educated in Nashville in more than one way. I'm also an African American gay male and presently single after being ditched for a newer model. What a waste of five years of my life. Naively, I just knew that our love would last forever. But does anyone ever really question his heart? Oh, by the way, I previously tested positive for HIV.

Years before the madness, I was surrounded by people similar to myself, people that were long forgotten and cast aside. Have you ever tried to actually put the square peg into the circle? Have you ever really tried to fit in where you didn't belong? Have you ever felt this way in your own family? I did, once for many years. However, that was before I found my new family: the circle.

I initially met some of the circle while attending Vanderbilt University School of Divinity while completing my masters. Everyone was unlike anyone else I had ever known. Yet, everyone appeared to genuinely feel concern for the others. Being someone with black skin didn't make a difference to him or her. Our tastes ranged from caviar to neck bones. We were a collage of misfits that demanded acceptance from the world as well as from ourselves.

The guy in my life at that time was my partner Antoine Stewart. We had the ultimate dream life, so I thought. You know, the Ken and Barbie thing except only there were two black Kens. We rented a small house on the north side of Nashville. For five years, we had it going on. We both were quite active at the Jordan Street Baptist Church. We kept our relationship on the down low, which meant we hide our secret. Or so, I thought.

Antoine and I often went to the Blair School of Music for the free recitals. Other than the taste for usual Snoop Doggie Dog, Mary Jo Blige, and house music, we also had a flair for classical music but could not always afford the tickets to the Nashville Symphony. We kept this fact from most of our black friends for fear they would consider us trying to be grandiose.

While I took classes in theology, Antoine was a dental student at MeHarry Dental College. Both of us struggled to pin point our careers. I pondered if I indeed wanted to minister to a flock. Why was I still going into a life where I wasn't accepted, I wondered. Although there were gays behind the pulpit, being open was out of the question. Somehow, the idea of counseling won out.

Antoine was from a small city near Detroit. Both of us came from meager homes where money was not always abundant. Our major common goal was to find out our own identities. In retrospect, I now wonder if we really had much more in common. But, before I digress further, I need to move on.

Of all my friends, Seth was the man! I had known Seth Mitchelson for what seemed forever. We became friends while students at Hillsboro High. Our friendship remained intact even after graduation from Vanderbilt years later.

Even in high school, his disciplined life aimed toward his goal of becoming a master pianist, but he also made time for a few others and me. Then he met Cleo Castleman when he was accompanist and she was a stage manager of a local theater production of *Pippin* at Vanderbilt University. I also had a part. I played Pippin, the son of Charlemagne, Emperor of the Holy Roman Empire. Life is full of irony. Finding my own corner of the sky has been as fruitless as Pippin's search.

By the time the musical ended, Seth and Cleo had become close friends. Seth brought Cleo along one night to a jazz concert in Centennial Park, and the three of us just seemed to click. Over the years, however, it became obvious to all of us that Seth and Cleo were closer than anyone else was in our circle of friends. I considered their relationship true love even then.

Cleo was the real woman in the circle that we all loved and adored. A true living doll! She was as beautiful as she was truly naïve. She was stuck in a loveless marriage to an old fart. I shuttered to think of his hatred for us. Nonetheless, she was still our girl. She always appeared to feel safe with the guys. But then again, why shouldn't she?

For the first time, I really felt as if I had found true friends, friends who had accepted me for who and what I was. You see, coming out of my closet was not a joy for me. After losing old friends and family members due to my disclosure, I simply stopped telling anyone else. I no longer went home for the holidays. Family gatherings became cold and traumatic. I felt as if I was a stranger in my parents' home. Years later, my parents still don't connect their phone lines with mine. Was it anger or guilt on their part?

I missed the closeness I shared with my family, but now, I found the love within the realm of the circle. My friends were my new family. Maybe, one day, I may find my God again.

Decades later, I wanted to capture my world in words. I wanted to record all that I could remember of my life over the countless years that the circle existed.. The happier times, you know, the Kodak moments. My conversations over the many years somehow gave me the courage and desire to share pieces of their lives. Somehow, I feel compelled to tell their stories. I want others to know them as I knew them. I wanted no stones unturned.

PANELS

My enthusiasm to complete this task rushed into my mind as strong as a summer storm. The unveiling of three thousands panels of the Quilt today in Centennial Park offered me a strong visualization of my reality of how death had encompassed not only myself but also the life around me.

My friendship with Cleo and my godchild Theresa weathered the raging storm. Although most of the circle had died before she became of age, Theresa held onto the countless stories told to her by Cleo or me. She said we were her uncles.

Less than a year later after the Renaissance outing, I found myself running back to Cleo and Theresa. After I turned into Centennial Park from West End, I saw the crowd. Rows of cars parked on both sides of the entrance drive that lead to the Parthenon. Cars were parked around the lake and at the amphitheatre. I also noticed people walking from across the street from the Sportsplex's parking spaces. Various groups of people walked toward the center of the park.

I eventually found a parking space near McDonald's and the Springwater Tavern. As I walked past the rustic tavern, I heard laughter. I closed my eyes briefly and thought about the past when I would go there with some of my friends to shoot pool or chug a beer over barbecue ribs. Laughter was still there, but it did not belong to my friends or me.

I cursed every step of the way as I walked up the slight incline. I really didn't want to come today. I was cold. I felt miserable. I had half-heartedly wanted the sky to rain. Instead, the sky was bare of any clouds. At that moment, the material appeared. Even as the people lined around the exterior, I still saw it.

The ground in front of the Parthenon, as far as the naked eye could see, was blanketed with countless square rows of fabrics. People were careful not to touch the exposed panels. Many onlookers watched as volunteers unfolded the sections. Their movements were reverent. The staffers slowly moved in unison to pick up the corners, back up, and then turn clockwise and set the block of the panels down on the covered land. Paths were created to allow walkers to read the individual names.

The park was void of any laughter or merriment. I just hoped I wasn't too late to read my list of names.

I didn't see Cleo at first. In fact, I hardly recognized anyone within the massive gathering. People were everywhere. I was getting quite frustrated and about to lose control when I heard a familiar child's voice.

"Mama, is it time to show my uncles' panels?"

"Soon, baby...it's almost time." Cleo grabbed the tiny arm of the little girl beside her. I watched as the child's eyes appeared glistened with anticipation as she looked into her mother's face. I watched as Cleo looked at Theresa with lingering eyes.

"Michal, I just knew you had stood us up."

"No, just running late...Man, look at all these people."

"It's obviously not too cold...God, I hope it doesn't rain." Cleo pulled at the collar around Theresa's sweater. She took her scarf and wrapped it around the child's neck.

"Uncle Michal, wait until you see what we did!" Theresa pulled at my pants.

"I'm sure, knowing your mama, you did a flawless job." I looked down into her big beautiful radiant eyes.

"I got my gloves on so I don't get them dirty. Mama said that we have to leave our pieces with the others...Do you think they are looking down from Heaven smiling at us?"

"Yeah, they are really proud of you. You helped give their life substance."

"Huh?"

"He meant that we have made something to remember them by."

"Oh, okay...good, 'cause I will always remember them...Uncle Michal, Mama said that she never wants to make another one. I don't mind helping. I like cutting out things. If Mama is too tired next time, will you help me, Uncle Michal?"

"Sure...I will help you."

"God, I hope there are no others to make...It was all I could do to make these...don't you even think about it, Michal."

"Yeah right, it's not like I sit and think about a panel in my name."

"Good, as long as we both know that, everything will be just fine."

"Mama, look at those panels! They have pictures of small kids like me! Did they die? Are they up there in heaven with my other uncles?"

"I'm afraid so..."

"But it's okay, Mama. I know they are playing with the angels in heaven."

"Out of the mouth of babes..." I said.

"Uncle Michal, I asked Mama to tell me something but she said she didn't know. Could you tell me why?" Theresa grabbed my hand and pulled me down to her.

"Sure, sweetheart. What do you want to know?" I knelt down.

"Were my uncles bad?"

PANELS

"No, not really bad, just crazy maybe." I laughed.

"Then why did God take them?" Theresa was locked on my eyes. "Mama told me I had the bad disease too, but I'm still here. Why did they have to die?"

"Maybe God wanted them for a reason and maybe you are here to give us hope…Each day, you open your eyes, we see God's love…It doesn't mean that they were bad or that God punished them, He just may need to work on them some more."

"Am I gonna die?"

"Naw, I'm gonna keep you here for a million years." I leaned over and picked her up.

"Oh, okay! Uncle Michal, now, don't you let anything happen to you. You the only uncle I got left." Theresa hugged my neck. "I will always love you."

"I will also always love you." I fought back the tears.

"Michal, it's getting really hard keeping up this face. I really don't know if I can read the names now. I need a drink."

"Yeah right. Cleo, you don't even drink."

"But I can always start. And baby, I don't know of a better time."

"Well, hello darlings…ooh, I just know that this little angel is Theresa. Oh my, look how she has grown…you are a big girl, now!" Our friend Sebastian's grandmother, the Duchess, was standing only inches from us. She opened her arms to hug Theresa. "Hello, Michal. Hello, Cleo."

"Hello, Mrs. Ingram. It's nice to see you again," I said.

"Oh, please, you can call me Duchess. That's what Sebastian always called me. And I know that you both were close friends of his. It's nice to see you both again. I just wished that it were under happier times. But, regardless, here we are!"

"Pardon me, Duchess, but have you seen Andrew yet? I know he was going to be here to display his friend's panel," Cleo asked.

"Have no fear, for I am here. Hello my sweethearts. Kiss. Kiss. Kiss. I would have never missed this moment for a million dollars…oh, who am I kidding, give me a few thousands and my ass would be grass." A very flamboyant aged man stood beside me. "You must be Michal? Hon, I have heard some marvelous things about you. Maybe I can find out later if any is true!"

"I'm sorry, but you are?" I asked.

"Oh, baby, just call me Andrew…in fact, you can call me anytime."

"Andrew Adstock! Behave yourself before I run you out of town myself…it's getting late, we better stop talking and head on over to the podiums." Duchess turned and walked away as we followed.

"Are you ready?" Cleo asked.

"No, not really. I kinda wished I hadn't signed up to read the names…there's something eerie about calling out the names of the dead."

"If that's true, why did you volunteer twice?"

"It's called lack of sanity."

"I hear you…but we can do it," Cleo assured me. "Theresa bounced out of bed before the crack of dawn this morning. She couldn't wait to get here. To be honest, I really don't think she is aware of the reason we are here. But, then again, I'm kinda glad she doesn't understand what's really going on."

"I don't know. I mean, after those questions she asked me, I sorta think she knows more than we think she knows."

"I was quite proud of you the way you answered her…I just can't do it. I just never know what to say…What do you tell a child about death? You can't just say someone has gone away because that child is gonna wonder when they're coming back…How do you tell a child the person is never coming back?"

"I don't know. I guess you just hope and pray that the good Lord will speak when you open that mouth again." I looked at Theresa. "She may be only six years old in age; however, what she had to live through just to make it to this day, made her older in wisdom. Can you imagine going through what she has at that age of your life?"

"Just look how energetic she is. Bouncing all over the place…She really was very proud when we finished the panels…I think she would have unveiled them the moment we drove into the park."

"Well, we must not disappoint her…Let's get the show on the road, folks!" I said. "Cleo, honey, you forgot to tell me about this Andrew fellow."

"Don't tell me you're interested."

"You need to get a grip…he's much too woman for me."

"See, that's why you're alone…you're too selective…who knows, he may be the man to light your world."

"And I may be the next Pope."

" Well, whatever…Lets get it over with." Cleo walked away after taking a deep breath.

We started walking towards the podiums. Suddenly, Cleo came to a sudden halt. Not expecting her to stop, I ran into her. She stumbled but did not fall.

"I'm sorry." I caught her.

PANELS

"Michal, I swear that I heard someone calling my name...it sounded like a man's voice."

"Oh no, its not that psycho ex-husband of yours, is it?"

"No, seriously, it sounded like...now you gonna really think I have flipped...but it sounded like one of the guys. When I turned around, no one was there."

"Cleo, maybe it was the wind."

"Huh, what are you talking about? What wind makes that kinda sound?"

"My dear, forgive me. I only said that because I didn't know what else to say."

She grabbed my hand and held it tightly. We ran to catch up with the Duchess and Andrew already at the podium.

Standing there, I could see across the park. The panels blanketed the earth. The panels were divided into sections covering the entire open field below the Parthenon. Each panel was 3x6 and sewn in blocks of eight panels. Volunteers carefully unfolded the materials and stretched them slowly to the ground. Each movement the volunteers took to unfold the edges appeared graceful and reverent.

Various colors and designs, some with pictures of people smiling, were displayed. Some panels were quite elaborate with specific characteristics of the individual while some panels showed only a name with their birth and their death.

People walked around the outer edges of the materials while stopping to read the names. I watched several pull tissues from nearby boxes and wipe their eyes. I could hear what sounded like stifled crying. I watched people embrace.

"I can't believe that damned fool is here protesting. I have half a mind to go over there and tell him what he can do with his signs." Cleo was irate.

"Of all days, this is certainly not the day. Where is his compassion?" I said after turning to where I saw a lone figure cloaked in a black cotton linen suit with a matching Stetson perched on his head. I knew who he was. The whole gay community knew this local fundamentalist preacher who always made his appearance at anything with an inkling of being gay. To him, we were all evil and doomed for the mighty fires of hell.

"You would think that if he was going to preach about the evils of Sodom and Gomorrah, that he would at least learn to spell it correctly before he put it on some poster."

"Cleo, my dear, I have known many religious fanatics in my lifetime.

Trust me when I say that usually a sense of compassion and intelligence doesn't always fall in line with those buffoons." The Duchess assured. "What I usually tell them is that my God tells me to love the sinners not the sin, which is why I love them."

"A few years ago in Atlanta, we did a human chain around a big time church after their preacher went on television and screamed that AIDS was God sent to all the fags from his pulpit. Hon, you better believe it hushed that little man up." Andrew bragged. "The lesbians shouted that they must be God's chosen since they are the least to be infected."

"I don't want Theresa thinking that there's anything evil about anything here today. It's not. Why did he have to come here?"

"Maybe he just has an attention disorder…you know…bad attention is better than no attention at all."

"Michal, perhaps you need to give him your card and schedule some therapy sessions with him." The Duchess smiled.

"Duchess, we would probably end up killing each other."

Above us, the icy sky appeared calm. The air was quiet. The wind blew cold on this particular New Year's afternoon.

Forgetting about the uninvited stranger, I watched as sporadic clouds of somber faces continued to gather around the delicately spaced pieces, fragments that depicted the lives of the fallen. Silent stillness encompassed the earth as individuals walked towards the center of the Parthenon.

Although most of the panels were displayed on the west lawn of the Parthenon, many panels were positioned on the front steps that lead into the massive structure. The enormous doors were open and Athena stood before me reaching to the sky of ageless wisdom. In my mind, she fearlessly stood guard over the fragmented fabrics.

I marched with the others with my head held high. I waited and listened as both the Duchess and Andrew read from their list of names. The names, the faces, and their souls forever engraved in the survivor's heart, at least I wanted to believe.

Standing in front of me, I noticed Cleo holding the pieces close to her breast. I also noticed that her eyes weren't watering anymore.

"Michal, as strange as it may sound, and I know it sounds mighty strange, but, at times, I wished that I could have felt their pain…I wished that I could have somehow shared it with them…Even now, I wish I could wave a magic wand across these pieces and they would be here in my arms instead."

" Cleo…I kinda know where you're coming from. I sort of wish the same

PANELS

thing, I mean, about them coming back…Now, I close my eyes and pray. Pray for that divine power to help me to let go without totally letting go."

"I felt so guilty working on Sebastian's panel before…before he even closed his eyes."

"Cleo, he was dying already. Whether or not you worked on the piece while he was still alive, wouldn't have made any difference."

"But.."

"No but's, Cleo. You didn't kill him. AIDS did!"

I glanced over at Andrew as he waited his turn. He now appeared rather sedated and numb. He wasn't flaming this time. Tears streamed down his face behind the Ray Bans' dark lenses.

Now it was my turn to read. While waiting to salute the dead, I glanced out at the multitude of the panels. Tears began to collect in my own eyes. I no longer saw the fabrics but the actual people represented. I wanted to scream. I wanted to run, run far away from this madness, from this hell.

My voice began trembling as tears clouded my vision. I took a deep breath. I had to be strong. I had to finish this moment.

"Anthony Tompkins…Ezra White…Gladys Williams.."

"Open the gates of Hell for your bastard children, Satan!"

"James Evans…Tim Meeks…Baby Marcus…"

"May they all burn in Hell!"

"Jessica Sims…Marcus Withers…Tim Simmons…Darcy…"

"Repent and save your soul from Hell!"

I searched around the crowd until I saw him. He was standing at the top of the hill. Armed with his religious posse and a bullhorn, he continued yelling his damnations. The preacher had returned. With the sun directly behind him with a raised bible in his right hand, this over zealous yelled as his meager group of followers chanted in response. Standing behind the park rangers, they were careful to keep a safe distance from us.

"Go on, read the names. Ignore the bastard!" Someone yelled from close range.

"Yeah, screw him!"

I continued reading and he continued blasting me. The more I tried to ignore him the more he blasted away.

"Deshawn Williams…Mario Jenkins…Crystal Gibbens…Baby Joshea…"

"Repent or you shall suffer eternity in Hell."

" Linda Swanson…Lenny…Casey…Rich…" I dropped the paper. Oh God, no! It was Richard's name. My heart stopped cold. "I can't do this anymore." I turned to Cleo. "I just can't do it!"

"What's wrong?"

"Cleo, Richard is one of us! Have you forgotten that? I just can't do it."

"Michal, you can…ignore the bastard…don't even give him a thought. Just remember why you are here."

"I'm sorry." I turned away and ran from the stage.

Leaning against the far column, I prayed to God to please help me. I prayed to God to forgive me for hating these people for bringing this reality…my reality…home to me. One day, there will be a panel for me and there's not a damn thing that I can do about it.

Later, as we strolled through the countless rows of blocks of panels, we talked about our feelings. Around us, in every direction, I heard muffled crying. Still, other people came and stood before the podium. They listened while others read names.

"I'm sorry…I really thought I could do it…but seeing his name was more than I could take."

"It's okay, I know. That was one of the hardest things I have ever done in my life…I wonder if people really understand what this is all about?"

"I feel like a bumbling fool. I screwed up…something as important as that, I lose it."

"Well, that asshole certainly didn't make matters any easier," Cleo reassured. "Where the hell is Act-Up when you need them?"

"I really thought I could do it. But when I saw Richard's name…I saw his face. I heard his laughter."

"Michal, you are not alone. I almost lost it a few minutes ago when I saw the children panels…the smiles on their faces trying to hide their God-forsaken pain and misery," Cleo whispered.

I took notice to how she was looking at Theresa. Was she still afraid of the virus returning inside Theresa, I wondered?

"Yeah, I can imagine…Hey, did you see how everyone got so quiet when Kathy Mattea was singing?"

"Yeah…something about hearing voices calling us home."

"Cleo, she was singing so passionately as they raised the blocks off the ground…it was almost as if she felt our pain."

"Did you know she takes a few panels with her on her concerts?"

"No, I didn't…I do remember seeing her at the first Walk for AIDS. Ever since then, I have been in love with her and her music. It's so real!"

"You mean that I have competition? I'm supposed to be the only woman in your life."

PANELS

"Cleo, of course you're the only woman for me." I smiled. " You know, she really put herself on the line speaking for us. I mean, not too many good old boys would understand what this is all about."

"That's what makes her so special...being able to love and not fearing the unknown."

"I hope the panel I made for Jonathan will be displayed with the rest from Georgia. Maybe then, I can have final closure and continue on with my life." Andrew joined us.

"Andrew, is that possible, I mean, to finally have closure on something far too painful to forget?" Cleo said.

"Something I learned years ago was the truth behind the adage of time healing pain. If you look at it in this perspective, compare it to coming out of the woods: it will take you just as long to leave from the woods as it took you to go into the woods." The Duchess lightly patted my hand. "There are no short trails to take but the same path. However, you exit with more experience and knowledge of what to expect. But, then, we sometimes stop to dwell on something still in the woods which slows us down." The Duchess' voice appeared calm.

"I guess it wouldn't be so hard if only I hadn't lost so many friends," Cleo whispered. "But I still have my Michal, don't I?"

"That's why we have to hang in there together, for each other." The Duchess clutched Cleo's arm gently.

"It's funny how strange thoughts can cross your mind at the weirdest times. I was just remembering something that Sebastian had once said about situations. He would laugh and say, 'Have you ever noticed that every time your life is screwed up, you are there.'"

"He certainly had a way at looking at life. His grandfather was just like him. When Sebastian lived with us, he and his grandfather would often engage in long thought retching conversations like two old men."

"Is there any real sense to death? What are the criteria for selection? I'm no smarter than anyone else but I'm still alive," Andrew said.

"Michal, this is the guy I was telling you about. Andrew and I met at a support group for survivors. Andrew was the primary care giver to his best friend Jonathan. He had died less than a year ago after fighting his only battle with pneumonia."

"Baby, that group helped me when I was at my lowest...Hell, we had to take straws at who would cry next. I knew I would just love Cleo the first moment I laid eyes on her." Andrew laughed. "Too bad she's not a man"

"Anyway, you couldn't handle me if I was a man." Cleo smiled. "As Andrew told his own story, my eyes just glistened with familiar understanding."

"Honey, Jonathan absolutely loved him some Pattie Labelle...chile, to him, there was no other rhythm and blues singer worth listening to..." A smile of restored definite pride beamed across Andrew's face. "But, honey, that night she called, I thought I would just die. I was half asleep and almost curse the poor girl out 'cause I thought some trick was playing a joke...but anyway, it was the real thing...you see, some time ago, I had sent her a letter regarding Jonathan."

Tears filled his eyes as he told us how Pattie had promised him that Jonathan would never be forgotten as long as she had anything to do with it. *The ultimate gift*, he thought.

We began to circle back to the front of the Parthenon for the dedication of the new panels. Our friends would now join others in the Quilt.

Sweat rolled off my brow as I anxiously awaited the union. As Cleo and Theresa watched their own creations breathe their own life, Theresa let out a proud yell. We watched as warm but unfamiliar hands manifested the panels and placed the pieces delicately side by side forming their own block. As the block was lifted, I gasped for air.

"Michal, isn't it amazing how something so soft and cuddly could be so strong with emotion?"

"Someone once said something about the Quilt being the loudest quiet advocate in the world...now I think I know what they meant."

"Standing here looking at all of this reminds me of a banner I once saw at that church where Richard's memorial was held."

"You mean Edgehill, don't you?" I asked. "Did you know that was once a garage?"

"Yeah, I think Richard told me that once...but, Michal, the colors were gloriously brilliant...as Bradley would say 'flawless fabo.'...I saw it as a light that surrounded a lone figure...man. I imagined myself being that lone figure standing below the illuminating bright rays of yellow, encircled with the expanding rings of purple, lavender, orange, peach, and red against that beautiful dark blue sky..." Cleo paused.

"In my mind, all of you guys were being drawn into God's almighty loving hands but, somehow, I felt that everyone was waiting for me to join in."

"Oh no, don't tell me I am gonna have to spend eternity with Bradley and David!"

PANELS

"You will, and you will love it! We will party until we get the boot."

"Did I tell you that I have started going there?"

"Seriously?"

"Yeah, I kinda enjoy it. They don't make me feel like trash…they told me I was a 'cog.'"

"What, may I ask, is a 'cog'?"

"A child of God…Cleo, do you have any idea how long it's been since someone told me I was anything to God?…I can see why Richard used to rant and rave about that place…they make me feel good about myself."

"Speaking of Richard, guess who may be here today?"

"Kari?"

"Yeah, isn't that great! "

"Cleo, you're lying. Is she really going to be here? Man, I haven't seen her in years. How is she doing? Did her brother come with her?"

"Yeah right, no, she is coming alone. I had written her about the panel I made for Richard. I was actually shocked when she called me."

"She was his heart. Richard only spoke of her, never anyone else in that family."

"Well, considering what they put him through when he came out to them, could you blame him? His own family. I wonder if they even know that he died."

"I asked Kari that…and the impression I got was that they could care less. He was already dead when he left home."

"That really pisses me off. People look at us with hatred without even knowing us. Richard really missed his mom…you know, he once told me that the first time he went to that church, there was this older white-haired black woman that he locked eyes with…he said she reminded him of his mother. He called her 'Ms. Laura.'" I paused. " Richard said he knew he had found a home there after this woman nodded with a smile. He told me that he felt accepted."

"Does this mean you may start preaching?"

"Who knows, stranger things have been known to happen."

Cleo appeared to have wanted to say something but one look at the Quilt, her words disappeared into silence. I just knew deep down that her passion was ringing loud against her heart.

The material flapping in the wind brought us back to reality. Filled with vast impregnated emotions, we quietly watched as eight panels were divided and carefully attached to form larger twelve-foot square sections. Stitched painfully together from vast tears and grief as well as love for those who have moved ahead to the outer perimeter of a life. Panels stood bold with emotional purposes that I felt included the individual's hope.

I was impressed by the fact that the finished three by six feet panels created a remarkable impression of one's life. Similar to the power of life, once a name has been stitched onto the fabric, the cloth takes the form of someone's previous existence. It served as a tool for those of us still dealing with the sudden removal of the fallen to continue to visualize the now silent laughter, their faces, and their souls.

"Occasionally I find myself popping a pill and calling it a day. I refuse to deal with this shit around me...Many of my friends live or should I say merely exist in various stages of dying...People do die, you know." Andrew was visibly shaken.

With the sight of Jonathan's panel being raised to the sky, Andrew fell to his knees sobbing. Instinctively, Cleo cradled his head in her hands. I felt a sense of awe as I saw the matted singing angelic figurine with the name 'Pattie' stitched below Jonathan's name.

Once again, we found ourselves preparing to read more names. Once again, I barely made it through my list before my own eyes began to water. I stepped out of the way to let Cleo read from her list.

Slowly, with an unsteady gait, I watched as she unraveled a crumpled piece of weathered stationery. I saw her hands trembling and her eyes were closed. As her eyes opened, I noticed her eyelids trembling. Cleo read each name slowly. Her pain obviously did not overwhelm her this time. I was amazed at just how emotionally strong she appeared. Others waited calmly for her to finish her tribute to her friends' lives. She repeated our friends' names again.

Someone had quietly approached Cleo. The stranger was a woman with a smile of comfort. She also reached out attempting to console the Duchess as tears fell from her porcelain face.

"I'm so glad to see you both!"

"Same here...Michal, I want you to meet Beth Wilkerson...Beth, this is Michal Cameron...Beth is one of the shoulders I cry on in our support group."

"Pleased to meet you, Michal."

"Thank you for being there for Cleo and the Duchess." I said as I extended my hand. Her hand was very soft and warm as the color of her eyes.

"Unfortunately, I know all too well of the heart's discomfort in seeing

PANELS

someone dying...I watched my brother John suffer until the end. But, my indestructible faith in God allowed me the strength to give him permission that would allow him to finally complete his lone journey with my forthright love," Beth said.

"My sentiments exactly...I would have never wanted my Sebastian to suffer any longer than he had to...I, too, feel that God is taking care of him...but, somehow, I rather not believe that his journey was by himself." The Duchess smiled.

"You're probably right." Beth said. Her voice seemed sincere and not patronizing.

"I noticed you have numerous signatures on your panel."

"Yes, Michal, the signatures are from all people that not only had known him but also somehow had their lives touched by John."

"That's really beautiful...how did you get them to sign their names?"

"Cleo, that was easy...I merely told others about my brother. Talking about him really helped me deal with his death."

" I think all I do is cry."

"It's okay to cry. It's okay to hurt over the loss of your friends."

"That's probably true, but I think I have cried enough...Yes, I miss them. But I'm tired of crying...my tears have turned to anger. I'm ready to fight but not sure whom to fight."

"Michal, fighting may only work briefly, but the physical void is still going to be there. As I said before, I made my panel for John to help me deal with him leaving me. I still need to talk about his death to others. Maybe, his life will not have been in vain."

"Yeah, I understand what you are saying, Beth. But if I thought that by crying, my tears would wash my hurt completely away, I would flood a river, to know that I had done everything possible for my friends." Cleo brushed her hair from her face.

"You guys, ask yourself what more could you have done? Could you have actually prevented their deaths? Probably not, but you could be there at their sides when they needed you the most, and you were," Beth said. "Take pride in knowing that you gave your friends their flowers while they could still enjoy the fragrances."

"Cleo and Michal definitely followed through with that job...they gave my brother bouquets of flowers while I gave him nothing." I turned around and saw another fallen friend's sister Kari standing behind us. "You guys proved more of a family to him than his own family."

"Kari, thanks for coming."

"Thank you, Cleo, for telling me about today…when you told me what you was doing, I knew I had to be here." Tears formed in the crevices of her eyes. "You know, he was a good person with a damn good heart."

"Yeah, he was."

"Kari, don't you ever say that you did nothing for your brother…you were there when he needed you. You never turned your back on him."

"Michal, I could have done more. Damnit, he was my brother!"

"You're here today, aren't you?" Beth took Kari in her arms and wiped the tears away. "That's all that matters."

The sun was setting over the Parthenon. The shadows became faint. The sky was painted with a backdrop of purple and pink hues in the horizon. There appeared a sense of calmness and serenity. Staff and volunteers began dissembling the Quilt for storage. People began walking away from the park. Voices echoing from the sympathetic crowd became soft soothing chants that whispered.

Somehow, I felt that our hearts would eventually accept that although sadness was indeed present that love itself never dies. We walked away but definitely not alone. I began to understand that the love that I had once shared with my friends merely becomes imprinted on an indestructible surface: the survivor's heart.

Night was quickly drawing near.

Sebastian was my personal therapist so to speak. Both he and Richard appeared older in their actions than the rest of us. Both always tried to protect us from all harm and at times, us. No matter what time I called, he was always there for me.

Although he was quite nurturing to us, he, himself, didn't always have a shoulder to cry on. I remember Sebastian telling me of his own experience with his family. Isn't it ironic just what we choose to remember from our early childhood? Sebastian swears he recalls the conversation between his father and the Duchess.

"You know, before I began living with the Duchess, I used to feel abandoned. Thrown away like yesterday's garbage. My own dad standing in front of me telling the Duchess that they didn't need me. But, the Duchess didn't take his lame excuse and blessed him out for bringing me up in their hellhole of a marriage…" Sebastian paused.

PANELS

"So, where was your mama while this was going on?"

"Oh, she was still in the car. Probably drunk, who knows. That's how I best remember her, always with a pint between her lips. Other mothers wore perfume and smelled like flowers, my mom smelled like some damned brewery...Anyway...the Duchess went off on my old man telling him that our family didn't walk away from each other...there I was, maybe seven or eight years old, hearing that shit about how he felt about me."

"So, how did you get with your grandparents?"

"They went to court and saved my poor ass soul...It wasn't too hard since my folks were ready to give me up for adoption...Michal, the rest is history."

"Do you ever see your old man now?"

"Naw...You would think that since the Duchess is his own mother that he would at least drop by to see her. But, hell, he doesn't even do that...I'm not worrying about it anymore...that wasting good energy for bad, and baby, he ain't worth it."

"Do you hate them?"

"Naw, well.. I won't lie. Yeah, I used to hate them but now I feel sorry for them. I used to wish that his ass would lose it all on Wall Street and my mom would become allergic to alcohol. No such luck...If I say so myself, they missed out on a grand opportunity to have me in their life."

"How long did it take you to get over it?"

"I'm not really sure I am completely over it...maybe I'm suffering from post traumatic stress disorder." He laughs. " I still have flashbacks of my father telling me he's sorry and walking to his car and driving away while I held onto the Duchess's hand. Tears were falling down my face as the car sped away...I remember looking into the Duchess's eyes and making her promise me that she would never leave me...and you know what? She never has."

I once asked Cleo how she actually met Sebastian. She told me that she was introduced to Sebastian while sharing a political science class in the Calhoun Hall.

"I always considered him to be quite attractive...a hunk."

"Cleo, was you not married at the time...what were you doing looking?"

"Oh, is it that way now? Men can gawk broads all day but let a woman glance curiously over at a man, and she's evil." Cleo laughed. "Anyway, if my memory serves me right, you also thought he was tasty."

"Yeah, but then insanity left me."

"Whatever! Anyway, he always ran from class. He would walk right by me as if he was in a fog. Sebastian always smelled great. Baby, I never knew what cologne he wore, but it always left me wanting more…He really didn't speak to anyone in the class. I knew he a bit of a loner…but he was still a cutie."

"So, how did you guys hook up?"

"Well, one afternoon after class, I zipped by 'Fido' in the Village for a cup of brew. That place was packed with people. You know how they go there to study or read the papers…anyway, while waiting in line, I heard this familiar voice behind me. Honey, before I turned around, I knew it was him by his cologne."

"Yeah, he loves his cologne. He spends more on his fragrances than I spend on my clothes."

"No comment! Anyway, the waitress asked me what I wanted and I told her a *'Dalmatian'* and a chocolate chip cookie. All of a sudden, this voice asks me if I'm sure I'm ready for the sugar rush. I turned around and he was just standing there smiling from ear to ear. So, I asked him if he had a better selection. You know, I was really trying to be really coy about it."

"So, did you sort of remove your wedding ring?"

"Maybe…anyway, we ended up sharing a table together. I mean, we had to since the place was so crowded." Cleo smiled.

Within the circle, Sebastian appeared to love each of us but in different ways. He told me once that he saw reflections of himself within us that made him both comfortable and uncomfortable. Whenever he spoke of his parents, he would also mention to me that he envied a few of us for our innocence and our ability to forgive unconditionally. Some of us gave him a sense of total assurance. He said we brought back his forgotten laughter.

Over the years, I began to learn more about Sebastian. In private, Sebastian was an introverted oppressed poet. He described this avenue as being the only instrument to battle mankind, his often silent words.

On the surface, Sebastian often displayed irritable and vindictive responses. He would appear bitter towards the world. I always felt that without us, he was forever the loner. In the midst of pity, he said he felt as if his life ended the existence of the happiness in others.

With the void of his natural parents in his life, his grandparents had refused to further downcast any of the necessary love that he longed for. He appeared to worship his grandparents especially his grandmother. He nicknamed her "Duchess." To him, she possessed the grandest southern airs spiced with daring wit and grace.

PANELS

Over the many years of our friendship, I soon realized just how he refused to allow anyone else to penetrate his inner structural sanctum. In contrast, he would wear a gentle but rather stoic smile masking his pain.

In later conversations, he would disclose more of his relationship with his grandmother. The "Duchess" and Sebastian had shared intimate moments of his youth. She was always there in the middle of the night whenever he awakened wet and shivering with perspiring fears from his nightmares. With her, he knew he was never alone.

Amidst the various clutters of wooden sculptures in his bedroom were books that filled the cedar boards. He was well versed in literature as he had always used his reading as an escape. According to Sebastian, the literary world offered him much freedom to be himself without ridicule.

His stubbornness prevailed miserably at times. Duchess had long taught him to never give up on his dreams and to fight to believe in their strengths. But, as I would learn later from him, Sebastian had a painful past he wished he could have forgotten.

"When I was a senior in high school, a bunch of us would get together on the weekends and go parking…in the back alley of a bookstore…you know, the seedy ones. Man, you won't believe the traffic of old farts trying to get one on…"

"Man, you guys went to a peep show?" I asked. "Wow, what was it like?"

"Hell if I know. We were jail bait, couldn't get in if we wanted to…we would sit in cars and watch those perverts run inside like somebody was after them…somebody would have brought weed or our friend "Jack." We sit around talking. Mostly lies, I'm sure. Somebody would be lying about some crazy thing they did. Some would brag about their tricking…I know I lied my ass off. I didn't want them to know that I had never even touched another man."

"Sebastian, you're telling me you was a virgin your senior year?"

"Yeah, I guess that's what I was…hell, I didn't even know what I wanted at that time…so I played along. Man, I got stoned out of my mind."

"You, Mr. Conservative, got blasted off your ass? Yeah, right!"

"I'm afraid so…but, you know what? That was the last time I ever let myself lose all control."

"Man, I can't imagine you wasted. You are always in such control. Hell, we always depend on you or Richard to drive our drunken ass home."

"Sometimes, being the boss, you have to pay the price."

"Meaning?"

"Meaning being wasted got me raped!"

"What! How? I mean where did it happen?"

"I was sitting inside a car. I think. We were all drinking "Jack" straight. That I know...I felt myself getting stoned. I think I tried fighting the liquor. Too late...my head was spinning and strange shit was dancing in my mind...Like a bad dream, the door opened suddenly and I was grabbed out of the car. I was being pulled away while I faintly heard my friends laughing."

"Was it the cops?"

"I wished it had been...but no, it wasn't...I hit the ground and passed out." Sebastian closed his eyes. "I finally woke up in hell. I couldn't breathe...I felt pressure on my head...something was forcing me down...I wanted to vomit...I tried turning my head away from the vomit and putrid smell, but I couldn't move...The light hurt my eyes when I tried to open them." Sebastian took a breath.

"Oh no, what did you do?"

"I couldn't do anything but lay there...out of the corner of my eye, I saw the bastard...some long haired blond guy that I had never seen before...all I could remember of him was a tattoo of a wizard on his right arm...wait a minute, why am I telling you this?"

"Because you can..."

"Do you realize just how embarrassing this is? I vowed to myself that I would never tell anyone about this night...I just want to erase everything about it from my head." Tears rushed down his face.

"Sebastian, it wasn't your fault."

Sebastian closed his eyes. "I winced at the pain as the brute grabbed me by the nap of my hair pushing me down to his dick...I gagged at the smell of his filth and stench...I tried pulling away but the asshole slapped me harder across my head...I could feel my blood trickle down my face clouding my sight, except I could see his round pale face smiling at me...I looked into his face seconds before he plowed his fist into my mouth. I think I blacked out."

"That cold hearted bastard!" I didn't know what to say at this point.

"When I came to, he was gone...my whole body ached as pain shot through me. My left wrist was bleeding and still tied over my head to the bedpost. I tried rolling onto my left side but I hurt too damn much. My ribs were swollen...the insides of my legs were stripped with scratches still bleeding...Somehow I got free...I found the bathroom and vomited on the basin after I saw my face. I just stood there. Shocked, I didn't utter a sound. I had to make sure I was alone...my bottom lip was cut open, my backside felt as if it was ravaged by some crazed animal...My body started to shiver...all I could do was let out a scream."

"Didn't someone hear you?"

"If they did, no one came...you know, I could never decide what was worse: knowing the assailant who had left me for dead or not knowing the bastard's identity...For years, I kept the pain so embedded deep down in my mind, I thought I would go crazy. Maybe it was God's way of punishing me for what I am sexually attracted to. I wondered. I used to wonder if my attraction to older men was maybe my desire to mend fences with my old man."

"Sebastian, you know that is not true. God is not evil. Man, you mean to tell me, that you have carried this on your shoulders?"

"Actually, no. I regretfully told two of my childhood friends. Their reactions were quite perplexingly indifferent towards me...it appears that they both felt I had brought this rage on myself...Needless to say, we are no longer friends."

"Did you ever tell your parents?"

"Hell no! I kept this from my grandparents as much as possible although I felt certain that they somehow already knew."

"So you think your grandmother found out?"

"Probably, but, nonetheless, between the 'Duchess' and myself, nothing mattered unless we spoke openly about it...Silence is our ever-bridging bond."

When Sebastian first met Bradley, he would say that their meeting was possibly fate. It was a cool autumn night with brisk winds snapping through clothing. The dead leaves fell to the earth after discoloring and detaching with help from the wind.

For five years, Sebastian was intimately involved with Daniel. They had shared a home and raised their two spoiled golden retrievers: Anita and Sandy. The only thing missing from this happy home was the white picket fence.

Their relationship with each other often fluctuated from being at odds to being positively hopelessly romantically involved. Your basic gay Lucy and Ricky even with the madness.

Right after Daniel had tested positive, Sebastian said their sex life was put on immediate hold. Daniel, according to Sebastian, didn't want to take the chance of possibly infecting Sebastian. Sebastian said he realized the reason but still felt slightly rejected. Their intimacy became rare and limited.

"Sebastian, how do you control yourself? I mean, I doubt if I could live with someone and not want to touch him…have you been to the lake?"

"Michal, I won't lie…my eyes still wander when I see something tasty, but the idea of me tricking at the lake ain't for me. Besides, I really love him…I would never do anything like that to him. Sex isn't everything, you know!"

"You know there are supposedly safer ways to you know."

"Yeah, I know…but he's not willing to take that chance. I will survive."

"Sebastian, my dear, you can't tell me that you guys have gone from being like too rabid rabbits to being…oh, I don't know of anything so asexual…like two earthworms." I threw my hands in the air. "And no, Ms. Gloria was not talking about no sex to survive."

"Michal, you are so wicked, but I love you anyway."

One cool night in March, Daniel didn't come home. Sebastian stared out of the open window into the darkness. Wind rustled the oak leaves, the air smelling of damp earth and spring flowers. Daniel should have been home by now. So, where was he? Fear crawled over Sebastian like a rash. The words *sick* and *hurt* bounced in his head.

Turning, Sebastian went to the telephone and dialed a number. Cleo picked up on the second ring.

"Hello!"

"Cleo, this is Sebastian…Have you seen Daniel today?"

"No, I haven't. In fact not for several days. Not since you guys were here on Sunday."

"He hasn't come home yet…I'm starting to get…"

"Don't worry, Sebastian. He's probably caught in traffic after work. You know there are a lot of jams on the interstate with the construction going on…hey, honey, to ease your mind, Seth, Michal, and I will form a posse to help find him. Okay?"

"Thanks, I appreciate that…do me a favor and leave a message if you find out anything."

"Honey, don't worry, we will find your man for you."

I had turned down my bed when there was a knock at the door. It was Sebastian. He was upset and crying. It was over. Sebastian told me that Daniel's voice matched the apathetic words, words that sounded distantly cold and clearly empty. Sebastian described Daniel's voice as being void of certain feelings of the slightest passion. There was no quivering in his tone as he tried to explain that he needed more out of life than a relationship.

"I waited two more hours after I called you. Daniel still wasn't home so I went looking for him…I drove a few blocks over to Percy Priest Dam…Michal, my inside felt like it was exploding…I was sick at my stomach…Daniel was in another man's car. *No, God. Let it not be true!* But God wasn't listening to me."

"Sebastian, I'm sorry to hear this…Are you alright?"

"I wanted to kill him. I wanted to kill that bastard…Daniel was sitting at an angle facing some strange man. He didn't even see me get out of my car. I just sat on a boulder and stared."

"Did anything happen? Did he ever see you?"

"I doubt it…He was too busy working his ass…Can you believe this shit? After all I have done for him. This is how he pays me back…"

" Did he ever come home?"

"Yeah, finally…I was laying across the sofa in the den. He came in the room. He sat down across from me…It was all I could do to not hit him…He had that smirk on his face that I wanted to slap into yesteryear."

"Sebastian, honey, you had more restraint than I could have had. Did he ever say where he was?"

"Yeah, get this; the hospital! I looked him straight in the eye and told him that he was a bald face ass liar…I told him that I saw him tricking at the dam."

"Well, alright! Speak the truth and it will set you free! What did he say to that?"

"Daniel looked across the coffee table at my ring that I had just taken off. Daniel told him that he no longer felt that he was in love with him but that he still loved me."

"Did you slap him? I would have…"

"No, I just looked at his pathetic ass…I just wanted him to get the hell out."

"I hate to say this, but you really can't say that you didn't see this coming. I noticed that you guys had been apart for quite awhile."

"Thanks, Michal. Thanks for the great words of encouragement." Sebastian appeared cold. "What's to say?…Why should I say anything?…Daniel obviously made his choice…I can't make him love me."

"Can you guys be friends at least?"

"I'm not sure I want him as a friend…I'm not even sure I know who Daniel is anymore…I thought I did but obviously I was sadly mistaken." Sebastian looked away so that I would not see the mounting tears.

"Sebastian, you know sometimes people grow apart."

"Five years, damn it, five long years...Was it the relationship itself that is smothering him...or was it me? Why, now all of a sudden, did he decide to break things off? Was his living with me been nothing but a complete lie?" Sebastian was crying. "Stupid asshole me, I just thought that after he tested positive, that maybe we would be there for each other...no, not the answer...Instead he wants to cruise that damn lake for quickies..."

"Now, Sebastian, you know that simply because someone is positive ain't a good reason to stay in a relationship."

"I didn't tell you that he called all of you crazy psychos and that I was sleeping with everyone including Cleo."

"That boy got a mighty truck load of issues...He was only trying to relieve his guilty conscious by saying you were having us."

" I told him that he knew damn well I'm wasn't sleeping with anyone!...I did tell him that maybe I should be sleeping with y'all, at least y'all were more loving to me than he was."

"You go boy! What did he have to say then?"

"He really got pissed then. He said that he just knew I wasn't a saint like I put on and that I was probably humping one of my patients."

Sebastian told me he closed his eyes before he became enraged with anger. He turned quickly without warning and shoved Daniel's face into the wall. Sebastian said as he glanced into the strange face that he tightened his gripe around Daniel's clutched neck. Daniel didn't try to defend himself.

"Sebastian, that was kind of low saying you doing it with your patients...actually I can understand that crack about us."

"You can...how?"

"Honey, it's called jealousy. Pure unadulterated jealousy...that the same kind of shit that Antoine laid on me. They can't accept the fact that we can love each other without doing the nasty...If you looked even harder, you would have probably seen Antoine out there cruising."

"Why would he be jealous of our group being friends?"

"Why is the earth round and revolves?"

"Michal, I just lost it...I have never hit him before in my life. Hell, I never hit anyone in my life"

"What the hell did he think by asking if you would want him as a friend? Friends don't screw over friends."

"I was so mad and hurt that I slammed him again against the wall and his

PANELS

face hit a glass picture that shattered to the floor...I just snapped. I just wanted him to get the hell out."

"Is he still there?"

"Nope, he took out like a bat out of hell."

"Are you okay? Do you want to stay with me tonight?"

"Naw, I 'll be alright...I'm sorry to bother you this late."

"Are you trying to start another fight? Listen, if you need me, you call me. You are always there for us. Let us be there for you...now, I'll ask you again, do you want to stay over?"

"Seriously, naw, it's okay...in fact, I'm going to get drunk to celebrate."

"Yeah right, Sebastian, this is Michal you're talking to and I know you don't drink especially when you're pissed...whatever you do, if you need me, I'm here."

"Thanks, Michal...I love ya."

"Love you too. Goodnight."

"Goodnight." He left.

The next morning, I was somewhat relieved that he was at work. I was not expecting to see him looking so disheveled and scruffy. Sebastian surprised me and actually went out to get drunk. He told me how he ran several red lights going nowhere fast. He said that he was crying so hard that his tears clouded his vision. He told me he wanted to punish Daniel for ever telling him that he had ever loved him.

"Where did you finally go?"

"The Cabaret," Sebastian whispered.

"On a work night, you got to be kidding...what was it like?"

"Actually it was quite festive and packed. I had to drive around the block twice before I could even park."

"Did you have a good time?"

"Nope, I had a ball! I almost didn't get in."

"Why, was it that packed?"

"No ID...I couldn't find my license at first...Did you know that Peaches is still there? That enormous burly black man scares the hell out of me...He and Patrick were standing underneath that damn sign about no one being underage being admitted. I was in never never land, totally spaced out when he touched me. I almost jumped out of my skin."

"Was the music jumping?"

"Baby, Santana was spinning his ass off. People danced on the stages, on the floor, anywhere they could move, they moved."

"Was my girl Tiffany Lynn there?"

"Yeah, that gal was too hot! She came out doing "Got to be Real" in that one piece beaded outfit, you know the one…She looked flawless!"

"Did you tip her?"

"Yeah, I did…you know what she did…she threw her leg over my shoulder and started hunching on me."

"You know you loved!"

"Maybe…maybe I didn't."

"I know you…and I know Tiffany. I know she has the hots for you!"

"Now, you know that we are just friends, nothing more."

"You don't have to convince me, umm. It's nothing to me."

"You'll die when I tell you whom I ran into over at Linda's bar."

"Who, pray tell, did you see?"

"Well, I was standing flirting with Linda about her being so beautiful and so flawless that I could eat her up."

"Yeah right, and what did she say?"

"She just laughed as always and asked me what I wanted to drink…that was when he came up."

"Who came up, alright already, the suspense is killing me."

"Seth's brother, Bradley!"

"You're lying…you know you're lying."

"Okay, whatever…he offered to buy me a drink…get this…the drink was called a slow screw against the wall. I asked Linda if that was a drink and she said yes. So, I tried one."

"Oh, you're a big liar. Seth said his brother doesn't buy drinks unless he wants to…you didn't, did you? Did you go home with him? You sleaze bag."

"Believe what you want to…I know he bought me a couple of drinks…and you can relax, nothing else happened."

"Yeah right, don't make me call Seth and have him spill the tea."

"Hmm, now who's jealous?"

"So, does he look anything like the pictures?"

"You sure are interested in him…actually his picture doesn't do him justice…He's flawless! I mean, obviously he's a gym bunny. No fat anywhere." Sebastian smiled. "Then we danced for hours and hours. At least it seemed like hours. Being so close, I couldn't help but smell his thick black wavy hair…hmm…and his body. His eyes made me melt all over the place…then like Cinderella, our ball was over and the damned house lights came on"

PANELS

"Can he dance?"

"Can he dance? Baby, he had moves like no other...I got excited just watching him peddle his ass on that floor...I was smiling from ear to ear, loving the fact that others were watching us. He's a damn good dancer."

"So, who went home with who?"

"My...you're nosy...for your information, no one went home with anyone."

"Why?"

"Well, for one, I'm not a whore and two, he is Seth's brother...I have already heard the talk." Sebastian smiled coyly. "Anyway, that was the last thing I needed. Oops, gotta go, group is starting." As he briskly walked away, he stopped and turned and faced me. "You remember how pissed I was last night, well, Bradley told me he just loved men with a lot of fighting anger in them!"

I mouthed the word "bitch."

The circle had considered Cleo extremely beautiful. She was our Spanish porcelain doll. Her silky raven black hair shimmered down past her sleek sultry shoulders. She is quite tall and lanky. Her piercing green eyes often penetrated into other's interior. Her surface sweetness always caught victims off guard. As she lost her innocence to the bitterness of the world, she became a survivalist.

"You know, I wasn't always this evil vixen."

"Cleo, you are far from being anywhere near being a vixen. You're too sweet."

"Michal, don't be too fooled...Edward found out I'm not so sweet and delicate, didn't he?" Cleo laughed. "I was originally christened Juliana Ramirez-Rivera. But, don't call me that. I prefer to be called Cleo. I was born the middle child of a poor peasant farmer in the tiny village of Santillana del Mar in Spain...Do you know where that is?"

"I take it to be in Spain."

"Well, you're close. Santilla del Mar is on the northern coast of Iberia, at the rim of the Bay of Biscay. It's really beautiful there. Seasonal weather from Atlantic's rains and snow kept the hillocks and hollows virgin green."

"Don't tell me you lived on a farm with Old McDonald's animals?"

"Don't laugh...yeah we had yard animals living with us...the insistent crows of the roosters and I remember all too well of the clopping sound of the hooves on the aged cobblestone. I remember it well because I could never sleep…anybody and everybody's donkeys and cows running wild on the streets with goats."

"They really didn't live with you, did they? I mean, the animals."

"Oh no, you see, in our village, farm animals stayed on the ground floor, small animals like chickens lived on the top, while we lived in the middle."

"Excuse me for asking, but didn't it stink?"

"No, my sisters, my mom, and I worked hard to keep the area clean."

"Well, that's one way of keeping your animals at home. Board them!" Bradley joined in.

"Did you learn English in school?" Sebastian asked.

"Actually, the American English was taught to me by my older sisters. We would play games that involved English. I remember once playing with some Americans. They had different board games where you had to read cards…later, without being embarrassed, I would stand in front of my mirror and try to say those words over and over and over…I watched my mouth forming these strange words…we also look through old magazines discarded by tourists." Cleo laughs. "You Americans were not always as clean as our animals!"

"You spent your days learning this language?"

"Of course not, we were all busy taking care of the animals…work has to be done on a farm. Something you guys don't know anything about. No, I would practice and read after my chores and dinner."

"So, how did you make it over here? How did you meet Edward, the Terrible?"

"Well, I was standing alone in the garden weeding. My thoughts were on the beautiful singing of the birds. I began to softly sing with them. I was humming some old ditty that my mother used to sing to us when we were so much younger."

"And the old buzzard flew in for the kill, right?" Sebastian smirked.

"Be nice. No, but he was standing nearby looking at me smiling."

"Omigod, I knew it…he's a stalker…old pervert!"

"Hush, David. Let her finish. So, Cleo, what did you do after you noticed him staring a hole in you?"

"Seth, I was startled…I turned quickly and ran into the house."

"You should have shot his ass, right there on the spot…I think you could have gotten away with it…just say he was trespassing," David piped.

"You are so evil." Cleo laughed. "You may be right, but I didn't shoot him. I probably couldn't have even if I had wanted to, no gun, only sticks."

PANELS

"Honey, don't you remember what they say about 'sticks and stones may break a bone'?"

"David, I can see you will never get Ms. Congeniality!"

"Hell no, I want the crown...screw being Ms. Nicey. She don't go nowhere."

"Ms. Diva, let the girl finish her story before I turn grey."

"That's alright, Seth. Anyway, then, this man enters my house with my father standing at his side. My father had this really sickened smile across his face. My father beckons me to his side."

"Girl, you were traded down the river to that dirty old fart for more goats." Sebastian laughed. "But did you really have to marry him?"

"Oh, believe me, I had quite a bit apprehension about marrying someone I didn't know nor loved. But my sisters, my grandmama, and my mama, all pestered me to do it. They thought that it would be a good passage to America. But I knew it was wrong. I never loved this man and I really doubt if he ever really loved me."

"Honey...wait a minute...just how old were you when you jumped that broom? You had to jump alone 'cause he's too old to even try," David whined.

"I had just turned seventeen."

"I knew it...child was jailbait...someone call the law!"

"David, don't you have a drag number you need to practice somewhere?"

"Ohh, Mr. Man wants me to leave. By the way, I don't do drag because I'm a great illusionist. You, my dear, are the leather drag queen, the wannabe!"

"Now, now...we must not get too grand here...Seriously, Cleo, why are you in school instead of relaxing in the limelight of your new wealth?"

"Seth, good question...I soon realized that I was pretty to look at but I must also remember to keep my mouth closed around his business associates so that they won't know just how stupid I am."

"His words, I'm sure...damn bastard..." Seth sipped on his cooling coffee.

"Sweetheart, you're much smarter than you appear." Cleo smiled.

We knew all too well that Edward was much older than his young naïve bride. He was well in his fifties. He may have taken her virginity but not her love. As years progressed, they both would begin to realize their irreconcilable differences.

Secretly, I always found Bradley Mitchelson to be tremendously sexy. Although I did lust after him, I didn't have the guts to approach him aside from our friendship. He was a radical extremist. He was the man I adored. He was the man I wished Antoine were. Unlike Seth, Bradley was not a practicing Jew.

As Bradley physically matured, he became quite beautiful in all aspects. His charming but equally manipulative personalities made others including myself melt under his ever so smooth passionate tone while forgetting any of his flaws. He was a superb actor on the stage of life, a real scene-stealer without a conscious.

Style was always crucial to him. Bradley was a slave to fashion with the matching perfect body to die for. Constantly, his opened and sensual clothing draped his figure effectively. His ponderous arms outstretched displayed the firm flexing carved muscle of a desired body builder. The tight washboard stomach with the titillating trail of thick black hair that streamed down his squared pectorals that were worshiped by others. His legs were strong. Each muscle glistened into sharp carnal definition.

With Bradley's dark Mediterranean appearance being so desirable, I knew that men often tried to please him with expensive gifts. He appeared as a hunter that did away with his prey as quick and brisk as the stalking had ended. Unlike most of us, Bradley felt that the concept was senseless for gay men to try to sustain fruitful relationships.

Bradley's arrogance often made me angry with him. His philosophy battled mine to no end.

"You know, you guys put too much trust in others," He would say.

"Bradley, no man is his own island."

"Perhaps, maybe that it is true…that's why each of us will either sink or swim if we don't look out for ourselves. It's not being selfish but a will to survive in this cut throat world."

"A person can survive in this world without stepping on others."

"Michal, my dear, maybe that works for you…but it doesn't for me…you can't depend on others and you shouldn't. Stay loose and aloft, I always say. Anyway, that's why you're in social work and I'm not."

Bradley was never really close to his parents. His actual mother died while giving birth due to RH factor complications. He was only two years old. His only sister to be born also died.

After years of boarding schools and the assistance of an aged bachelor uncle, his father Benjamin finally remarried Elois, a widow left with four small children. Seth was one of them.

Bradley, at first, refused to accept this new family. Still refusing to

PANELS

compromise his standings to any extent, Bradley lived with his great uncle until his uncle's death. Resentment spiced with petty jealousy was abounding in the novel household. Angry verbalizations with occasional fighting. According to both Seth and Bradley, most evenings the family spent together were cold and empty. The advent of fall and winter brought relief because of school while summer renewed the hellish tortures. Bradley and Seth fought each other relentlessly.

According to Seth, the year he and Bradley turned fifteen, a tremendous singular change took place that proved phenomenal in nature. It was as if both boys had stood in front of a mirror and discovered that their own individual crumbling reflections of their exposed inner selves were the same. The similarity made them uncomfortable.

Without Seth's knowledge, Bradley confided in a few of us of one possible turning point that he and Seth had experienced during their earlier attempts at bonding. Their love for each other was never a given; it was earned.

Bradley described it as a dreadful hot blistering summery day with the air being stifling muggy, a true southern summer of sorts.

"I had just returned home from playing a few sets at the Westborough Racquet Club. At first, I thought I was the only one at home since I didn't see any cars…so I started to take off my clothes as I walked up the spiral staircase…I had to stop a few times to gaze at the gorgeous hunk in the reflective glass."

"I thought you said you was by yourself. Who was this hunk?"

"Richard, my man, I was the hunk!"

"You know, Bradley, you are one conceited child."

"Why thank you, Sebastian, I'm not really conceited, just quite sure of myself."

"Bradley, get real! Finish the story," I said.

"As I started to say, I was admiring my muscles and I took my moist hand and ran it down my bare chest and…."

"Bradley!"

"Chill out! Anyway, I had this strange feeling that I wasn't alone in the house…I didn't hear anyone come in."

"You were too busy making love to yourself."

"Sebastian, you really are a jealous queen, aren't you? Well, anyway, I started creeping to my room. I would stop and listen…my heart started beating faster…I won't lie, yeah I was getting scared…I didn't know what I would find...then, I heard a sound. It was coming from Seth's room. A clicking sound...I thought someone had broken in at first then I realize it was his room. Someone was in there rummaging around. He ain't got nothing valuable in his room, I thought. So I crept to his door and listened. Someone was definitely in there."

"Why didn't you call the cops?"

"Michal, I guess I wasn't thinking right...I was actually pissed off thinking someone had broken into my house."

"Were you scared?"

"Hell yeah! But I had to find who was in there."

"So what did you do?" I asked.

"I closed my eyes, took a deep breath, opened the door, and ran in."

"Child, you could have gotten your fool head blown off."

"There he was...standing with his back to me...before I could say anything, I saw that motherfucker holding a gun to his temple!"

"Omigod! No, tell me he didn't do that!" Richard was shocked.

"What happened next?"

"I ran to his side and knocked the revolver out of his hand...but he just stood there looking dumbfounded...the asshole didn't fight back."

"Thank God you got there in time."

"Yeah, otherwise we would have no Seth...just your vain ass!"

"You wish you could have more of me anyway, don't you, Michal?"

"Dizzy queen, get back to the story...what happened next?"

"I was so pissed at him for trying that shit that I picked up the gun and started beating the hell out of him."

"You what!"

"Then he tried to get the gun back and we started wrestling on the floor...somehow I kicked the gun over to the door. When I wasn't looking, he clocked me with his left. That really got me. So I pounded his face with my fist until he stopped...then, for a brief second, we just laid there."

"No body else had come home by this time?"

"Naw, at least no one came to us..."

"Did he say anything to you?"

"Nope, he just laid there crying on the floor...whimpering like some hurt dog...I crawled over to the gun, picked it up, and left his room." His voice softened. "Please don't ever tell him that I told you guys that. Please."

"Bradley, you have my word," I promised. Sebastian and Richard echoed the same.

"He was obviously depressed about something. Do you know what it was?"

"Sebastian, I didn't know at the time, but I soon found out by accident."

"Alright already, stop talking in riddles. What would drive him to want to take his life?"

"Other than having you as a brother?" Richard joked.

"Do you really want to know?"

"Yeah, we do."

"You guys do me a favor and go look in a mirror."

"Bradley!"

"Just do it! That's all I ask."

"Okay, so what's the point?" I asked. "All we see are ourselves."

"Right…come on, you head shrinkers, think about it. Looking into a mirror, you see what others see, right? "

"I'm lost…just what are you trying to say?"

"Okay, I'll tell you…Seth began to see himself as others saw him. He didn't like what he saw. He fought against it and lost…the only way out he knew was death."

Bradley paused. "Seth hated being gay."

"Damn!" Richard broke the silence.

"Is that why he tried to shoot himself?"

"I think so, I never asked…I just know that something went off in me when I saw him with that gun to his head."

"Maybe you did it out of love for your brother," I said.

"Maybe…maybe you're right…I guess I did kinda get used to having him around. I really couldn't relate to those other goons."

"You know, I used to wish I had a brother…or even a sister for that matter. My parents decided one was definitely enough," Sebastian said.

"I guess it has its good points…you can usually blame them for your screwups."

"Bradley, I really don't doubt that you did just that." Richard smirked.

"Did he really tell you he hated that, that he hated being gay?"

"Not, not really…Michal, you know how private he is. He doesn't talk about his problems, you know that…I only found out he was gay by accident."

"What do you mean? What kind of accident?"

"Maybe I better stop now before I dig my grave deeper…he would kill me if he knew I was telling you guys this."

"Too late, spill the rest of the beans. Like Michal asked, what accident?"

"Well, once I eaves dropped on the phone call he had with some woman named Penny. She worked at some center…and something about a 'One in Teen group.'"

"Yeah, I know her…that's the Center you're talking about…but that doesn't mean that he's gay."

"It only means that he had a nosy brother," Richard piped.

"I love you too, Richard. Anyway, that's not the accident."

"You know, Bradley, it takes you hours to tell anything."

"Details, baby, details! You should know that about me by now…anyway, he got to where he would leave and not tell anyone where he was going."

"So, does that make him gay?"

"Michal, shut up! Anyway, a old running mate of mine, Marshall, was sitting in his car waiting for me. We were going cruising, you know. Or maybe you don't know. Anyway, Seth came home. Well, Marshall had seen him before and asked me who Seth was. I told him he was my brother and that he was musical monk."

"You not talking about that brute with the curly locks of California white blond hair? Yeah, I see him at the gym…not bad eye candy especially with those sensual steel blue eyes…I didn't know you knew him," Sebastian said.

"Yeah, he is cute but not as cute as I. Anyway, Marshall flipped out. He told me that I was holding out on him…"

"How, what did you not tell him?"

"At first, I didn't know what the hell he was talking about…well, Marshall proceeds to ask me all these questions about Seth…He was really getting on my nerves…but before I went off on him, he tells me that he had been with Seth."

"What!…was he serious?" Richard asked.

"As serious as a heartattack…baby, you could have knock me over with a boa after Marshall told me that…Of course, I said he was lying until he told details about Seth that no one else should have known."

"So, knowing you…you probably went back to Seth and blabbed it to him, didn't you?" Sebastian asked.

"Naw, this was too good to do that."

"So, what did you do?"

"My, you guys are some nosy queens." Bradley paused. "I did the next best thing."

"Which was?"

PANELS

"One night, I followed Seth to the park."

"Honey, Nashville has thousands of parks! Which one?" I asked.

"Please don't say Cedars," Sebastian said.

"You got it, yep, it was Cedars…I waited in the bushes and watched him sit on a picnic table…I still didn't believe he was cruising…so I waited to see what would happen next."

"Is that all you was doing in the bushes? I know you too well."

"Yes, my dear Sebastian, I was there for another reason."

"So, what happened next?"

"Well, I was sitting there pissed off because I had wasted my time when it happened."

"What?"

"This guy walks up to Seth…looking at him from head to toe but then he walks away…then he walks back. You know that damn game acting like you not interested. Don't' you do that, Michal?"

"Whatever. Just tell your story."

"Finally this trick takes a seat right next to Seth. Seth doesn't move but this jerk moves closer to him and even put his hand on Seth's leg."

"Did Seth move away?"

"No, he sat there…he didn't touch the guy back…then all of a sudden this moron pulled Seth into his arms."

"Don't tell me they did it right there on the wooden table…can you imagine splinters in the ass and trying to explain that?"

"Richard, are we speaking from experience?"

"No, Bradley, that's your scene not mine. What happened next?"

"While that pervert was holding Seth, I came out of the bushes. I called Seth's name."

"Baby, I bet he freaked out big time seeing you."

"You know he did…I caught his ass totally off guard."

"What did he say?"

"He looked me straight in the eyes and had the nerve to ask me what I was doing there."

"What did you say?"

"I smiled my pearlies, put my hand on his shoulder, and told him obviously the same reason he was there."

Bradley's playground was corporate America. He was an investment broker employed with a old traditional established ultra-conservative firm. Upon his completion of his MBA from the Owen School of Management at

45

Vanderbilt University, he was hired with unlimited conditions. He was the golden boy that brought his clients much money.

My biggest issue with Bradley was that he compared his financial acquisitions with his sexual conquests. Numbers mattered, nothing else. He often admitted to being selfish. He wore that trait as if a badge of honor.

Seth, on the other hand, was quite the opposite. Earlier in his youth, he excelled magnificently across the ivories. Seth became preoccupied with his music career while placing his sexual needs on the non-existent proverbial back burner.

Seth was the quietest of the entire lot. While we toyed with our playthings, Seth was busy becoming a disciplined musician. After graduating from Blair School of Music, he had aspiration of studying at Julliard in New York. His inner world of musical notes and lyrics created his imagination, his chosen form of escapism. Music allowed Seth the avenues to openly express what he feared verbalizing.

Seth invited us when he would occasionally perform on whatever stage he played on. The choices were wide ranging from the honky tonk beer joint corners of hell to the grandeur of the Nashville Symphony.

Later in life, we would learn that Seth had long established himself as a renowned pianist whose music was once described as "capturing the virgin pain." His composing talents were sought later in life to write pieces such as requiems for friends.

He loved literature, especially the classics. His favorite writer was E.M. Forrester. Seth once told me that he felt Forrester's novels not only captured his true essence but also allowed him to be himself. Isn't it imagination!

Cleo told both Sebastian and me once that Edward treated her as some delicate emerald.

"At times, I felt so damned imprisoned...you know, things that sparkled but were otherwise silent."

"So, he purchased your rights and I'm sure you were supposed to follow him around like some lovesick puppy...never question authority but be a good little soldier and obey."

"Sebastian, are you saying that I should buy into this type of control?"

"No, not really...I just hoped that you realized that no one should ever have that much control over anyone."

"Maybe Sebastian's suggesting that you and he run off and live passionately forever and a day," I joked.

"That would definitely surprise a few people including the Duchess."

"Why? Is it because I'm not an American?"

"Be for real! No, trust me. That has nothing to do with you not being an American…Hell, in fact, my family would accept you even if you came from another planet just as long as you are a woman."

"She is woman, hear her roar and Sebastian hear him moan."

"It would be their ultimate dream for me to settle down with a real Martha Stewart instead of Tom of Finland wannabe."

"I'm afraid that I don't understand what you are trying to say."

"Baby, don't grieve it. It's simple…we're gay boys living in a very het world." Sebastian laughed.

"And the het boys are all jealous of our perfect flawless bods."

"Oh, how bloody narcissistic." Cleo joined the laughter.

" I just know she didn't go there…calling us narcissistic when her palace of a home is named 'Casa De Los Homboys.'"

"It's 'Casa De Los Hombrones' to you…so, what's wrong with that?"

"Nothing wrong with that…girl…but if I'm right, doesn't that roughly translate into something about a house of the giants?"

"Ah, I see someone didn't stay asleep in Spanish class."

"Nah, I really enjoyed the class…"

"Yeah, right. He probably had a male teacher."

"Michal, you are so jealous…anyway, I speak a little Spanish."

"Oh, yeah! Say something." I asked.

"Si, señor…or in your case…señorita."

"For your information, señorita is a woman. I'm a man."

"So you say…señorita!"

Cleo realized the powers of her dangerous beauty with those commanding mint green eyes. She had the height with alluring style. No one could have ever imagined her being a field girl. Her skin was as delicate as a porcelain doll.

She was always full of some mystery that her eyes seldom revealed. As she matured, so did her volcanic anger.

Cleo was destined for the stage. Initially, her survival appeared to have depended wholly upon Edward's directions and support. While married, she enrolled in formal music classes at his insistence. Edward remained impressed with her voice.

"I couldn't do like my mama did with my papa…I hate to admit that I don't

think I could ever love Edward as my mama loves papa."
"Surely, Eddie boy don't want you to be his doormat?"
"Sometimes, I sit and think about leaving him…and going back home."
"What! And leave us…how dare you even think that."
"Yeah, Seth would be right behind you."
"You mean, that neither of you would miss me?"
"Don't be foolish…of course we will miss you. But we don't have to worry about that because you ain't going nowhere. Now, are you?"
"Michal, don't be so sure…You guys just don't understand the hell I go through…We go out to dinner and sit in silence…I hate going anywhere with him especially those boring ass business dinners. I simply smile and nod my head. I must not say anything because it might embarrass him."
"You never embarrass us."
"Yeah, you guys make me feel like I'm somebody with a voice."
"Don't make us have to go to Eddie boy and straighten his antique ass out."
"That's all I need, you guys to go to him for anything…you know he already despises the whole lot…He doesn't understand why I hang around you guys."
"He's jealous."
"Jealous that I might be sleeping with one of you?"
"No, jealous because he doesn't know you like we know you," I said.
"You see, Cleo, we see you as the beautiful person you are inside and outside. We don't want anything from you except you."
"Girl, we always knew that your old man detested the mere sight of us. Why do you think Bradley and Tiffany give him such a hard time? I don't waste my breath on his ass. He's not worth it. We are here for you."
"Just remember, that you will always be loved and adored by us."
"I so hearby name you 'Honorary Queer' of the circle."
"Why not queen?" She laughed.
"Honey, there is already too many of them already running around thinking they are grand."

Cleo was indeed close to us but not as close as she was to Seth. Watching them interact gave me much to wonder about. They were practically inseparable.
Cleo had initially met Seth during one of his many piano recitals at Blair.

PANELS

She was quite impressed with his playing but bothered by his shy standoffish mood when she approached him after the performance. Without receiving the response she had hoped for, she quietly faded away into the audience.

A week later, Cleo and Sebastian met me at the Gas Light for a few drinks. There he was tickling the ivories. His head was raised above the piano and his eyes appeared focused directionless. As Sebastian handed Cleo her wine, she nodded in the direction of the piano

The piano rested on the raised portion centered across the black and white tiled floor above the main floor. There were a few small intimate tables that nestled around the outline of the piano's edges. Against the piano were wooden stools where patrons sat closer around the pianist. A rather large glass goblet graced the middle of the baby grand Steinway for tips.

On the right side of the stage were large billiard tables within inches to a vintage ornate jukebox. On the left side, patrons sat in intimate conversations while relaxed on over stuffed cushions near the fireplace. Some played backgammon.

The room in its entirety was decorated with large baroque pieces of antiques. There were enormous planters filled with fresh cut flowers.

"I know him…I met him last week…at the recital…he's the one I was telling you about."

"You mean the one that ignored you?"

"Yeah…that's him…isn't he cute?"

"Whatever, he's not my type."

"Yeah right, he's breathing, aint he?"

"Whatever, you really prefer those quiet types, don't you?"

"I guess. Just look at him."

"Cleo honey, I hate to burst your bubble, but I kinda think he may prefer the other sex."

"There's something about him that seems so familiar. I can't place it, but I feel a strange closeness to him."

"It's called lust, honey, that's all."

"Cleo, he's probably seems familiar because he's probably gay. You know, you are attracted to them…and please spare me that theory of us being fragments of a total being and that he may be one of your fragment type."

"Laugh at me if you will. There's something about him that draws me to him."

"I told you it was lust."

"I don't know, Michal…I sort of agree with her, I think he is kinda cute myself." Sebastian smiled.

After some people left the piano, Cleo ran to the stools. We were close behind her. The piano player continued to play as if he hadn't noticed anything. Instead, he began to play another song as glasses clinked and drunken laughter sounded around him. His eyes remained closed as his fingers moved about the keys. He appeared truly engrossed in his own world.

He began to softly play a tune that was quite familiar to me. It was a tune from my old disco days, one that Sylvester and Pattie Labele had immortalized: "You Are My Friend." I became caught up in my own bit of nostalgia and felt a little mellowed. Suddenly, I was brought back to reality by the sound of another voice joining. It was a feminine voice. Cleo's voice.

Both singers appeared to sing with that certain definition from their hearts that appeared to understand the lyrics without doubt. People stopped talking and glanced at the stage. Couples held onto each other and some swayed in the wind of the music. The piano player opened his eyes and saw Cleo. He continued playing while giving her approval through his eyes.

Tears formed in both Cleo and his eyes as they continued to proclaim words of searching for that special friend for all of the love and understanding and realization that the person was there beside them all the time. They closed their number with an outstanding roar of a standing ovation with shouts and jeers for more.

As their friendship developed, Cleo confessed to me later that she had eventually loved Seth more than just a friend. He was more than just her personal confident. He was her lover but in far different perspectives than the others. She said she knew that Edward realized this fact but could do nothing to change her feelings.

Seth, on the other hand, became overly protective of Cleo. He worshiped her. He never once betrayed any of her most inner thoughts nor would she his. Over the years, their passion entertained each other daily.

Hello, my name is Sebastian Ingram. After learning that my friend Michal was indeed writing some form of a memoir of our circle of friends and of our rather distinctive relationships, I asked him be sure to include Gregory. Gregory was the first.

I only assume that since Gregory and I shared a large portion of his last days together that Michal thought I should be the one to write about it.

I must admit that I find writing about our moments to be somewhat a bit

PANELS

awkward especially since I'm not quite sure as to what to write. Somehow, I feel that I am betraying his confidence in placing his life on a petrie slide waiting for the microscope.

And yet, I recognize the beauty of his transition. I prefer to say "transition" instead of death. To me, death has too much finality. Shall I begin?

It was the last day of the week of our graduation when we all met high atop the Polaris to celebrate. Everyone was present, everyone that mattered, so to speak. Edward had escorted Cleo but soon left shortly afterwards, much to our joy.

We were searching for tables near the stage. We all wanted to be close to Jamon. The jazz singer was someone we all knew. Her sultry voice continued to mesmerize the audience. Her long sensual fingers gliding down the microphone stand made her polished nails glisten as beams of light bounced off.

Suddenly the music changed. Percussion instruments began to sound. The song now had a Caribbean beat to it. Jamon began singing about finding another person in her life after her last lover had been unfaithful. She closed her eyes while gyrating to the beat. We started singing the chorus with her.

"I bet you never thought I go that far, I bet you never thought I'd break your heart."

"The story of my life, get a man, lose a man, get man, and lose a man!"

"David, honey, it's probably because they don't know what you are."

"Oh, do I see someone at your side? I think not...Ms. Thang, don't do me!"

"It's Mr. Thang to you." Bradley corrected.

"Girls, girls, girls, chill out!" Michal said.

"Señorita, may I have this dance?"

"Which señorita are you referring to?" someone asked.

"The real one, of course." Bradley reached for Cleo's extended hand.

"Yeah, let's dance. I like this number." Cleo left the table.

Bradley took her into his arms and pressed her close to his chest. From a stranger's point of view, they really appeared to be in love. She had her head on his shoulder as she lightly caressed the nap of his hair. He was kissing the top of her head. Both of them had their eyes closed. I noticed Seth glaring at them.

"Just look at them...Ms. Ginger Rogers and Mr. Fred Astaire."

"Well, alright girl, you better ballroom dance...I just gotta have them pumps…honey, she better not take them off in here."

"David, you know your feet are too damn big for those little shoes…it's for the petite not the full figured woman like you."

"Ms. Thang, you didn't have to go there…I will have you know that I'm more petite than your fat ass. Don't do me!"

"David, chill out. You know that I love ya."

"Hmp…Whatever, so you say…anyway, I'm gonna steal them damn pumps."

"Seth, why are you talking so much?" Michal asked.

"What?"

"Man, you have been sitting here so damn quiet I had to get you to say something."

"Leave him alone, Michal, you see the man is pissed at Bradley dancing with his woman."

"Ooh, Oh no, Ms. Thang ain't wanting the impossible!"

"Shut up! There's nothing wrong with me…I'm just quiet, is that a damn crime? Does everyone in the group have to be so obnoxious as hell?"

"Ooh, somebody done touched a nerve."

"David, you are a nerve!"

"Richard, honey, I won't say what you are…'cause you know I know…so don't make me spill the tea on your righteous ass."

"I'm going to really miss this madness." Gregory smirked.

"So, gang, here we are, all dressed up and scared out of our minds," Bradley said as he returned to the table. "No more help from our mommies or daddies."

"Don't forget that one of us is married and will still get help," Michal said.

"Oh Gregory, do you really have to leave us at this tiring time in our lives?" Bradley asked through his sparkling wine glass.

"Gang, I will be back…It's not like I will be gone forever…" Gregory assured us. " We have a pact, remember!"

"Omigod, not that damn St. Elmos crap!"

"David, honey, you will be alright."

"No, Sebastian, honey, you will be alright. Ain't nothing wrong with the diva!"

"Let's make a toast…as we sit here and evolve around watching Nashville's skyline, let's promise to always return to this point in our lives where we are together once more." I held my glass high.

"Here, here," everyone chanted as we clinked our glasses.

PANELS

Gregory Lawrence was originally from the East Coast near Pittsburgh, Pennsylvania. He was an only child. Gregory was a devout practicing Catholic and an avowed gay man with what he considered conflicting staleness.

Gregory had always been extremely attractive with his definite clear-cut dark Mediterranean features. His raven night hair danced upon his shoulders. His facial structures with the defined high cheekbones. He was indeed manly: virile and full of vim. We all loved him except for Bradley. Bradley saw him as an adversary to his own beauty.

He was always quiet and always appeared in heavy thoughts. He was always in control of himself. To be honest, I was in love with him but dared not speak the truth.

After graduation from Vanderbilt University, he was offered a position in business administration in Atlanta. Gregory was the first to actually leave from our family. Some of us, including myself, had a bit of initial resentment for his leaving us. Being the ever-independent soul he was, his personality allowed for no simple sentiments. I questioned, once, if he was actually close to any of us.

It was almost eight years before any of us had heard from him. Surprisingly, I was the first to receive the phone call. But it wasn't from him. Someone else unknown to me had called me late in the night. I had just turned off my light and pulled my pillow to my face when the phone rang.

"Is this Sebastian Ingram?"

"Yes, this is he."

"I'm sorry for calling you so late. It must be 11:00 p.m. there...Mr. Ingram, you don't know me but I'm taking care of a friend of yours."

"I don't know who you are talking about."

"Do you know a guy named Gregory?"

I paused. "Yes, is his last name Lawrence?"

"Yes, sir...He's very sick...he's dying."

"What the hell do you mean he's...Omigod, no! What happened? Why is he dying? How did you get my number?"

"Mr. Ingram, I found your number in his things...I thought I call you since he said you was a close friend...I just thought you would want to know before it was too late." There was a brief silence. "Mr. Ingram, are you still there?"

"Yeah...damn...what happened?"

"I'm sorry but I can't tell you over the phone."

"Why the hell not?" I was becoming annoyed.

"I think he needs to be the one to tell you."

"Where is he? Why didn't he call?"

"He's at home…on Myrtle near Ponce…I just left him…he's very weak and tired…Mr. Ingram, I would really appreciate it if you didn't tell him that I called you…he talks about you and some others in Nashville often…I just figured he wanted to see you before it was too late. Time is not being very generous to him." The savagely rough voice said. "I'm sorry to bother you, goodnight, Mr. Ingram." The phone went dead.

I replaced the phone back onto the cradle. I was wild-eyed. I lay in bed unable to sleep. I didn't know who this stranger was that had entered into my life. Somehow, I began to trust his words. I tossed around trying to sleep but it was useless. My mind was full of unanswered questions. His face would not leave my mind.

Over the years, I had only spoken with Gregory briefly during the holidays. Our conversations ceased being intimate. I really didn't know much of his current status. I closed my eyes and remembered the last time we embraced. I had to know what was going on with him. I had to go to him.

Standing outside Hartsfield International, I flagged down a taxi. I felt as if I was in a total fog. I heard nothing from the driver except to ask where I was going. I reached in my pocket and took out the crumpled sheet of paper. I recited the address that I had scribbled the night before.

Looking around the skyline, I rested my head on the neck of the seat. Reflections of the past danced around in my mind as I remembered a few of the silly escapades we did. I smiled. I still felt somewhat uneasy, but I still smiled. I really had no idea of what to expect.

The fast talking cabbie attempted his tourist spiel until I grudgingly told him that I had once lived in the Buckhead area near the St. Phillip Cathedral on Peachtree. I wasn't trying to be rude. I was too emotionally occupied with concerned worry to carry on a hackneyed conversation. Instead, I stared into space waiting for the truth to unfold.

The cabbie stopped minutes later outside a white-shingled house on Myrtle near Ponce De Leon. The overgrown weeds appeared out of place in comparison to the adjoining manicured lawns. The weathered cracked porch was bare. The rose bushes appeared withered with whatever remaining life slowly draining into the earth. I stood on the curb with my bags as the cabbie sped away.

I took a deep breath—twice. I walked towards the porch. The white wooden door had paint peeling and the wood was rotten. As I knocked, the

PANELS

door made a clapping noise signifying the wariness. Seconds later, a small silver haired man wearing spectacles appeared at the door.

"Yes, may I help you?"

"Aren't you Mr. Lawrence?"

"Yeah, and what can I do for you?"

"Mr. Lawrence, I'm Sebastian...a friend of Gregory..."

"Oh, then come on in...he's in the back room."

He stood aside as I walked into the house. The house was dark with windows half drawn. If I hadn't seen the portrait of Gregory on the wall I would thought I was in the wrong house. Nothing else in the room spoke of Gregory.

There was a pleasant aroma of herbs and spices being cooked. Clinking of tin pans permeated the delicious air. Running water broke the silence.

"John, who is that at the door?" a female voice asked from behind the old man.

"He says he's a friend of our boy..."

"Well, tell him to come on in."

"I did and he is already in."

"Hello...my, your face looks so familiar...but I can't rightfully place it...My name is Joan Lawrence, Gregory's mother and this is John, his father...and you are?" Joan extended her hand to me.

"Sebastian Ingram...My name is Sebastian...Gregory and I went to school together at Vanderbilt in Nashville."

"Oh my dear Lord, yes, I know I knew you. How are you doing? Are you hungry?" She paused as she wiped her hands across her apron. She sees my bags. "Come on in and sit down. Are you traveling?"

"I've just arrived into town...I'm here to see Gregory."

"Well, honey, he's sleeping right now...he had a fitful night, just tossing and turning...I really hate seeing my baby in so much pain...Did you say you were hungry? I just finished making lasagna...come on in here, put your bags over there...Now, John, go show this boy where to wash his hands."

"Ma'am, that's okay...I really don't want to be a bother. I was going to grab a bite at the hotel after I saw Gregory."

"Hush, honey, there's no need for you to get that awful food at that hotel. This is home cooking. There's plenty here for all of us...any friend of my boy is a friend of mine. After that last scoundrel left him, I was starting to wonder if any more of his friends would even come by. That damned bastard!"

"Joan!"

"Well, I'm not sorry, John. You know as well as I do, that wasn't right what he did to my boy."

"Joan, not now. Not in front of company."

"Well, he's bound to find out anyway. But that's okay. My boy Gregory has gotten down on his luck before and has always bounced back up. He will again, I just know...then they will be running back to him."

"Joan, now just calm down. You know you gotta watch your blood pressure."

"Now, you do as I told you. Go wash your hands. Dinner is getting cold." Joan disappeared to the kitchen.

"Where is Gregory?" I asked as she abruptly rushed away. Without missing a beat, she waved her arms to the direction of the back room.

I noticed the back room where the door was partially closed. A muscular black man stood briefly in the threshold. I felt his eyes staring at me. Was this where Gregory was sleeping, I wondered. My stomach knotted and tightened.

I slowly walked down the hall to the door where the light was brighter. I could see where the room was sparsely filled with only a bed, a small table, and a few upholstered chairs.

On top of the small wooden table were both a radio and a 13-inch television. A game show was on. The sound of the television was mute while the radio played softly. As I came closer, I saw him. In the middle of the floor was a massive bed filled with several pillows that appeared to outline a thin figure in the midst. A pair of swollen feet was propped separately while resting on stacked pillows and eggshell cushions. His feet were covered with purple blotches and open sores.

"You must be his friend?" The black man asked. I knew this voice but I didn't know him. "Gregory is sleeping now."

I stood dumbfounded. I couldn't speak. I felt the room start to spin. What's going on, I wondered. I fell against the doorframe and closed my eyes. I didn't want to see what I saw. I wanted to see my friend sitting up in bed laughing. I didn't want to see this damn emaciated shell of a man.

"I'm sorry...maybe I should come back later."

"If you wish...but nothing will change...no matter how long you stay away."

"Who's there?" Gregory began to stir in bed. His eyes slowly opened. "Who's here with us, Duncan?"

"I believe his name is Sebastian."

"Come closer...I won't bite...let me see if it's really you."

PANELS

"It's me, Gregory. It's me." I mumbled.

"Well, hell, if I knew you was coming, I would have made myself pretty for you."

"You look okay."

"You like the look…I call it pre-transience…Sebastian, you're a damn liar. You know that? I look like shit." Gregory attempted to laugh but coughed instead. "Who else is with you?"

"No one. I came alone."

"How does that song go, alone again naturally."

"Yeah, naturally."

"That's okay…I'm used to it by now." He pats the side of the bed. Motioning. "Here, sit down…I promise to be good."

"Gregory, I'm sorry but I have to ask…what the hell is going on here."

"Sebastian, welcome to my nightmare…its called Kaposi's Sacroma. KS to be short and it hurts like hell." Gregory stared directly at me. "Besides the fact that I have other complications of AIDS, I guess I'm doing alright."

"Why didn't you tell me sooner?"

"Why should I? And have you run for the hills like my other so-called friends. All except for Duncan…No, I didn't call you. I didn't want to bother you."

"Gregory, damn it! You always have to be such a dick on being in control. You would rather lay here and die alone."

"Whoa, just one fricken minute. Honey, this is not Guyana. In this hell, people do die alone." Gregory glanced over at Duncan. "Anyway, how did you find out?"

"That's not important. What matters is that I'm here now."

"Well, bless your little heart. I'm sure you will be well rewarded for caring for the dying at judgment day."

"Gregory, don't be a dick."

"This is my dark angel of mercy, Duncan…I would introduce you guys but I kinda think you probably already know each other."

Duncan glanced briefly in my direction. I lowered my head. He need not worry. I wouldn't betray his trust. Before I could answer, the clanging of the pots and pans in the kitchen along with his mother's singing reminded me that we were not alone. She was walking down the hall to tell us that dinner was ready.

Later that night, after Duncan had left and his parents retired to the front room, Gregory and I talked for seemingly hours before he began to tire. I stayed with him until he fell deeply into sleep. I carefully crawled beside him, kissed him gently on his lips, and went to sleep as silent tears filled the crevices of my eyes.

The next morning, someone lightly tapping me on my shoulders awakened me.

"Breakfast is ready..." Mrs. Lawrence smiled. "You can wash up in that bathroom. I already put out some fresh towels."

"Thank you, ma'am. I'm sorry. I didn't mean to pass out on his bed."

"Honey, that's alright...he's sleeping better now than he has slept in many a days. I'm glad you came." She paused. "Did he tell ya?"

"Yes ma'am, he did...I just wish that there was something more I could do for him."

"Sweetie, listen to me, being here is doing him a whole lot of good." She stopped to look at Gregory still sleeping. "Now, git up and git ready for breakfast. We ain't got all day...It will soon be time for supper."

For the next few days, I stayed at his side. I left only long enough to call back to Nashville to make arrangements for clients to be covered. For once, I was having my own crisis. Michal was quite helpful and also quite inquisitive.

"No problem, we can manage your case load until you return. Now, if we get some real headaches, I'm sending their ass packing to you in Atlanta."

"Hopefully you won't have any real dilemmas."

"So, are you going to tell me?"

"Tell you what?"

"Don't play Della Dumb ass with me...you know...what is going on with Gregory?"

"It's not really for me to say."

"Com'on, Sebastian, this is me...level with me, is he in some kind of trouble?"

"Yeah, I guess you can say that."

"Is he in jail?"

"No, but he is, hell...what is this, some kind of a damn Spanish Inquisition?"

"Sorry, I just thought that if there was something I or all of us could do then we would know what to do."

"You know, Michal, sometimes not knowing is best."

"Sebastian, damn it, you are really getting on my last nerve. What the hell with all these riddles? You're not the only friend he has." I could tell he was becoming irate. "I will call him myself and ask him what the hell is going on."

"Good...you do just that...I gotta go, he needs me."

During my stay, Duncan and I shared caring for Gregory. I have never changed a diaper for a child let alone a grown man. My clumsiness was quite obvious. I think I was more embarrassed than Gregory was. We constantly joked and laughed to avoid giving any consideration to what we were doing. I can proudly state that I have learned to put a diaper on without it being inside out!

"Duncan, the moment I saw you, I knew you was the one that called," I whispered as we watched Gregory sleep.

"Maybe...maybe not. Who knows," Duncan said.

"Why did you call me?"

"Why did you come?"

"Because he's a friend of mine and I love him."

"Good, you just answered your own question...you see that dude over there?" Duncan pointed to a picture hanging near Gregory's head.

"Yeah, who is he?"

"That asshole is Gregory's heart: Patrick...I can't stand the bastard. I despise the air he breathes...just let him set the first foot in this house and I will put all of my size 13 shoe up his ass."

"I take it that Patrick is Gregory's ex? Why is the picture still there?"

"Gregory wants it there...Gregory looks at that damn picture of that two bit whore every time his eyes are open. I really think he thinks that bastard is coming back...Gregory throws a hissy fit when you touch the frame."

"Did he just leave?"

"Yep, he practically grew wings and flew out of here...first time Gregory was sick...running high fevers and sweating like hell all over his bed...his sheets were so soaked that you could wring them out...anyway, I came by here after I saw that bitch Patrick at the Alcove...that whore was drunk and rubbing up against anything that walked...when I got here, Gregory was on the floor at the front door...man, at first I thought he was dead 'cause he wasn't breathing."

"What did you do then?"

"I called 911 and they took him to Grady Hospital...when he came to, he was so worried about his Patrick...Wanna know how Patrick showed his love; he moved the hell out of here and even took all the money out of the bank...man, you know that ain't right."

I shook my head. "How is he surviving?"

"For many years, Gregory managed an after-hours joint called the Alcove. That's where I met him. He gave me a chance when no one else would even look my way. I mean, that man is beautiful inside and out. He's fucking real…anyway, the club started having benefits for him. Couples of local dragqueens put on shows and give him their tips…man, everybody loves this man. For a few times since I have lived here in Atlanta, I have really seen the community take care of our own." Duncan was crying. "He doesn't deserve this shit!"

"Does he have insurance?"

"Yeah, kinda, even though he ain't working no where, the owners of Alcove still pays his premiums…and then there's this group of mega bucks gay doctors helping out…man, I really didn't think people gave a damn about others."

There was a light knock on the door behind us. As we turned to look, I saw a gorgeous man standing before me in a suit. Sporting a thick bushy frock of red hair, he captivated me. I felt somewhat aroused by this stranger. I found him alluring. I so wanted to passionately melt into his massive arms.

"Please do come in." I flirted. "My name is Sebastian and yours is?"

"Andrew Welding…you must be the friend from Nashville. I'm so glad that you came. I'm confident that Gregory is indeed pleased with your gesture."

"Well, if I had known that I would have met a hunk like you, I would have come sooner." My own words seemed foreign even to me. Duncan was making loud noises as if he was trying to clear his throat. My heart began to race as the stranger came closer towards me.

"Oh, good! Sebastian, I see that you have already met Father Welding…He's our priest." Mrs. Lawrence said as she entered the room behind the guest. "Father Welding is such a dear…always stopping by to check on my boy. Now, we must get out so they can pray together."

I froze in embarrassment. I wanted to die! Priest or no priest, I wanted this man to give me my last rite and I'm not even Catholic! Outside the bedroom, I caught Duncan by the arm.

"Why did you let me make a fool of myself?"

"Man, for a quick second you wouldn't even felt the earth move…you was too busy drooling over that man. I tried to warn you." Duncan chuckled as he walked down the hall towards the kitchen. "By the way, I wish you could have seen your face. It was priceless!"

Gregory would have his equal share of good and bad days. When he wasn't throwing his guts up, we would walk him around the house and even outside when the weather permitted. He was still very weak but strong with faith in himself.

One beautiful warm day, Gregory and I decided to leave the house and go to Piedmont Park. His mother wasn't too keen on our idea. Gregory hadn't been out of the house except to go in for doctor's appointments. However, cabin fever was definitely taking its toll. Without much more fanfare, his father handed me the keys to their car. Before she could utter another word, I had Gregory's wheelchair folded and in the trunk and Gregory sitting in the passenger seat. Off we went.

It was on a Sunday afternoon in the summer of 1982. There was a jazz concert scheduled. Gregory loved jazz. He appeared to perk up at the mere thought of going to hear live music. Reluctantly, Joan prepared what she considered a light lunch. I thought it was quite hearty myself.

We parked on a side street near Piedmont. Gregory was too tired to walk so I pushed him over in his wheelchair to a remote slightly inclined area that faced the band shell. Crowds of people were storming around us scampering for space. Some even stopped briefly to stare at us without saying a word.

I spread the blankets on the ground. I slowly eased Gregory down onto the ground. I folded the chair and placed our food and drinks at arms reach of Gregory.

Reality wasn't deemed necessary until the alarm beeped from the container that housed his numerous pills broke our peaceful turmoil.

"Sebastian, you really amaze me." Gregory was trying to rest his sunken head onto his thin hand.

"How so?"

"You see things but you don't see things."

"Huh, I don't get ya."

"Have you ever been around anyone as sick as I am?"

"No, at least, I don't think I have. Why?"

"I don't know if it's your naïve nature or your pity for me, but you don't appear afraid of me."

"First of all, it's not pity…Second, why should I be afraid of you?"

"I'm laying here across from you looking like death warmed over and you don't even flinch. Hell, those quacks at the hospital run in stare at me like I'm some damned specimen just waiting to be dissected. Hell, the gay boys are just as bad as some of the straights. Just look at the sea of all those muscle pretty boys. Great eye candy but none of them have a clue what's going on around them...I catch them staring at me like I'm some damned freak...a real oddity, definitely not something to take home to meet your friends."

"To be quite frank, I really don't know what the hell is going on with you....But, I guess it really doesn't matter."

"It's ironic...I once refused to ever think about it. Yeah, I had heard of some strange shit going around killing us queers but I knew I wasn't a possible candidate. I didn't whore around...but now, look at me, I'm a breathing test tube statistic."

The clinking sounds of bicycles came closer from behind breaking our feelings of being alone, a couple with a toddler resting on the darted.

"Do you have any idea how you got it?"

"Yeah, a mosquito."

"Excuse me, what do you mean?"

"It's about as senseless for me to try to determine just how I was infected by drumming up my past sexual encounters, my drug use, and so on. I may never know."

"Could Patrick possibly be the one?"

"Umm, I see that someone has been talking to you. I would hate to hear what Duncan or my mom said about him."

"He's well adored," I lied.

"Yeah, as much as Herpes...I don't know, maybe, maybe not...Duncan and my mom thinks that I still love him and that's why I keep his picture near by bed."

"That smirked smile tells me differently, am I right?"

"You got it, Ace...I have been down the road of heartache too many times. I have been hurt and I have hurt others, maybe not intentionally...I look at his picture every time I open my eyes because it's my way of saying 'you bastard, I'm still here.'"

"It's out of anger, then?"

"Yep, and this anger fuels my life another day." Gregory grimaces as he moved his legs.

"Your folks seem so loving and understanding."

"Yeah, I got them trained well, don't I?...Actually, my old man is having a real hard time with it. I can tell he wants to cry sometimes, but he would never allow that. He has to be that freakin' Rock of Gibraltar. My mom is busy cooking enough food to feed a damn army. You see her. She starts supper immediately after breakfast."

"I know I have gained a few pounds since I've been here...but I'm not complaining."

PANELS

"Sometimes I feel smothered by my folks and even Duncan. I know they mean well but I have no space. I have no time to myself. They so afraid I going to fall out and they won't be there to hear me. Sometimes, I wished that they would go back to Pennsylvania. "

"They only are being concerned about your crazy ass."

"Yeah, I know. But it still gets on my last nerve. If you tell them I said this, I will kick your ass…but often, when they would get on my nerves, I would act like I'm sleeping to get them to shut up." Gregory looked mischievous.

"Does it work?"

"Yeah, it works too good. They act as if I'm in some deep coma and starts to talk about me as if I wasn't there…nothing bad, just things they can't say to my face…I guess I should be glad that I have them in my life…I know I'm glad you are in my life."

"I'm just me."

"Sebastian, you have never been able to accept a compliment. I wish I had a mirror to show you how you are blushing. Can't a friend tell a friend that he loves him?"

"It depends on whether a friend or really a friend…"

"Is it my drugs or did you just say something really stupid?"

"Don't you remember the scene in 'Torch Song' when the little boy is trying to describe Harvey's relationships? Anyway, I'm glad you feel that way."

"The hardest time I ever had playing possum was when my dad was talking to me while he thought I asleep. He said that he didn't understand the life I chose…like I really have a choice…anyway, I have always known my dad to be a proud man that was embarrassed having a queer as a son, especially his only child. He loved hunting and fishing. I could fish but hated hunting. He saw a deer as food and I saw a deer as 'Bambi.' He was interested in the military, I'm a conscious objector. You know, all the common threads of a father son relationship."

"Trust me, you don't want me to go there when it comes to father of the year recipients," I said. "At least he is with you now."

"Until the bitter end, right?"

"Don't think that way."

"Why the hell should I not think that way? What other ways are there for me to think? Sebastian, in case you haven't noticed, I am dying. My ass is on borrowed time. Each day I open my eyes I thank the Lord…but one day, my eyes will be closing as the last rites are read."

"I won't deny you that...but I will say that you are not dead yet. You can still enjoy what's left."

"It's a bit too late to take out installments, it's strictly cash on demand."

"The sky is so clear. The stars are bright. I used to look in the sky and imagine seeing a shooting star...If you had a wish, what would you wish for?"

"I just know you thought I was going to say my health back. But I won't be selfish. If I truly had a wish, I would wish for others to see me as I see myself. See beyond my lesions and purple spots. See me in themselves. Realize that they must never cease loving themselves even if they should fall in the same direction of my path."

"There is always hope to the end."

"Sebastian, have you noticed how I never tell anyone 'goodbye'? Gregory paused. "I always say 'see ya later.' Telling someone goodbye is so final. Telling them that you will see them later implies that you will see them again, which I hope will happen."

Eventually, Gregory felt well enough to converse with others in our circle. He told them. Gregory appeared to never have felt ashamed of his illness nor had he wanted anyone to pity him. As fate would have it, Bradley was the first to call him back. Gregory later told me of the rather eerie apprehension he had noticed in Bradley's nervous tone. Although Bradley had promised to come to visit him as soon as he could, Gregory knew he would never see Bradley. Gregory said he understood.

Seth and Cleo called, mocking anger, stating that they were piqued at Gregory for waiting so long to remember them in his busy life. Gregory told me that all of them ended up crying over the phone. The reunion of the hearts as they reformed their past commitments. They were coming to Atlanta the following weekend.

Gregory's lesions multiplied ignoring his positive jest. The raised areas caused by the Kaposi's sarcoma were extremely sensitive to the touch. We took turns carefully rubbing vitamin E oil into the raw crevices of his skin. I showed others a way to wash his hair when he was too weak to move. I had longed admired his thick velvet hair that once cascaded down his back. I tried to hide my hurt at seeing Gregory's face becoming so sulkily shallow. Still, I stroked Gregory's hair delicately as I reminded myself of his former beauty.

I noticed that Gregory rarely spoke of his pain. Instead, he wanted us to talk about ourselves, our feelings. He was still a very caring and loving person. Often, he would lie awake in great pain in the middle of the night refusing to upset anyone's moment of tranquility especially his mother who always came running abruptly to his side.

Gregory was constantly being admitted to hospitals for complications of his disease. His external lesions were being constantly bypassed because other conditions imitated Kaposi's sarcoma. Eventually, his pain became so unbearable that the doctors injected an open line pump of morphine for his discomfort. Sometimes his speech was slurred and he was often disoriented.

It was a balmy summer night. Cleo and Seth were scheduled to arrive into Atlanta in two days. I rode with Mr. Lawrence to Ansley Mall to pick up the recent prescriptions. We took our time with some liberty walking around the store. All of a sudden, we heard our names being paged across the store's intercom. We hurriedly went to the service desk. A woman with a lowered face suggested that we return home.

Mr. Lawrence began to cry. His body started to tremble. I tried to assure him even though I had my own fears to contend with. I drove in silence as he stared into space.

As I rounded the curve, I saw a police car parked in the driveway. In front of the patrol car was a Grady ambulance. Before I could do anything, Mr. Lawrence cried out Gregory's name.

I parked the car on the grass and helped Mr. Lawrence out of the car. His body was still shaking. Someone was holding Mrs. Lawrence as she flailed her arms madly about in the air. Mr. Lawrence ran to his hysterical wife and held her close to him. Both cried.

I looked at Mrs. Lawrence's face and my heart pumped harder. I ran past them all the way to the back room. Duncan was standing near the window with tears falling down his face. His body shook quietly.

A uniformed officer and two ambulance attendants stood over the bed as another officer completed his paperwork. The zippering sound of the body bag being opened made me tremble. I felt faint. I sat on the side of the bed watching them lift my friend onto the stretcher. I couldn't cry. I was too angry to cry. Gregory had said his goodbye.

Duncan came to where I was seated on the bed. He sat down beside me. After Gregory was placed inside the bag, Mr. Lawrence came and stood at the side of the bed. He reached over and grabbed his son's clenched right hand. He opened the fingers and we saw an impression of a crucifix in the palm of Gregory's hand. Mr. Lawrence stood back as the bag was zipped. I buried my face into Duncan's chest. We rocked back and forth, watching them take our friend away. The entire room smelled strongly of flowers, specifically roses.

PHIL MICHAL THOMAS

The next day seemed so endless. The Lawrences were busily completing the arrangements for Gregory while I drove to Hartsville International to pick up Cleo and Seth. I stood numb. I tried not to betray myself to them or anyone. I tried to smile but it wasn't meant to be. Cleo knew the moment she crossed the terminal and faced me.

"Oh no!" Cleo closed her eyes. "When did it happen?"

"Last night...we had just left him for a few minutes."

" How are you holding up?" Seth embraced me.

"As well as can be expected, I guess." My eyes became moist. Damned tears!

"I'm so sorry...We tried to get here sooner...We should have been here with you guys." Cleo wiped my face.

"You're here now...that's what's important. You are here when I need you the most."

The portrait that had graced the living room over the fireplace showing the beauty that once was possessed by Gregory was used at the altar. In front of the portrait were various colored burning candles that surrounded a golden-laced delicate designed urn. Gregory's wish was to be cremated and his ashes spread around the spacious mountains near where he grew up as a boy in Pennsylvania.

A recording of his favorite singer Wynnona Judd filled the sedate air with the songs he had carefully chosen. People crowded into the pews of the Catholic Cathedral while many friends stood around the walls.

The very man that I once sought after now stood before me in reverent form. Father Andrew Welding began the memorial mass for Gregory Andrew Lawrence. The parents, having said their last goodbyes, sat mesmerized by the kindness of his words. Behind the family, the rest of the gang from Nashville and I sat. Some of us cried while some of us simply stared at his portrait.

I noticed that Duncan was standing in the back amidst strangers. He was standing against the wall, alone. I felt that he above all others deserved a place near Gregory's family. I left my seat and asked him to join us as we celebrated the transition of Gregory from this world to his new world. Joan turned briefly and gingerly patted Duncan on his shoulder. His eyes were filled with tears. None of us wanted to say goodbye.

The next day as some of us were preparing to leave Atlanta, Duncan appeared in the lobby of the hotel where we were staying. Cleo, Seth, and I were having coffee at Micks' Cafe when he approached us. Through swollen eyes and a confident smile, he proceeded to tell us of a way to keep Gregory's memory alive.

"I don't know if this would be of any interest to you but there's this national project that some folks are doing in San Francisco to honor people that have died from AIDS. It's called the Quilt." Duncan grabbed a chair from another table and joined us. "I would like to send them something for Gregory."

"I think I have vaguely read something about this Quilt thing. Is this the same group that put on a display in Washington on the Mall?" I rose in my chair.

"Yeah, that's the one. Some folks went from here to go see it. I couldn't afford to go, but I wanted to so bad."

"You just tell us what we need to do to help you." Cleo placed her hand on his shoulder. "You were a good friend to him and to us."

Within a few days, we joined with his parents and other friends and created a panel for our fallen friend. His mother kissed the finished panel. On a mountainous backdrop, the words were simple: *Gregory Anthony Lawrence, My Brother's Keeper.*

Several months collected and past while we gained control of the life around us. Gregory's death left a resounding thud on our spirits. Through his death, we began to see ourselves a bit differently.

The years stopped at 1986. One brisk evening in October, I met Richard for coffee at the Elliston Soda Shop. This small quaint eatery, a throw back from the days of the small tabletop jukeboxes, had gradually become the gang's usual fortress. There was one large Wurlitzer near the kitchen. I expected it to play Peggy Lee's "Is That All There Is" any moment even with the posted out of order sign. Stainless steel tables for four crowded sporadically between the counter and rows of booths. Meat and three place where hot buttered cornbread or muffins are available. Slow service but incredible home cooking.

"What ya have, honey?" The slender aged blond waitress asked as she poised her pen on the ticket ready to strike at the first word of food.

"Actually just coffee." Richard raised his head.

"And you, honey, what ya have?"

"I just wanted coffee...but a piece of pie sounds mighty tempting right now," I said as I glanced at the glass covered pie bins behind the counter.

"Well, I guess you can have both." She smiled, still poised with the pen.
"You know that key lime pie is the boss." Richard shifted in his seat.
"Yeah, but I think I want something richer."
"We got chess pie." She nodded toward the pies.
"That's the ticket. I'll have slice of chess."
"Honey, you want ice cream on top of it?"
"No, too many fat grams already. Just the coffee and pie." The waitress took our menus and hurried off. Before the next words flew from my mouth, she had piping hot coffee in front of us. She dropped dairy creamer on the table and left.

I heard the door open behind me. There was a jingling of an attached bell that announced arrivals and departures. Richard rose back in his seat with a look of disappointment.

"Whazzup! My Nubian bro or is it my soul sister?" Bradley grinned as he walked up from behind me. He startled me. He almost made me drop my steaming coffee..

"What!" Richard almost looked as if he was in disbelief.

"Man, you know. Hows it bes?"

"Bradley, if you don't mind, will you speak normal?"

"I guess he's trying to be cute," I said. "Maybe his drugs are kicking in."

"Richard, you and Michal have got to be the whitest black dudes around," Bradley said. " Man, I bet you croon to that Lawrence Welk dude. Y'all in here drinking this white boy's piss water when y'all should be out there with the homeboys downing some Malt."

"Whatever...why are you tripping?" I refused to shift over in the booth to allow him to sit. Perhaps he would go away, I wished.

"It's like this, my little Mandingo warrior...you need to have pride in who you are...stop acting like you are white." He proceeded to edge his way in.

"Just because I don't sling that nubonic shit doesn't mean that I'm not proud of who I am...I know who I am, obviously you don't know who you are."

"Why can't you be cool like David?"

"Why can't you be sensible like Seth?"

"Please spare me, I have a life...but ya alright with me. I got yo back." Bradley laughed. "We cool."

"You know, Bradley, you are one great guy until you open that mouth of yours and your ignorance spills out."

"Hey, its no big thang, you're still my nig!"

PANELS

"Your what!" Richard reared back as if waiting to strike.

"Hey, dude, chill out...ain't nothing but a thang." Bradley left as quickly as he had entered.

"Good riddance." Richard mumbled as the waitress placed the chess pie in front of me. She nonchalantly poured more coffee and was off to the next table..

"He's a great guy but one that I have to take in small doses. Otherwise, I may want to strangle him."

"I hear that. I don't hate him but he and Diva David grate on my last nerve...I really thought they had learned something from Gregory. But those children have not slowed down a bit."

"Richard, behaviors always gets worst before they get better." I sipped my coffee.

"Yeah, I hear ya. But time isn't always promised to us."

Within every friendship, there is always that person that forever remains calm during the turbulent storms. Richard Gulley was that friend. He was the oldest member of the circle. He was the paste that kept us together. He was our father, so to speak.

Richard became a self-made man. He was a go-getter. He set out to make himself someone that others had to contend with. Richard survived the struggle to achieve a formal education at Vanderbilt while working various and numerous tedious jobs. He paid for his own tuition without any assistance from his family. He believed in himself and often suggested that we do the same.

After he graduated, he went to work as a systems analyst for American Express. I used to tell him that he acted so much older because he didn't take time to relax. His response was always the same: you must never stop climbing the mountain if you can help it.

Richard was born in Kentucky. After his father retired from the military, his family settled in the quietness of suburban America: Muncie, Indiana. His home was nestled only a few feet away from Ball State campus.

Over the years, I learned that Richard was raised in a moderate black middle income Baptist family. Both of his parents worked. Richard was the middle child with a younger sister named Kari and a older brother named Robert. He absolutely adored Kari.

From his years in the Baptist church choir, Richard possessed a well-trained beautiful voice. Richard said he was so active in his church that his mother often spoke of him becoming an elder or even a minister.

"Tell me if I'm stepping on toes…but you seemed out of it lately. What gives? I shifted my back against the wall. "If you don't want to say, just tell me and I will leave it alone."

"You're very perceptive, my dear man." Richard lowered his cup. "I got really bummed out at Gregory's service. Seeing his folks sitting with their heads held high as if they were proud at who their son was."

"You have lost me. I don't understand what you are saying."

"Michal, I would have given anything to have my folks be that supportive. I heard from Sebastian how much his people carried over him. Gregory was not only gay but he was dying from the gay curse and his folks didn't flinch an inch."

"Yeah, I did notice. I can relate to your pain. Ain't no way that our folks gonna act that way if that should happen to us."

"Hell Michal, I doubt if mine would even show their face in public if I was dying from AIDS."

"But we won't worry about that, will we? We are gonna take care of ourselves and not let that bitch of a virus bite us." I stared directly into his eyes filled with rising tears. "It won't happen to us, Lord willing."

"I always felt close to the Lord and to my God. I can still remember some of those hymns we used to sing. My favorite is 'His Eye Is on the Sparrow.'" Richard paused. "It always gave me much comfort."

"Was your old man religious?" I asked.

"No, not really…actually he was a hardcore military man…he only went to church to shut Mama up…usually end up sleeping during the sermon. His god was Uncle Sam."

"So your mom was the church lady, huh?."

"Yeah, kinda like that one on Saturday Night Live." Richard laughed. He raised his coffee cup to the sky. "She was a bible totting woman from way back."

"What about your brother and sister?"

"You mean, did they go to church? Kari did, but Robert was a heathen. Lucifer's own child…he was the player, even after he got married, he still had women on the side. Dad loved him because he was a man and they could play soldiers together."

"So, I take it that you wasn't close to your dad?"

"Baby, that's one mountain that Moses didn't even touch…That man lives and breathes the war...Out of three brats, only two made it to the military. Guess who didn't? Yours truly. I couldn't fight in someone else's war especially not for an establishment that didn't believe in me."

"How did that go over?"

"Not very well. But that was to be expected...I mean, his basic philosophy of war meant making a man out of the boy. If you're black, this was the only way to see the world. Blacks needed the army to stay out of jail...He was a drill sergeant that forgot the war was over."

The waitress was back and about to pour when Richard covered the rim of his cup. Without missing a drop, she aimed for mine. The bell on the door sounded again. The waitress looked behind me and grunted. Curiously, I turned my head to see the new arrivals. A trio of scruffy androgynous youth paraded in and took refuge at the front round window table. I doubt if there were any non-pierced orifice not taken by a piece of silver. Dingy tee shirts barely reached their slopping loose vintage jeans. Their whole mannerism appeared rebellious but in a rather passive way. Were they our past, I wondered.

"Did he know you was gay?" I gathered my thoughts back to Richard.

"Yeah, I told him...but much later. One night, somehow the conversation started about some black soldier that was discharged dishonorably because he told he was gay. I told them that I thought it was unfair for the army to do this man like this after he spent many years in uniform."

"Man, I bet they didn't like that."

"Not at all. In fact, dad said that the guy should have been shot for being a faggot and disgracing the country. To this day, I really don't know why I did it. Maybe it was that pissed off snarl my old man gave. I really don't know but the next thing I knew, I was standing there in front of Robert and Dad telling them that I was gay."

"Are you serious? Man! My old man would have flipped his curls if I told him I was gay. I would have felt the back of his hand so hard against my jaw! How did your old man respond? Did he go berserk on you?"

"Man, did he ever! You would have thought I had slapped him silly. My old man and Robert decided to show me just how much love and affection they had for me...They whup my ass. Honey, we were falling into the front yard fighting."

"Are you serious? What did your mom do?" He had my full attention.

"Just what any God fearing military wife would do...Mama stood and watched her son get one hell of a ass whupping. That whats she did. Man, I was bleeding so much in my face that I couldn't see. But I had to fight back. Or they would have killed me."

"Okay, I can understand your old man throwing a fit, but your entire family. What gives?"

"You know the rule…. it's not okay being black and queer."

"Yeah, I used to hear that broken record over and over from my folks. Why? It's not like we are the only two on this planet."

"You know how it is, we blacks feel that we are already damned anyway merely because of our skin color, at least that the crutch that some of the brothers have. Now add a touch of fairy dust, and you are double whammed."

"And it's a hell of a whammy."

"Well, you already not being accepted because of your color, then you risk additional hell because society as a whole doesn't accept the gayness. So, you are screwed…and in some gay circles, you ain't accepted in their circles either."

"Yeah, Sebastian and I had this discussion just yesterday about whether or not being gay was selective or genetically inborn. What do you think?"

"Ask yourself, if you could change yourself in order to fit in with the norm, don't you think you would gladly change? Believe me, at times, I would have gladly given up this life just to be accepted. It's not easy lying to yourself acting like you're somebody you're not. You gotta be true to yourself and others no matter how they treat you."

"Damn! I never thought about it like that. But, you're right to some degree"

"More than you can imagine…so, my folks went to war on my ass."

"No one tried to break up the fight?"

"Kari did. She went off on them. My GI Josephine sister fought them like a man trying to get them off me. They finally gave up and went back into the house…I lay on the ground scared shitless as Kari wiped the blood out of my eyes. Next thing I know, Mama was throwing my clothes out the door and Dad was telling me to get the hell off his property before he shot me. Since I wasn't moving fast enough for him, Dad came and grabbed Kari off of me and pushed me into the street while our neighbors watch. Doesn't sound much like Walton Mountain, does it?"

"Have you ever gone back?"

"The dead doesn't visit. In their eyes, I'm dead. You see, the only good queer is a dead queer."

"How old were you when this happened?"

PANELS

"It was the day after my fifteenth birthday. Not many places back then for a young boy to go without money or a job." His voice started to crack. I took my hand and covered his. His hand was cold and clammy.

"So, what did you do?"

Richard took a deep breath. He was slow to exhale. His body raised and then he spoke. " You see that street beggar on the corner with the sign? Poor bastard is dirty and all scarred. Yesterday's treasure but today's trash. Worthless...that was me at one time. I wandered the streets of Muncie. I became a native of the land of shantytown."

"Man, you were only fifteen years old! How did you live on your own? Are you saying your folks really didn't come looking for you?"

"Like I said before, in their eyes, I was dead already. They no longer had a son named Richard. I died the moment I said I was queer."

"What about Kari? Didn't she come for you? What about your other friends? No one did anything to help you?"

"Michal, no one really gives a damn about a little black boy wandering the street. I simply became another face in the horizon...but things did change a tad later on...some of which I wished hadn't happen, but it did...I survived it!"

"How did you manage on the streets? Weren't you scared?"

"You better believe I was scared. Hell, I was terrified. I mean, you are talking to someone that was once afraid of his own shadow, never ever slept away from home, but now home was the streets."

"What did you do?"

"Before they start charging us rent here, let's leave. I really need some fresh air." Richard edged from inside the booth, threw a few dollars on the table. He picked up the food ticket.

"What's my part?"

"Don't worry, I got ya back. Anyway, a free meal for free psychobabble is worth it." He cocked his head back and smiled while he paid the cashier. The bell clanged as we went out onto the street.

The humidity was scorching. Immediate puddles of sweat formed around my brow. The nightlife on Elliston Place was almost nil. The rats weren't even scampering around the overflowed garbage on the street. Maybe this was good for us, less distraction. We headed west towards Centennial Park.

"You know that hymn I told you I loved: "His Eye Is on the Sparrow"? I know that God was watching over me when I was out there. In fact, he was working overtime protecting my ass...Oh, I met me some real live characters.

There was Jerry that would cut his own mama's throat for a buck. Half of the people on the streets were loonies that used to live in the city's crazy house. You learned to watch your back and sleep with one eye opened all the time...they stole from each other religiously. You were your only friend. Some of them would drive you and Sebastian to suicide."

We stopped walking and listened to the bells ring from the Carmichael Towers. The dull ringing broke the quietness of the night, although momentarily. Casual walkers conversing behind us broke our trance. Richard took off walking again. My short legs were no match for his long lanky legs.

"So did they ever try anything with you?"

"Baby, they had some real issues. But, in a strange way, they were really okay. Kinda screwy, but okay...One woman, I laugh when I think of her even today. We called her Big Bonnie."

"Was she a big fat woman or something?" I was still trying to keep in step with him.

"Yeah, she was on the heavy side but that wasn't why we called her Big Bonnie; this woman had one of the biggest heart of anyone I have ever met in my life. She was a large white woman with dull unkempt red hair. In her sixties, I think. She always walked proud in her torn shabby dress. Baby, she had holes in her clothes all over from head to her swollen flat feet...she named me 'Music Boy' because I was always singing something. She became my mama...you better believe she watched over me like a hawk."

"You was just a boy, how did they accept you?" I had to stop to catch my breath. I pulled at the back of his shirt to stop him. We sat on the brick wall outside a church. Across from us was a vacant lot where a Catholic school once stood. Now the lot housed weeds and the openness.

"Not very well, at first...I mean, these were people that would fight over a rotten bag of food or they would dive into dumpsters outside restaurants for the garbage...you'd be surprised at how much good food gets thrown away...not given away but thrown in the garbage. After a while, you learned what dumpster you would hit on what day...most of them teased me about running away from home...they called me a wimp and shit...I didn't dare tell them why I was there...they already hated me being there. At first, I felt out of place. Then at night, everyone would huddle around and shoot the shit, kinda like a family. Big Bonnie was my mama!"

"Why did she like you?"

"I really don't know except some of the folks did say that she always talked about her rich family and her boys that she had to leave behind."

PANELS

"She came from money? What was wrong? Why did she have to leave?"

"Big Bonnie was a drunk...I really don't know if she actually left on her own or if she was forced out."

"Oh, sounds like she's right from the movie *Madame Ex*."

"Kinda, I mean she never talked about her family and when you asked her about them, she got pissed off...her favorite saying was always 'Make it all right again in the mind.' She would stare into space and then clumsily dance wildly about the street."

"She sounds sorta philosophical."

"Naw, she was usually taking her usual swig from any available bottle of liquor." Richard laughed. "Honey, she would act like she just had that wine of the gods."

"So she treated you like one of her boys."

"I guess...one time, I was picking off some chicken from some bones I found. In the bag was a partially eaten ear of corn. Big Bonnie sat down beside me and I gave her the corn. Her eyes sparkled like new money as she took the corn. She sat her wine down between us. She hugged me and devoured that corn...after licking her lips, she pulled out a small child's red and white plaid shirt she found on the streets. She just looked at it and smiled, still smacking her lips from the grease."

"What was she going to do with that shirt? Surely, she didn't think you could wear it."

"Oh, it wasn't for me...she said it was for her youngest boy...she stopped talking and I felt her shoulders shaking. I tried to put my arm around her and told it was going to be all right. She told me, no, not for her. She whispered through her tears how she missed her family. She told that everything she had was gone even her boys that she loved so much...All of a sudden, she pushed me away and grabbed her bottle. She turned that bottle up and drained it to the last drops. She looked over at me and told me that it would make it all right again in the mind."

"You could have easily turned into a drunk or even an addict. Did you ever hustle? I mean, I would understand if you had to. You know, trying to survive and all."

"I thought too much of myself to do that. Even if I had wanted to, Big Bonnie taught me how to survive by panhandling. She was a real pro and knew the best spots to work...As for me hustling, I didn't know how to be with anyone. Yeah, I knew how I felt but I still had never done anything with a single soul...I just knew that I would make it."

"Man, you were so brave. You were living on the streets, young and dumb, so naive. You're lucky you wasn't raped or even killed."

"Well, one out of two isn't too bad. At least, I wasn't killed." Richard jumped down onto the pavement and started to walk away.

"What are you talking about? Someone did rape you on the streets?" I grabbed him by the arm making him stop in his tracks.

" Let's just say that Sebastian isn't the only one that found the cruelty of man love."

"I don't understand."

"You know how they say that most molesters are either family members or friends of the family?" Richard paused. "It was a friend of the family."

"Is it something you can talk about? I mean, does it still hurt to think about it?"

"Not anymore, in fact it's one of things in my life that pushes me forward and not backwards...I have always wanted to kill that bastard because of what he did to me, but over the years, my hatred turned to, believe it or not, feeling sorry for his worthless ass."

"So, what happened?"

"For several days, I would see this old blue Chrysler circling the block...at times, it would just cruise by me, never actually stopping...At first, I used to hide from the car thinking it was either my brother or father coming to beat my ass again...But it wasn't them...Big Bonnie cursed at the car telling them to go ahead and take a picture of the freaks 'cause it would last longer...all of a sudden the car stopped only a few feet away; I was getting real nervous. I didn't want them to bother Big Bonnie. I knew I had to do something but didn't know what and the others weren't around to help us...Big Bonnie leaned over and picked up a brick from the road. She was going to knock the hell out of them."

"Who was in the car?"

"I didn't know at first...She told me to pick up a trash can lid to clobber their ass but I picked up some broken glass...I was beaten enough already and I wasn't about to take another ass licking...My blood started boiling. We were ready to fight!"

"So what happened?"

"Just about the time I was going to strike, a voice called my name...A voice I knew."

"Was it your family?"

"Naw, it was a dude that knew me and my folks...He opened his car door

PANELS

and asked me to get inside…Big Bonnie was so pissed when I went near the car…She went off on me…After I saw who he was, I tried to tell Big Bonnie that it was alright…oh, no, she went completely berserk telling me that I was leaving her like all the others had left her. I couldn't get her to listen to me so I just got in the car and left."

"Maybe she was trying to tell you something."

"Maybe…anyway, it was a guy that I knew as Jack—Jack McNeil to be exact. He lived on the other side of Muncie…I had always heard that he was a closet queen although he dated some women around there."

"Oh, a regular down low dude?"

"Yeah, keep it under the sheets and no one will ever know…But at that time, I didn't care about his reputation, I was just tired of living on the streets. I eventually moved in with him."

"He became your lover?" As soon as the words left my mouth, I looked directly in the face of a stranger walking in our direction. He mumbled "faggots" and spit on the street as he past us. I turned around and blew him a kiss and called him an asshole.

"Not that way. He let me sleep in the other cramped bedroom…I would try to keep the house sort of clean while he was at work." Richard acted as if he didn't hear any of the words being passed.

"What did he do for a living?"

"He was a professor at the university. I think he taught English or History…I thought everything was cool; I had a place to stay and he gave me my space. But I was still missing my folks, mostly Kari. I used to cry myself to sleep thinking that my life would be like that for the rest of my life…everything was great until it happened."

"Until what happened?" I stopped in my tracks and grabbed Richard by the sleeve of his shirt. He turned and faced me. This time, he wasn't smiling.

"I soon realized that Jack used to cruise the parks. He wanted to trick with anything and everything. He never touched me and he didn't try anything for the longest…I wanted to go out myself and try to meet somebody my own age, but he wouldn't let me."

"Okay, you didn't have sex and he wouldn't let you be with someone else; were you a some kinda prisoner?"

"Yeah…you see I know just how Cleo feels with Edward watching her every step. Jack did me the same way…I had no company to come over; it was just the two of us. After, of course, he finished his tricking." He appeared somewhat uneasy and continued to walk away.

"What did he want from you? You didn't see anyone at all?" I caught up with him.

"Nope, not a soul...except for the time when Kari surprised me with a visit."

"How did she know where you were?"

"She told me that two gay friends told her...Man, I didn't even know she knew anyone gay. I mean, she never told me."

"Did you ever think she might have always known about you?"

"Probably...but she never said a thing...anyway, I was cleaning his bedroom when I heard this soft tapping on the window pane in the front room. I crept up and peeked out the window and there she was. Standing between the rose bushes. She was calling my name."

"Was she alone? Was anyone with her?"

"Well, to be safe, I did look out to make sure she was by herself. Thank God, she was by herself."

"So, did you let her in or what?"

"I opened that door and she was inside in a New York minute...I was so glad to see her that I cried. She cried. Hell, we both cried...My world wasn't over after all."

"Oh, sounds like a perfect Hallmark movie." I held my arms out and played my imaginary violin.

"You can be sarcastic all you want. It don't bother me...Kari stood there and looked at me like she hadn't seen me in years...She did tell me that I looked like something dragged in from road kill."

"I told you about wearing that butt ugly blue mascara in the day light. Ain't too pretty on ya."

"You'll be alright one day...anyway, Kari walked all over the house asking me if we were lovers. Before I could say anything, she pointed out that the house reeked of Jack and that made her feel creepy...She didn't say she was upset with me having a lover; she just didn't want it to be Jack."

"I think I'm going to like your sister. Why don't you fix me up with her?"

"You're not her type."

"Why?"

"You are not her type because she prefers men and not women!"

"That's not what you thought that night you slept with me."

"A moment of charity is always good for the soul."

"Whatever!"

We both stopped at the curve. While I waited for our chance to cross the street, Richard darted into the traffic headfirst. Horns blew in sequence as I ran to join him.

The lights on West End sparkled and blinked around us. Joggers ran their perfect strides appearing totally oblivious to all but the cars. Richard and I both stared a bit longer at the moving physiques and smiled. Suddenly, Richard ran around the park sign which stated in large letters of being closed at dusk. He placed his finger to his lips and made a shooshing sound. "Gotta be quiet or the parkies will get us thrown in jail."

"Why, are you afraid of running into some old flames?"

"You know I love you…what's your name again…Anyway, where was I. Oh, so Kari is talking up a storm asking me all these questions…I was sort of nervous thinking that Jack was coming home any moment…I was getting scared and practically jumped at every sound made outside…We talked about why I thought I was gay…Kari really made me cry when she told me that she loved me regardless of whom I slept with."

"I take for granted that the others didn't feel that same way about you."

"No, I was still dead in their mind…we talked for a long time until she looked at her watch. She had to leave before Marvin went to work."

"Who's Marvin?"

"Her boyfriend."

"Was he cool about it, you know with you being a little gay boy?"

"Kari said he was…I found out later that he really was cool about it. He was from California. Okay dude. No hang-ups."

"So, how did he get involved?"

"He saved my life. He dashed me away on his fleeting horse…"

"Excuse me! What are you saying?"

"You know, like the damsel being whisked away by the knight in shining armor…One night, Jack came home. He was stumbling over everything including me. Stupid me, I tried to lead him to his room so he could pass out in there…This mother knocked my ass down on and got on top of me…the bastard tore my clothes off me and…forced that amyl nitrite shit up my nose I couldn't breathe with my face in the pillow…my head started spinning after I got a whiff of it. My blood started rushing to my head. He slapped me hard across my face a few times…I think I passed out."

"Tell me he didn't take it further, you know?"

"Yep, he became my first."

"That bastard!"

"All I know is that when I finally opened my eyes, his fat ass was on top of me. I couldn't breathe. I was too scared to move. I didn't want him to wake up. I cried asking the Lord to just take me…I cursed my life…I hated life."

"How did you get away?"

"Jack eventually rolled off me. I got up and went to the bathroom. I tried being very quiet…I just stood in the shower for a few minutes. I was listening for him…I have never been as terrified in my life as I was at that time…I turned on the water. I wanted it hot. The hot stream of water started to scorch me but I didn't care…As I closed my eyes, he yanked open the shower curtain and grabbed me…He grabbed me by my neck and dragged me across the house to the front door…I tried fighting back but it didn't help…The front door was already opened when he shoved me outside. Naked, I was naked…That bastard threw me down the steps and then threw all my clothes at me."

"Omigod, what did you do?"

"Nothing I could do except put my clothes on and get the hell away from there."

"No one stopped to help you?"

"Nope. See, this was on the other side of the tracks. This happened all the time. Fights, stabbing, you know the drill. No one wanted to be involved."

"At least you got the hell out of there."

"As soon as I put my pants on, I ran down the street where I knew a phone booth was."

"But, who could you call? Who would come?"

"I really didn't know at first who to call. I was shaking bad. I kept on looking behind me thinking that he was coming after me…By the grace of God, I found a quarter in my pocket…I called Marvin…I was hoping that Kari was there."

"Did anyone answer?"

"Yeah, thank God, Kari did!"

"Is this when Marvin came over and kicked his ass?"

"No. Marvin never touched him…but within minutes after I hung the phone up, Kari was there…my baby sister was there to my rescue…She and Marvin put me in his car and took me to their home."

"Did you tell her what happened?"

"No…not right off the bat…I think I remembered telling both of them after I had a shower and had some food in me…To this day, I will always remember Kari telling me that she will be always be there for me…And you know, she has."

PANELS

In reflection on past conversations with Richard, I now realize that those he loved did not always tell him the truth. A lover had taught him an unfortunate lesson: you cannot trust the one you love. If I had known then what I know now, I could possibly have saved a life—Richard's life. In the valley of love, unfaithfulness is never a stranger.

Daniel Brooks, Richard's lover, was indeed someone I never could trust. When I looked into his soul, I realized that he wasn't a just man. Nevertheless, how does one tell a close friend that the love of his very existence is not the one for him?

Daniel had turned Richard's heart into a spiraling whirl of conflicting emotions. I never really understood their common interests nor their drive to be together. I must admit that I was once attracted to Richard when we first met, and I may have been slightly jealous of Daniel. But Daniel was so different from Richard. Richard was warm and affectionate while Daniel was distant and cold. He lived behind a heterosexual façade, thinking he was discrete, without the slightest suggestion of queerness. The circle felt he was sadly mistaken. We accepted him only because we loved Richard.

One Sunday afternoon in June, we all gathered at Cleo's home for a community champagne brunch. Seth and Richard were in the kitchen preparing eggs Benedict, chicken with shrimp- basil sauce and roasted rosemary pork loin with wild rice. Simmering on the back burners were baby carrots with walnuts and honey and O'Brien potatoes fragrant with herbs. David had just finished making baby lettuce and herb salad with a tart raspberry vinaigrette. He retreated to the balcony:

"Ms. Betty Wannabe Crocker and Ms. June Cleaver done ran my ass out of the kitchen." David flailed his hands around. "Gimme some of that bubbly. Mama has worked her magic and is tired."

"Everything smells delicious!" Cleo shifted Theresa in her lap. "When do we eat?"

"Times are a- changing. Just look…the women folks are sitting around waiting for the men folks to cook their food. Ain't that something!" Bradley paraded around the table nibbling at a few morsels.

Sebastian was placing more food on the table. The centerpiece was a mélange of fruit in a melon basket surrounded by trays of fresh vegetables, chess pies, tricolor pasta salad, potato salad, and assorted cheeses and pates. The aroma spiced the air and teased our starving souls.

Our thirsty bodies were enticed by the bar spread with glasses and drinks. Mint juleps, bloody Marys, Chablis, and Corbel.

David posed as a grand dame on the balcony waving to the strangers on the street below. His high shrill voiced taunted any who didn't wave back. Bradley and Sebastian were discussing the politics of the day. Each voice rose occasionally with authority. Cleo rocked baby Theresa as I continued to pour the bubbly in raised empty flutes. The room was filled with laughter and good talk.

Suddenly, the baby grand came to life. Seth stroked the keys of the Steinway and Richard stood behind him and began to sing. I knew the song, a spiritual I was raised on. Richard's smooth baritone filled the room. His eyes closed, his head held high.

"Oh dear God, we are having us some church up in here!" David swirled from outside. "Can I get a amen up in here?"

Theresa jumped from her mother's lap and ran to the piano. She danced around the room while she clapped her hands. Seth looked down at her. He stopped playing just long enough to pick her up to sit beside him. Theresa giggled and beamed up at him.

The tempo changed to a jazzier number. Richard moved over to Theresa and started dancing with her, her feet dangling in the air as he held her in his arms. The music ended when Sebastian announced that brunch was ready. We gathered around the table, and Richard blessed the food.

"Does anyone need anything before I sit down to eat?" Cleo stood holding Theresa.

"Honey, sit your bony butt down! If these chillums need something, they know where to go get it." David nodded to her chair.

"We probably know that kitchen better than you anyway." I laughed.

"You got that right. To me, a kitchen is only another room in the house." Cleo positioned Theresa in the chair beside her.

"Did I tell you guys where I am working…actually volunteering?" Richard poured orange juice in his glass. "After Gregory's death, I started to volunteer with Middle Tennessee Cares. I'm modifying their computer network to combine several different data systems into one main line"

"Richard, is that why you are flying solo today?" Bradley pointed at Richard's side. "I don't see anyone hanging onto you."

"Shut up, Bradley and pass the eggs Benedicts." David reached over the table. "Y'all can almost cook as good as me. Even got that little child eating."

"I'm surprised she ate the chicken since it's not a leg." Cleo wiped

PANELS

Theresa's face with a moist napkin. "So I take it that Daniel has some issues with you not being around."

"Yeah…I can't believe that Dan is giving me such a hard time. It's not like I'm hanging out at the lake or some bar." Richard stopped eating. He toyed with the baby carrots.

"Maybe he just wants to spend more time with you." Cleo sounded concerned.

"Yeah, but it's not like I don't see him." Richard still not eating.

"You know, you had this little problem before with him when you guys first got together…he didn't want you to spend so much time with us." Bradley reached for the rolls.

"Yeah, Richard, is he jealous or something?" Sebastian asked. "Pass the tricolor salad, please."

"Anyway, I'm proud of you. You are doing something that's unselfish. You are giving a big part of yourself to others who are dying. I couldn't do it," Bradley said.

"I prefer to think of them as people living with AIDS, not dying."

"Actually, Richard is right. The mind set has a lot to do with their healing process," I said. "A positive outlook may lengthen their lives."

" But what kind of life? I remember seeing those pictures of you and Gregory before he died…I couldn't do it. I couldn't live that way." Bradley appeared fidgety.

"Bradley, that's because you are so damn vain! There's more to life than looks." Sebastian sat upright. His face red.

"So you say, I just know it ain't going to be me."

"Forget Bradley, back to you, Richard, what are you going to do?" David rubbed Richard's back. "Gimme some more wine, my glass is suffering from dehydration!"

"I don't know…but I do know I'm not going to walk away from folks with AIDS. Enough people have walked out of their lives already."

"So, you gonna give up your man to stay with those that ain't got much time. What gives?" Bradley asked.

"Bradley, you know, you are really a sad person. I hope to God you never have to experience what they have to…But what really pisses me off, is the fact that there are many assholes like you that feel that same way."

"I don't know why you getting so pissed at me, I don't give a damn what you do with your time…it's your man that has the problem…so you need to tell him that…anyway, I gotta go, some of us still have a life." Bradley rose from the table, almost knocking his chair to the floor. He left in an angry frenzy. After a moment or two, the rest of us ate our food.

"Ohh, I believe Ms. Bradley got a piece waiting somewhere in the woods…or at the cliffs at the lake." David cocked his head toward the now empty chair..

"Richard, I don't know why you let him get to you. Bradley ain't gonna change. He will always be an asshole, a selfish one at that…Just talk to Dan," I piped in.

"Yeah, talk to him. Surely he's not that insecure that he is afraid he will lose you. I mean, look at yourselves, you guys have been together, what three years?" Cleo tried to be reassuring.

"Four!"

"Is four years something to just toss out with the cat?"

"I love cats."

"You know what I mean, smartass…talk to him. Find out what really is bothering him." Seth paused. He reached for the wild rice. " Surely, it can't be your working with the terminally ill."

"I will talk to him. But now I better hurry home before he starts beeping me."

"Honey, do you need me come and straighten your man out for you?" David flirted. "You know I will."

"Naw…that's okay. I'm sure it's really nothing. We just need to talk it out. We have always opened up to each other in the past." Richard smiled. Somehow, I felt he was trying to reassure himself more than us.

"You know, the only thing missing are the ribs, turnip greens, and skillet cornbread. Baby you talking about some good eating." David smacked his lips.

"David honey, you know what they say, you can take the girl out of the country but you can't take the country out of the girl," I joked.

"Michal, you betta be glad there's a chile at this here table or I would have read you to filth." David rocked his head back and forth. He reminded me of those rear window dolls with the spring action head.

"Theresa, these are your uncles." Cleo pointed at each of us. "You gonna love them, madness and all."

Within a month, the beeps ended as well as the relationship. Dan had met someone else. Rumors had it that Daniel started the fling weeks before he told

PANELS

Richard. For his healing process, Richard increased his volunteer hours.

In other conversations, Richard confided that he missed the religious connection. He missed the closeness of his own family. He told me that he would lie awake tormented by the sorrow and desolation of his heart.

"I was raised in the church. All I knew was the church...now, I hate the church."

"You don't really hate the church, you hate what people in the church have done to you."

"I guess you're right...God doesn't hate me...but listening to these voices in my head telling me that I have forsaken God is driving me crazy. I still love God and still want him in my life. I am worthy...I am worthy."

"Always remember that our God is indeed a loving God. Think about some of the songs you heard in church growing up."

"You mean the hymns?...My favorite was 'His Eye Is on the Sparrow.' However, I can't sing that song anymore. I'm not happy and I'm certainly not free..."

"Is there not a church that you would attend?"

"Surely you jest. Honey, you have no idea the hell some of those churches have put me through...Oh, don't get me wrong, all you have to do is look in the choir stands and you will see more family members than you can imagine, swaying in their robes...but they are also trying to be down low. Just look at your ex...I'm sorry, I can't be that way."

"You don't have to have a church. Remember the scripture of 'Where two or three are gathered in my name, I am among them'?"

"Yeah, I know it."

"Who knows, maybe you will one day experience it."

"Say, Michal, out of curiosity, why didn't you get a church and preach?"

"Maybe one day I will...Remember all things are possible in His name."

Several days later, Richard called. There was much excitement in his voice. He rambled something I couldn't quite understand.

"You'll never believe what has just happened to me!"

"You found a new love in your life?"

"Nope, something better!"

"Richard, there's nothing better than a new love.'"

"Oh, yes there is!"

"I give up, what is it then?'

"I found one."

"One what?"

"A church!"

"You are this excited over a church. Honey, what gives?"

"It's a reconciling church...I went last Sunday for the first time. It was totally unbelievable!"

"I doubt that it was that unbelievable."

"Okay, dirtbag, tell me the last church you walked in where they had a gay flag hanging for everybody to see that wasn't a typical gay church?"

"Yeah right. So, where is this totally unbelievable place and what's its name?"

"It's right here in Nashville...it's called Edgehill."

"Hey, I have heard of that church...So, what's it like?"

"Well, it's definitely not your run of the mill traditional place...the people are so real there!"

"How did you find out about it?"

"Remember that older couple Eddie and Alan that I was telling you about? The ones that took care of AIDS patients in their home for free? They told me about the place."

"Those two guys that you said have been together for twenty-eight years?"

"Yeah, those two. You know, I gotta really hand it to them...Here they are, two guys that should be living it up. They live in this nice cozy house. Beautiful antiques. Alan painted while Eddie restored old furniture. Instead of enjoying a life of leisure, what do they do? They bring in the homeless to live until they die...and don't ask nothing for it. Michal, now that is true Christians. They don't sit back on their asses and dog out others. You know the kind."

"Surely you don't know anyone of that caliber, not in the church!" I was sarcastic.

"Please...Michal, now don't get me started...I get more hell from those so-call Christians than I do the drunken sinners on the streets. They praise the Lord one moment and then cursing up a storm the next."

"You can say amen to that!"

"Even to this day, when I think about what they did for a guy named Lee, I get teary eyed...You see, Lee's favorite holiday was Christmas...But this particular year he was getting weaker and weaker as the days drew on...I really didn't think he would make it to Christmas. I sorta felt that Eddie nor Alan thought he would make it. So, we decided to celebrate Christmas early...They decorated their house with fake snow and garland. The house smelled like baked ginger cookies and pound cake. They even had presents wrapped and placed underneath the tree. All of this in November!"

"Did you play Santa?"

"No I didn't, smartass…I would have if they asked me to…anyway, and we all started singing Christmas carols. Lee was brought in and propped up on the sofa. He was in so much pain, but he still had a smile on his face…you remember that preacher at Edgehill? Well, he and his wife Brenda were there. You should have seen Lee's eyes, baby, they were twinkling like stars…Then we gave him his gift. It was a sweatshirt that he had wanted. He had wanted all of us to sign his shirt…"

"I thought he died later."

"He did…later. His life ended on New Year's Eve…Afterwards, I watched as Eddie and Alan bathed his limp body as tenderly as they would a newborn child…The radio was on. Jim Croce was singing 'Time in a Bottle.' We dressed Lee into his Christmas clothes. He really looked good wearing that sweatshirt." Richard paused. "Then they came and took him away.'

"This minister guy really means a lot to you, doesn't he?"

"I guess he does. Maybe that's why I really love that church."

"So I take it that this place is without those heathen hypocrites?"

"I may be naïve but I don't think they could handle that church…Michal, I'm serious, the place is wonderful!"

"How on earth did they persuade you to go there?"

"Well, it took them a lot of talking to me…I would go over there to see my buddy Lee. We would visit for about an hour and then I would leave an hour or so later, you know, to give him time to sleep…But instead of leaving, the two guys would often invite me out on their sun porch for something cold to drink…anyway, somehow the conversation got started about religion and churches…At first, I didn't say anything. I didn't want to offend them by telling them that I thought religion was a crock of shit. So I shut up and listened until I had had enough, then I would leave…This same scene went on and on…I finally opened my trap and told them straight up what the church had done for me."

"Oh no! The gates of rapture opened up." I laughed.

"Not exactly, they listened and didn't get pissed off at me. At least they didn't tell me if they did…then one of them said that he totally agreed with me because he also had hell to pay when he came out…then they told me. Honey, their faces actually lit up when they talked about that place."

"Edgehill?"

"Yeah, They just kept on talking about how wonderful it was and how receptive the members were...Being black, I questioned if I would be welcomed...Eddie said it was the least of my worry...that they didn't see color."

"What was the catch?"

"There wasn't any...So, I figured that I would go by there one Sunday before church, to see what everything looked like so that I could tell them that I had gone. Maybe they would leave me alone if I tried it; at least that is what I hoped. I drove by the church that following Sunday. I saw that old vintage bus they talked about before I even saw the building. Honey, I ain't never saw no church with purple doors in my life!...No one was there at that time. I thought, this is good now I can leave and they would never know I didn't stay...You are not gonna believe this, but as I was driving away, the car brought me back to that church. This time, people were there."

"What did you do then?"

"I took a deep breath. My heart was beating so hard I thought I was gonna pass out. I touched the door handle and went inside."

"Did pieces of the ceiling come crashing down on your head? Did the Heavens open up and rain locust upon the earth?'

" I think I see why your tired ass ain't preaching...You got major issues, man."

"Yeah right. Com'on, admit you was scared going in that place."

"I was, at first. But after I looked around, everything seemed okay...It was kinda set up odd with no pews or a choir stand. Everybody was dressed in causal clothing...it was kinda different."

"Wait a minute, isn't that a Methodist church?"

"And? What's your point?"

"Aren't you Baptist?"

"I was when I was younger...anyway, it doesn't make any difference. That church is like a melting pot that has a little bit of everything going there."

"Way different from your Baptist church, I bet?"

"You betta believe it...but it was alright...I sorta felt right at home...Bro. Bill stood in the middle of the floor. Nothing fancy, no three pieces, just a turtleneck and a large silver cross around his neck...People sat in stackable chairs placed in a semi-circle. Some looked over me and smiled but it wasn't a stare...I sat down in one of the back seats...As I looked around the room, my eyes locked tight on this older black woman seated across the room. She was beautiful and elegantly dressed. Her hair was pure white as clouds...Her name was Ms. Laura...I think she had enough bangles on her arms to give everyone in the church one...She smiled at me and nodded her head as if to say 'it's alright, now'...I got goose bumps. I really think I felt the presence of God in this woman...It was like I have known her all my life...But I had never seen her before...For whatever reasons, my eyes started to water...then it happened. Looking behind Ms. Laura, I saw it...Tears started running down my face."

"What happened? What was it that you saw?"

"They have this large banner of a flag with their name on it and the word 'reconciling.'" Richard paused. "It was the rainbow flag!"

In the past, the inner conflict with his love for his God had overwhelmed him. At this moment, with this new revelation, he was as giddy as a young naïve schoolgirl on her first date.

Richard had not walked inside a church in several years with the unfortunate exception of the memorial services for fallen friends. He told me once that he had long accepted the belief that the God he so loved had turned his back to him because he was gay. He told me later that going to that church was one of the best things that have ever happened to him. He finally felt accepted by God and even his own race.

One of my memories of Richard and this church was when he joined into their congregation. Several of us including Bradley were there for moral support.

The seating was as Richard had described: semi-circle rows with the mouth opened to face the minister. William Barnes, a kindred spirit of faith, stood before the diverse multitude at the communion table where purple advent candles burned. Dressed in adorning simplicity wearing a white formal shirt with tiny floral designs accentuating, he stood with a reassuring smile nestled on his face. Standing near the advent fire, his receding hair displayed. He was a tall man with a deep voice of definite authority and grace.

As I glanced around the room, I took notice to one of the banners. The designs reminded me of the panels we had created for the Quilt. I became mesmerized in the simple figurine that appeared to have been walking into the light of the sun or rather God's arms of compassionate love. Somehow, I felt like that figurine reaching out for understanding and truth.

Throughout the entire service, I noticed Richard wiping his eyes. Bro. Barnes spoke of life, comparing it in terms of fragments of a wrecked ship. He said that people tended to hold steadfastly onto the splinters of the ship just to keep afloat.

PHIL MICHAL THOMAS

When Richard stood to join Bro. Barnes at the altar, we watched as two older guys went and stood beside him. To his left, stood the black associate minister named Moses. According to Richard's description, I think it was Ms. Laura that approached him. She was indeed well dressed with a distinguishable head of white. As she balanced herself on her cane, I heard the numerous bangles clinging. There was another woman, a younger white woman that stood by his side. He told me later that she was Mauri, someone he had met at Middle Tennessee Cares. She hugged him. She made brief comments and spoke of his contribution at the agency. This woman spoke through her tears. As the minister prayed, all those around Richard placed their hands on his back. The congregation sang "Bless His Life"...Richard's eyes appeared swollen. He was crying.

I don't know why, but I wanted to cry for him as well. Some how, I felt he was doing okay.

Although I loved David as a friend, I often loathed his ways. David was the most flamboyant one of the circle. He was what you may consider as a "screaming queen."

The drama queen drop out filled with catty remarks and batty eyes. You know the type, the grandiose diva from hell.

David was the only friend that did not attend Vanderbilt University; he had received his formal training from the Jon Albertson School of Cosmetology. He was actually very good in the art of make up and style. Hairstylist by trade, the twenty-eight-year-old also performed as a female impersonator.

David was very petite with natural feminine features with the exception of his manly sized feet and hands. He grew his hair long and usually wore it in his trademark French twist. He had a beautiful face in or out of drag. Oops, did I say drag? He preferred to be called an illusionist. He considered drag queens as being street trash. His eyes would arch sternly when compared to a drag queen.

David was indeed the biggest flirt of the circle. Actually he wasn't. He played second fiddle to Bradley, his counter part in crime. Secretly, I think most of us envied both David and Bradley for having the guts to do as they pleased.

There is not an easy way to describe the first time I met David. Let's just say, he wasn't quite himself. I was to meet Richard and Bradley at the Cabaret one Saturday night. Bradley told me he had someone he wanted me to meet. He assured me that it wasn't some twisted blind date but someone he had wanted us to meet. This alone should have raised the flag since Bradley didn't make a habit of us knowing his other friends. David was always extremely honest and caring to all of us. He genuinely was kind. However, when he transformed into his alter ego, he became Tiffany Lynn. Converting into the sultry, sexual, sensual, and unforgiving diva of the stage. Her moves connected well with the art of lip synch. Emotions danced about the stage as she gestured the lyrics.

With the virgin mannerism of a true queen of the Nile, Tiffany Lynn set the mood. Tiffany also wore the face of being brass, an unequal bitch, innocent lass, graceful, and even a whore. She was not to be understood nor taken for granted for she was as mysterious as she was open.

Tiffany dressed only in the finest clothing. The delicate bugle beaded gowns were either borrowed or her own creations. David had an infamous history of buying exclusive designer gowns, wearing the gowns during the performances, and returning the slightly soiled dresses on the following day. Religiously, he aired the attire outside his enclosed patio to rid the bar's smoke or have the gowns dry-cleaned. Once the upscale boutiques realized his habits, they would refuse the items on return. No problem since Nashville had numerous designer boutiques to hit, he thought.

As David, he was attracted only to the rugged type. The real brute. The seedier the better with a spiced dark past. The bad boys. His preference was always black men. I eventually saw blackened eyes, swollen lips, etc, after some of his sexual quests. Richard and I once asked him why he was attracted to the unattainable.

One early morning after the Cabaret had closed, Richard and I drove David home after he had changed back to his boy clothes. His home was dark. We were alone. His brother was out running the streets much to my joy.

"You girls just don't understand…why should I want some wimp ass guy…I want a man…A true man…A man to love…" David placed his gowns in the hall closet. He pointed towards the kitchen. "Y'all wants something to drink?"

"Naw, I gotta go to work in a few hours," I said.

"Well, suit yourself. I'm gonna have me a cocktail." David poured vodka into a glass and splashed a scent of orange juice. " Like I said, I want a real man to love me."

"Honey, you are not the Rose, so don't go there…you are a nice looking guy that could find someone that would love you."

"Nice looking, hell! I'm flawless…Just look at my figure, women would die to have this…My unblemished curves are to be worshiped…I got more beauty on my big toe than some of the shapeless women I see…They all love me."

"Yeah, but we are talking about real love…love beyond that damned stage."

"Richard, my dear, before you do me, you need to look around yourself and see if your love is there. I don't think so. And you ain't on nobody's stage."

"David, you're right. I am alone because I refuse to go out and get somebody just to say I have somebody. I rather stay at home without putting up with the bullshit."

"Honey, you definitely got your wish. Not everybody wants to be a homebody like you. Just 'cause it's good for you don't mean it gonna be good for me."

"I just think you need to be more choosy of what you sleep with, that's all."

"Michal, sweetie, tell Ms. Pure and almighty here, that I don't sleep with my men, I trick with them. Then I send them home with their tongues hanging out."

"There's more to life than tricking…What are you going to do when you are too old for the stage? Have you ever thought about that?"

"Don't you worry about me and what I'm gonna do. You need to worry about your tired self."

"Now, girl, don't you snap at me! Have you thought about your future? I mean, Richard does have a point." I decided I needed a drink after all.

"Oh shit, now they got Ms. Polly Padre going after me…If I didn't like y'all damned asses, I'll tell y'all to kiss me where the sun don't shine…Y'all don't understand 'cause y'all ain't never been down my streets…Y'all ain't had to pick yourself up off the streets after being knocked down…Y'all don't know what it feels like not having a pot to piss in…Baby, I have got a dream where I'm somebody…I wake up and people treat me right…don't dog me out…but be there for me."

"We will always be there for you, if you only let us. Right, Michal?"

"You already know that. If you don't, then you should by now."

"Well, don't I feel like a white woman!" David threw his hair from his eyes.

PANELS

"What's the deal with you? Don't you see we only trying to help you? I know you can do better than this."

"Oh, I get it…Just 'cause I sleep with my own, I'm trash…But if I start messing with them little pretty white boys, I can have the world. Is that it? Richard, are you a better queer than I am just because you do it with those lily white faggots?"

"I didn't say that. You know exactly what I mean…Why are you being so trifling?"

"I really don't think he meant that you have to start dating white guys or that you are nothing for seeing who you do see, it's just the caliber of the men you like. That's all."

"The caliber of the men I like…I know you didn't go there…look at Bradley, I don't know a bigger whore than him, white or black."

"I guess I won't argue you with that. But, nonetheless, there are other choices."

"Well, you boys go and find me that perfect little white boy that is gonna love me the rest of my life…and while you at it, find one for your damn selves."

"David, why are you becoming so upset?"

"Look guys, y'all might mean well, who knows. It's just that I get tired of everyone telling me I'm shit…Hell, I know that Tiffany ain't gonna last forever. I ain't that crazy…But that's all I have right now…Prancing around on stage in front of people is something I like. I wanna do it. Not for the dollar tips, but for the moment…Hell, why am I telling y'all this, y'all ain't gonna never understand."

"David, I do understand…I do know what it's like to be out there scared shitless. You know how I came here not knowing a soul. No family, no one."

"Yeah, but at least you got the group."

"And you don't?"

"Now did I say that? Don't go putting words in my mouth."

"I care for you, much like the brother I lost when I told them I was gay…I don't want anything to happen to your silly ass."

"You know I once wanted others in my life…But I can manage by myself…don't have to put up with the bullshit of fake friends and family…"

"I know you not calling us fake."

"No, Michal. You and Richard are actually dolls…It's just hard for me to trust anyone…my own folks treat me like shit…My brother Eric is always high on crack. He steals every dime I try to have…. worthless ass won't work.

He's been in jail more than there's Doans pills. Even tried to kill...But, my folks like him more than me 'cause I'm the pervert. I'm the sissy...I worked my ass off going to do hair and buying them things I thought they want...But I'm still the faggot...Only one to graduate from high school, do you think any of their asses came to see me? Hell no! They were ashamed of my homosexuality."

"At least your brother didn't try to kill you when he found out you were gay."

"Hell no, instead he laughed at me...told me that he knew I loved him touching me...Yeah, my brother Eric used to rape me almost every night when I was younger. Yeah, right under the nose of my sainted mother and her new Baptist preacher husband. Now ain't that something."

Whenever Bradley and David were together, trouble was definitely nearby. Some of their escapades ended orderly with the result of only a small prank or two. A few of their pranks bordered on situations that I even felt uncomfortable with. Nonetheless, they managed to avoid any damaging repercussions.

One night, after the bars had closed, we all went to a popular eatery on West End. The eggs and steak diner was opened twenty-four hours a day. The food was greasy and the utensils not always without some morsel of dried food residue. The interior was small but quaint with wooden partitions of the booths slightly raised. The service was slow and the waitresses were all quite aged. If you were in a hurry, you need not stop here.

In the right corner of this very cramped room was the jukebox. The vintage player obviously had played far too many vinyls as evident by the loud scratching noise.

"Do you see anywhere to sit?"

"Michal, my dear, have no fear, for we are here...We should have no trouble finding a table with Ms. Thang here." Bradley smirked.

"Honey chile, all I gotta do is sit my flawless ass down by one of those jerks...Oops, I mean...jocks...and baby, watch them flee!"

"You better watch that, David. They may want you to do those nasties."

"Bring them on! Baby, bring them on...I might even enjoy it."

Moments later, two giddy teens got up from their table. While paying their check, one of the girls kept turning around staring at us. Fortunately, David did not notice her. I pulled at Bradley's arm and pointed to the empty table.

PANELS

"They were some messy chillums. Just look, they got jelly and shit all over the table. Just can't take breeders no where." David shuffled to sit down.

"Ain't they kin folks of yours?" Bradley asked.

Naw, my peoples knows better than this...My momma wouldn't take this shit...She would have yelled at them to come back and clean up...It's y'all white people."

"What y'all wanting to drink?" a middle-aged waitress asked. She rarely raised her eyes from the yellowed piece of paper that she was waiting to write our order on. Gray streaks escaped underneath her black wig. She was very pale and tired looking. As she leaned against the table, I noticed her legs covered with exposed varicose veins.

" I'll have a vodka and tonic."

"Does this look like a damn bar?"

"Well, not really...But since you asked, it don't look like no diner either."

"You are more than welcomed to take y'all asses across the street to Krystal." The waitress pointed out the window.

"Naw, Ms. Thang, we gotta stay here. I just gotta see your smiling face and eat this food that's to die for." David bats his eyes.

"Well, shut ya trap and tell me what ya want. How come you ain't in drag, you got fired or something?"

"Now Ms. Mabel girl, don't you go there...You know I don't do drag...That's for those little street urchins...I'm an illusionist."

"Look like a drag queen to me." She left the table smiling.

"You mean, you gonna let her get away with that?" Bradley asked.

"Honey, if she was somebody else, I would have laid down the law...but since she is gonna get me my food, I ain't gonna get her pissed off."

"I think someone has an admirer."'

"What are you talking about, Michal? Bradley looked around the room. "You know the eyes gotta be for me. Who else?"

"Hmmp, Ms. Thang, I have you know I got more beauty in my fingernail than ya got in ya tired ass." David brushed back his hair. "So, it must be for me!"

"I really don't think either one of you would want it." I pointed at the burly shabbily dressed man clad in overalls. He was sucking on a hand rolled cigar and staring right at us.

"Omigod, a damn troll...A real live farmer in the dell troll...I don't know, Michal. I think he's more your type." David swished around. "Honey, looking at you like new meat."

"David, sweetheart, are you sure you don't know him? Maybe he's old trade. I could have sworn I saw him leaving your crib this morning."

"Not in your wildest dreams, and baby I know they are some wild ones...anyway, I wish he stop gawking over here. He ain't getting nothing over here."

"David, calm down, girl. Maybe he just wants some little hot chocolate." Bradley laughed.

"He better look elsewhere...I don't do charity for the old and decrepit...and I wouldn't do it for his tired ass anyway....Just look at him, he looks like he ain't touch no water since it rained last week." David flipped his hair.

"Careful, the old troll might hear you."

"And...he might do what? He ain't that crazy to mess with this queen."

"Have ya decided what ya want yet?" Mabel was ready to write. "I ain't got all damn day."

"I don't think what those homos want is on y'all menu." The stranger at the counter chided. "Hell, I don't even think they know themselves what they are."

We, including Mabel, all turned around and faced this man. Sure, we had talked about him but not loud enough for him to hear us. How dare this stranger try to insult us. He didn't know us and we definitely didn't know him. Before I could respond, David sprung to attention.

"You know what they say about those big brutes that suck on cigars, don't you? Their lips are always perfectly formed to give the best..." David swirled facing the man. He grabbed his groin. "So, big boy, is it really true? I'm dying for you to show me."

"Why, ya little queer ass pervert...I ought to kick ya ass all over this place." The offended man rose from his stool, clenching his fists.

I tried to stand between them but David pushed me back down. I wanted the madness to end. It wasn't fun anymore. I was actually scared. Around me, the room was unusually quiet. People were staring in our direction waiting for the next pin to drop. Only sound was the sizzling of the grease on the short order grill. I looked over at Bradley for support. But he was sitting there smiling as if in anticipation of what could happen. He started edging David on.

"Listen here, you ugly two bit slimy-ass reject from Sunnybrook Farm, I'm more man in high heels than you'll ever be and more woman than you will ever have...so unless you have a death wish desire to be ball-less, you had

PANELS

better get the hell out of my face."

"Ain't no damned queer gonna give me a threat!"

The angry man lunged at David. As if in a slow rehearsed motion, David quickly caught the stranger by his assaulting arm and twirled him around. David had the man's back in front of him. In a flash, David pulled a seven-inch switchblade that he held against the man's jugular's veins. I was in total shock. I started to pray that David wouldn't do anything worse. I turned and saw Bradley glancing at the menu as if nothing was happening. My heart began to race. I didn't want to go to jail. I didn't know what to do.

The old man stopped fighting. He was breathing rapidly. His face was beet red with his veins protruding. Sweat was pouring off his brow. Suddenly, the door opened. While the door was opening and as more people were coming inside, David rushed the man through them out the door. I watched as the man's body sailed onto the pavement.

David closed the door. Wiped his hands off. He reached down and adjusted his ruffled clothing and sat down at the table with us. I kept looking out the window fearing that the man would return for revenge. He did not return.

"Obviously, the old fart didn't know who he was messing with, the grand queen diva herself." Norma, the elderly spaced tooth cashier, laughed. "For a moment there, I just knew I was gonna have to clean up some guts off my floor."

"Ya gotta do what ya gotta do to survive." David replied as he reached over to read from the menu. "Damn, he made me break a nail. Now, I'm really pissed, do ya know how much a set of Lee's Nails run ya?"

The gawking ceased as eyes were lowered back inside the other booths.

"This is the last time, I will ever go anywhere with you guys again. Y'all crazy!"

"Oh chill out, Michal, it's just a little fun. Nobody got hurt." Bradley stirred his coffee.

"Yeah baby, it's all good! I bet that cigar sucking farmer will think twice before he calls somebody else a homo," David assured.

During the formidable years of our circle, someone introduced *Messages from a Soul*. The belief was that we were actually fragments of a larger entity that created a soul. When you meet someone for the first time and feel an eerie acquaintance, you met another fragment. You both were only two pieces of a single spirit.

I have always felt the bond between us to be spiritual. As if by fate, as society misfits, we were together. We needed no others. Our relationships went beyond sexual; we took it to a higher plane. We had weathered many a storm without any faltering. Until Gregory's death—suddenly, it appeared that our bonding force quivered.

It was right after a weekly staffing that I realized that something was indeed wrong with Sebastian. Ordinarily, he ignored sarcastic remarks from our associates, but this time he didn't. Without any notice, he flew into a verbal rage. All eyes turned on him. I just sat there and stared at him even after he stormed from the room. Then, their eyes were on me. Don't look at me I wanted to say.

I began to wonder if Sebastian was losing his mind after seeing Gregory die. He had been so tight lipped over the whole experience. I wondered if he blamed us for not being there when Gregory died. How could he when he didn't tell us that Gregory was dying?

Later that night, I met Cleo and Sebastian for drinks at the Cabaret II. Gay bars, for whatever reason, always ends up being that safe haven for the lonely depressed souls. Not only did everyone know your name, it was a place where you could safely unleash your gaiety after hours of being someone you were not. It became the home away from home.

The bar wasn't crowded. The noise was at a minimum and the smoke didn't strangle me. The setting was intimate. I was to meet the others at the booths in the removed alcove in the back bar.

It was ten thirty and Raquel Scott was performing. I was standing looking through the glass doors to the show bar when Cleo grabbed me from behind.

"Hey, big boy! What are you doing tonight?" Cleo danced around me holding her wine. "You wants some company?"

"It depends on whose asking."

"Well, you know it ain't me…but I did see some cute eye candy over there." Cleo pointed toward the back bar. Sebastian was standing at the corner of the bar waving us forward.

"What kind of mood is he in?" I lowered my head to whisper.

"He's kinda in a foul mood, but that's why we are here, right? To cheer him up." Cleo spoke out of the side of her mouth. "Oh, beware. He's kinda got the gutter mouth disease."

"Something ain't right with this picture…do you know what's going on with him?"

PANELS

"Michal honey, you just got to find out yourself. I'm not a mule to carry anything."

"Okay, I will ask him."

"Good to hear that, Michal…then you can tell me." Cleo skipped to the booth where Sebastian waited for us.

"Well, if it ain't the holy padre. Am I getting your royal highass blessing out?"

"Man, what got in your pants today?" I asked as I slide across from him.

"Is everyone pissed at me for running out?"

"Kinda, hell, I don't know…you know how they are. " I motioned to Michele, the bartender. "Hey sexy, how about a rum and seven?"

" I guess I sort of made a fool of myself, huh?"

"Actually, I think you scared us…After you left, they all started looking at me like I knew what the hell was going on…So, what is going on?" I turned and paid for my drink. Cleo and Sebastian sat together and I sat across from them.

"If you don't tell him then I will." Cleo leaned against Sebastian.

"Tell him what? He ain't nobody special. He's just Sister Michal, the nun that don't get none."

"Calm down! I ain't your enemy. Get your claws back in before I defang your ass."

"I'm scared…"

"Scared of what?"

"I'm scared of dying."

"Okay, what brought this on?" I stared at him. "What are you talking about?"

"He's talking about Gregory leaving us."

"Oh, I see. You are still grieving?"

"Michal, you are so damned smart. Hell, I never stopped. What is so weird about it, is that I don't think it really is about Gregory but death itself…I mean, this thing has me in a choke hold. I can't sleep at night. I don't eat. I live like a damn zombie."

"Sebastian, you know you're letting depression kick your ass, don't you?"

"Yeah, but what can I do?"

"Sure sounds like cruise time to me." Cleo smiled. "How does Bermuda or Cancun sound? Hmm, just think about beautiful clear water and the beach! I can see all those hunks running around us."

"That's really not a bad idea. Sebastian, you know you got plenty of time."

"So, when I come back, all my hell will be gone, right? Is that what you're saying?"

"Be for real, Sebastian! You know perfectly well that's not what he's saying."

"Sebastian, we are your friends, not your enemy. We want to help you not hurt you." I stirred my drink.

"But what can you do that I haven't done for myself?" Sebastian raised his voice. Those seated across at the bar turned and looked at us. Sebastian rose from the table. "What the hell you trolls looking at? Get a life and get the hell out of mine."

"First of all, we can listen…obviously you not listening to yourself." I pulled at his shirt to sit back down.

"You know, you never did tell us much about Gregory's dying…you kept it inside and away from us." Cleo cocked her head. " I ain't the therapist here, but I do think you are letting it eat at you."

"I'm just raw inside where this stuff is nibbling me. I know something is bothering me, but I don't know what it is. I'm going crazy and there's not a damn thing I can do about it…Occasionally I sneak from everything and try to find solace sitting alone on remote cliffs around Percy Priest…Sometimes early in the morning before dawn…Just thinking…mostly about the past…I lay on the ground and watch the sun rise…It's so beautiful…I mean the blue sky with bruises of pinkish strokes in thick zapped lines…I lay still and listen to the quietness of the earth. Nothing but the sounds of the flying birds and the rugged wind swept waters washing unevenly against the graveled shore. The stillness comforted my solace." Sebastian stared in our direction although he didn't really seem to be talking to us.

"Omigod, don't tell me that I'm going to read one morning about a body washing up near the cliffs, am I?" Cleo asked. "Seriously, we do need places where we can release our thoughts and I know I don't have to tell you that. Why don't you try to remember all that mental health mumbo jumbo you give your clients and maybe, just maybe, start to believe it yourself."

"Yeah, I know…But it's still a bitch…I fight the damned silence all through the night to no end."

"Man, I didn't know you had it so bad," I said. "Why didn't you say anything before now?"

"And let everyone know just how I'm an apple turnover, a real basket case. If it ever got out that I no longer had control of my own life, I'm finished…That sort of thing kinda messes with my credibility with my few

PANELS

citizens of the land of the wacky."

"Hell, I'm not asking you to confess to the masses…I'm just saying, talk to us."

"Just suppose, that, you guys were the problem…Have you ever thought about that, Michal?"

"How can I think about that if I didn't even know there was an issue…so, are we the problem?"

"No, I guess not…it just that, my life isn't what I want it to be. I feel smothered and I really don't know from what." Sebastian cupped his face in his hands. "My life is so damned routine, I could scream! I'm drowning"

"Honey, you really got it bad…my life with Edward isn't nowhere near the Utopia. But, without sounding too corny, I learned from myself that you just gotta believe that things is gonna get better." Cleo brushed Sebastian's hair. "Tell me something…is it that you are just lonely and need someone to share your bed?"

"Please don't be bashful with your words, Cleo." Sebastian pulled back. "I need a man in my life like I need another…oh, I don't know what I need. It surely ain't a man. I have resolved myself to the fact I'd be alone the rest of my life, without a lover, that is!"

"Why are you so afraid of commitment?"

"Michal, who the hell said anything about being afraid of commitment? You're not listening to a word I'm saying…I just don't have the energy to nursemaid anybody…When I'm alone, I don't have to worry about trying to impress anyone. I can be myself."

"So, what you're saying is that you can't always be yourself even with us?"

"I guess that's true…but with you guys, I don't have to always be that perfect little good boy. I'm free to be a bastard when I need to."

"Which you do so well, I might add." I smiled.

"What do you get out of it when you hang out at the cliffs?" Cleo motioned for another drink. Michele sent over another glass.

"Cleo, it's sort of hard to explain, but when I sit down on the cold ground, I stare into the sky…the moon has already fell and the sun is breaking to be free…Everything is beautiful up there. Everything is peaceful with the quietness…why can't my life be like that?" Sebastian paused. "That just goes to show you that it is true what is said: have you noticed that whenever your life seems so screwed up, that you are always present?"

"Sebastian, honey, that just went completely over my head." Cleo appeared puzzled.

"What can I do?" Sebastian paused. "No, Michal, you tell me what you would do."

"If I had the answer, there would be no need for bars nor treatment centers...I just try to tell myself that all things will change for the better."

"Now, who's looking at life through rose colored glasses?"

"Seriously, I'm not kidding. Just believing that my life will one day change for the better really helps me to struggle along."

"Michal, your problem is that you are still stuck in all that dogmatic religious doctrine. You so want to be a preacher that you can taste it." Sebastian paused. "I, on the other hand, prefer to deal with reality not something I can't prove."

"Whatever...just look inside yourself, Sebastian. When all else fails you, what do you do?...The mere thought of AIDS has you scared and locked in some emotional prison. Although you may try to fight the fact, I really think that the cliffs provide that certain openness that eradicates your needless boundaries and maybe even your faith in God." Cleo shuffled her wet napkins under her wine.

"She got a point. You better listen to the old girl," I said. "Stop being so damned bullheaded and stubborn. Whatever it is, you ain't in it alone."

"Maybe you both are right...but, how can I not be scared when people around me are dropping off like flies...from something that I myself may have inside me?" Sebastian took a sip of his drink. Paused. "If either of you tell a single soul what I'm about to tell you, I'd swear that you was lying out of your ass...but I do feel closer to God when I'm at the cliffs by myself. I sometimes even imagine myself soaring alongside the birds in a dimensionless flight to the heavens."

"Well, you can imagine all that you want, but you better think twice about taking a flying leap into the clouds. You're not leaving us that easy." Cleo leaned back. "Joking aside, all you got to do is look inside yourself and know that God is always there for you, and not just at the lake. What do you think, Michal? "

"Thank the heavens that God is not like the mortal men on this earth."

"Can I get a Amen to that?" Sebastian laughed.

"Can you ever get serious?"

"Cleo, I am being as serious as I can be...the other day, for whatever reason I don't know, I picked up the *Diary of Anne Frank*. Even though I read this book years ago in high school, I never really gave it much thought. I couldn't totally relate to that story...Don't get me wrong, it wasn't right what

PANELS

Hitler did to those millions of Jews, but I just couldn't relate to it....until now. The Nazis imprisoned and killed Jews because they were different. I feel that AIDS has the same impact on me...Did you know that Anne Frank and her people had to stand quiet for hours for fear of being found out? Now, AIDS is making me stand quietly so that I won't be found out. God has cursed me because I am different.

"Sebastian, we are all hurting. None of us have that answer. I won't believe that my God, the one I love so much, would ever curse me with a death sentence. He's not that kind of a god."

"I agree with Michal. I can't tell you how you should feel or that what you feel is wrong. But, I can say that my faith has helped me tremendously...He's been there for me through hell and back with my marriage. I'm no one special. I haven't done anything in my life so magnificent that I should be spared. You just got to believe."

"One time, I really did believe in a lot of things...I would take pride in things, almost trying to be that perfect person...but, instead of strengthening me, the whole damned thing exploded around me..."

"Sebastian, we all want to be that special person, you know, the one that can never be...Remember that time when David tried to kill himself?"

"Yeah, do I ever. There I was, enjoying a buzz and trying to be romantic when all hell broke out."

"He really put a damper on that party, didn't he?" I laughed. "There he was, all depressed and no place to run. So, what did he do...he took the razor to both of his wrists."

"I felt like a damned fool telling that emergency room nurse that he had ran into a barbed wire fence."

"Well, we were young and dumb. But I could have strangled him myself after he told her that he ain't even seen any barbed wired fence." I smiled.

"For once in his life, we know he told the truth."

"Well, at least he got a free two week stay along with three hots and a cot...even if it was in the nut house!"

"Michal, I guess you know that I got chewed out royally by our kindhearted administrator last week."

"Yeah, I did hear something about it. I wanted to ask you about it but decided to wait until you brought it up."

"Is that why you so bummed out?" Cleo asked.

"Somewhat...plus all this other crap around me...I'm a just a regular Mary Poppins!"

"Since you brought it up, what did she have to say?" I was curious.

"Well, nothing that wasn't expected, I guess. I just sat there quietly and obediently while Dr. Lewis sat across her massive mahogany desk and pointed out my inabilities...You know, it really amazed me how she could look a person in the eyes and calmly tell them just how much a screw up they were. Her voice never faltered or even changed pitch...She really got style, you know..."

"Did she say anything specific?"

"Michal, please. I knew the moment I sat down that she had all the goods on me. She knew I knew, so why waste my time lying and pleading?...She reminded me of the countless previous conferences she and I had had...Her expectations and my inability to carry them out...Even at that point, I stopped listening to her."

"I know you are not trying to say you ignored her!"

"I just wasn't in the mood to hear her whining. I almost wanted her to say that I was fired."

"Man, you definitely like to live on the edge. What did she end up doing to you?"

"Yeah, did she fire you? Are you history?"

"Not yet, but I'm sure she's working on it...Hey Cleo, you could use some help at your gallery, can't you?"

"Sebastian, you know I love you with all my heart, but you don't know the first thing about art." Cleo laughed. "You wouldn't know the difference in impressionist versus surrealist. You probably think Picasso painted for Andy Warhol. You better stick with psychology."

"I may not have a choice if I don't get my act together...Dr. Lewis told me my attitude was filled with apathy and that I needed to analyze myself to see what could use some changes...if I don't improve, then my days were numbered."

"At least, she gave you a chance. Give her some credit."

"Michal, you don't know how close I came to breaking down and crying my eyes out. I wanted to tell her everything I was going through. I wanted to tell her about my nightmares and fears, but I didn't...I didn't think she really cared."

"Well, Mr. Stubborn-ass, we do care about you." Cleo rubbed his shoulder. "Now, we gotta get you to care about yourself...Now, let's go dance."

The next morning, Richard called. I was between sessions so I was able to talk to him briefly. I told him about the previous conversation with Sebastian.

PANELS

Richard wasn't surprised. He said he had wondered about Sebastian for some time. Sebastian had been extremely short with him for no apparent reason.

"So what do we do? Do we let him hang himself or do we try to rescue his tired ass?"

"Michal, besides his grandmother, we are actually the only family he has. We can't just kick him to the curb."

"Richard, I'm not saying we should walk away. But, what can we do if he doesn't want our help?"

"Michal, he's family. He will have to tell me to butt out and he would have to pray I abided by his choice. I'm not giving up on him, not that easily."

"You're right. We have been through a lot of grief and we did manage to survive."

"Michal, dear heart, we also have shared a hell of a lot of great times. Whatever is bothering him, I will find out…I don't care if he gets pissed off at me, I love him too much to let him rot in his own hell."

"Richard, you missed your calling, you know that? Maybe you should have been a preacher after all."

"I know you're being funny, but I really don't care…all those nights that I walked down those horrible cold streets, being homeless, but not really alone. I would sing my song about God's eyes being on the sparrow. Knowing that I wasn't alone in my struggle gave me strength to open my eyes every morning…" Richard's voice cracked. "Sebastian has to know he's not alone."

"Okay, I'm game. What's the next step?"

"What are you doing this evening?"

"Nothing, why?"

"Good, meet us at the Goldrush tonight around 9:00. Don't be late," Richard said. "By the way, I will have Sebastian there."

I returned the phone to its cradle. I thought briefly about Richard's last words. I really couldn't see him pulling this off. How was he going to convince Sebastian to join us?

The rest of my day was quite uneventful much to my pleasure. Several clients missed their appointments. The staff meeting was cancelled. I was literally free for the day. The hours seemed to stretch longer while the minutes crept on. I was dying from anticipation. Finally, it was the quitting hour.

The dark rustic atmosphere of the restaurant was practically unchanged from any of my previous visits. To my immediate right, the video wizards were honing their digital skills of weaponry. The clashing of the bells and flat rings sizzled the stale smoke filled air. The bouncer sat on the stool checking id. He was dressed in aged leather garments that partially covered his arms displaying his weathered tattoos of sniveling serpents.

He barely glanced at my driver's license as he continued cleaning his greasy overgrown fingernails with the glistering blunt side of his switchblade.

Jazz played in the background. The Crusaders, I think. The moderately loud music mixed with the challenging brass voices of conversations and the clinking of beer bottles. My mouth began to salivate at the smell of their overly spiced Mexican bean roll, my favorite dish whenever I'm here. A dab of sour cream on the cheesy beef topped off with a large jalapeno on the side. The dish was definitely not for the weak stomach.

Finally, I saw them. True to his word, Richard had somehow gotten Sebastian to come. Seated behind the red and white vinyl checkered tablecloth underneath the large portrait of Donehogawa, Keeper of the Western Door of the Long House of the Iroquois, both sipped on their beer.

"I see you found us."

"Yeah, all I had to do was to look for that portrait."

"That's my man! Even though the white man changed his name to Ely Samuel Parker, you know, trying to anglicize him, he still fought for respect." Richard's fingers danced around the lip of his beer. " For almost a half a century, this man battled with the afflictions of racial prejudices."

"Man, you missed a damned good show over there tonight." Sebastian slid across the seat. " Seth played the hell out of those ivory keys."

"No! Don't tell me this was the night Seth had his gig at Exit In. Please tell me it wasn't tonight!" I was pissed.

"Hate to tell ya, but tonight was the night. And baby, he shined like new money. Didn't he, Richard?"

"Michal, Seth played like he was possessed." Richard nodded. "They probably gonna retire that old keyboard once Seth finally eased up off it."

"Was his eyes closed?"

"You know they were closed. Does he know how to play any other way? You should have seen him. He was so freaking powerful!"

"Why didn't someone remind me?"

"Now, don't you go looking at me." Sebastian leered. "You should start reading your frigging emails."

"Was Cleo there?"

PANELS

"Be for real! You honestly think she would miss him performing? Baby was front row. A few inches more, her butt would have been on stage with Seth."

"What about Bradley? Was he there?"

"Bradley who? Richard, did you see anyone named Bradley there?"

"Yeah right! I know you are not referring to our Bradley, the one that always needs to be the center of attention…He would have had too much competition tonight."

"Michal…Seth played your song. I mean, he really played your song."

"Thanks, Sebastian. Thanks for really making me feel lower than sea scum." I shook my head. "He actually played 'Song for Guy' and I can't believe I actually missed it. He knows I love that song."

"Well, you missed it. You also missed some nice looking specimen." Richard patted my shoulder. "I thought I was gonna have to drag Sebastian out of there. He was salivating all over the place like some starved dog."

"Ms. Thang got her nerve…she's the one that was drooling over herself." Sebastian laughed. "Anyway, I don't do trade nor breeders."

"You're no fun…sounds like you got major issues," Richard teased.

"Issues, hell! I got enough to make a whole damned book." Sebastian dipped his chip in the salsa. "But, somehow, I think you already know that, don't you?"

"All I know is that you are having a hard time…that you won't talk to any of us about it…I'm not gonna lie. Lately, I have been feeling that something was bothering you for some time now, but I didn't know how to say anything to you about it except to be straight up…what's bugging you?"

"It's nothing. I'm just having a rough time right now." Sebastian cupped his face in his hands. "Nothing that won't pass."

"Cut the crap, Sebastian. You ain't been right since you came back from Atlanta…man. I know you like a brother, don't feed me that line of bull…Has Gregory's death destroyed you?"

"Maybe, maybe not. Maybe I'm just tired of hearing everyone's freaking problems and maybe I just need a break. Have you ever thought of that? I mean, look around us, all we see is people screwing up their lives. Not a damned soul ever listen to anyone…"

"Sebastian, when are you gonna learn that you ain't gonna save the world? When you are dead and gone, those same poor suckers are gonna do the same things over and over…Okay, I'll bite that that is some of your problem, but it's not all of it. What gives, man?"

"Can we just change the subject?" Sebastian shuffled in his seat.

"Naw, that's the problem…we have changed it too many times already."

"So, Michal…are you going to just sit there and say nothing while Richard attacks me? What kinda friend are you?"

"A friend that cares enough to take you out of your hell…You know that Richard is right…what can we do?"

"Nothing, there's nothing you can do…look, I gotta go. It's getting late…Richard, will you please move."

"No! Not until you tell us what the hell is going on with you…Just look at you, you look like a Amtrak wreck. You ain't yourself. Who are you?"

"I have asked you nicely to please move out of my way. I'm trying not to get angry and cause a scene."

"And do what? What if I don't move? What of it?" Richard was stern.

"Scottie, prepare to beam me up, quick! Now, boys, everybody needs to stay calm. Can't have no fighting here…at least not around me." I leaned back on the booth.

"If that's what it takes to get him to talk, then I'm ready to kick his ass…Sebastian, I love you too much to see you go through this hell."

"Look, I don't need your damn help…yours neither, Michal….Who the hell do either one of you think you are? You both need to climb down off your white horse of piety and leave me the hell alone!"

"Is that all you can dish out?" Richard taunted him. "Gimme more than that?"

"What the hell is it that you want from me?"

"Talk to us. Tell us what's wrong." Richard paused. "Gimme a chance."

"Remember when we all took that winter trip to Belgium? Remember that no one wanted to come back home?" Sebastian's eyes began to glisten with tears.

"What does this have to do with today?"

"Michal, damn it, let me finish, please!"

"Okay, you have the floor. Go for it."

"Y'all remember the look on everyone's face when we first arrived at the Metropole Hotel in Brussels scared to death that we didn't have enough money to pay for our week?"

"Yeah, that was a great place, wasn't it?" Richard appeared relaxed. "I can still remember that enormous Gothic oak bar with that hulk of a bartender that both David and Bradley tried desperately to cruise."

"Regardless of the fact that neither spoke a word of Dutch nor German," I said.

PANELS

"Don't forget Flemish...but, without missing a beat in translation, the bartender did manage to steer us to the gay bars without any trouble." Sebastian finally smiled.

"The only part of those foreign bars that I never did understand was paying the cover charge as you left the bar. Hell, what if you managed to drink all your funds and couldn't afford to pay your cover, what happened then?" Richard asked.

"It's a pity we never found out." I smirked.

"If I recall correctly, Richard, you went home with a Belgian soldier. Didn't even come back until later the next day." Sebastian laughed. "Was he trying to enlist you in his own army?"

"I will never tell...what about that rather young blond tyke that you met? I saw the signs on your face of true love...I bet you don't even remember his name, do you?" Richard teased. "Looking so dreamily into his eyes while professing your undying love and devotion to him. That is, until your Visa ran out."

"You just lost your bet...his name was Kevin...and before you even ask, that hulk from the Netherlands was Yos...now, what was that soldier's name?" Sebastian cracked a smile.

"Hell if I can remember." Richard laughed. "Remember when one of your many brief lovers took us to that beautiful majestic Corroy-Le-Chateau in the Namur province? I was so embarrassed at David for queening out so bad telling everybody that he wanted to marry the Marquis."

"They built castles to last forever...why can't they make life last forever...is that too much to ask?" Sebastian's voice dropped to a whisper. His eyes were wet.

"Those were definitely some good old days...a time that I learned a lot about myself and the world around me...I think it brought us all closer," I said.

"Spending all that time together in close quarters, I'm just surprised we didn't kill each other...we were all so naïve and stupid, but we all thought we knew it all. Couldn't tell us anything. We had all the answers." Richard drained his beer. Nodded to the waitress for another round.

"Let's go back there...to those days." Sebastian perked.

"Can people ever really go back to their past?" Richard asked as he gestured to the befouling waitress for another round of chips and salsa.

"So, Sebastian, is that what your problem is?" I finished my beer before the waitress returned with the next bottles.

"To be honest, that is my problem...at least the main one. I think that Gregory's passing made me realize that I'm mortal. That my own life can be taken away as quick as a breath of air...I see people in a far different way now."

"Baby, that's why it's important to live your life as if every moment counted...None of us knows when we will leave this place...and at the same time, we shouldn't continue to dwell on waiting for old man death to come a knocking at our door." Richard paid for the drinks.

"Isn't it ironic how we used to cruise around Centennial Park, see those old trolls trying to pick up those dumb Twinkies, and we said we didn't want to be one of those old queens. Remember?" I swished my beer around. "And now, we decided that being an old queen isn't so bad after all."

"I don't know...I mean, I don't know if I want to be one of those old dollies that sit in rocking chairs straining through bifocals at young trade...But then again, I don't want to be the next one planted either." Richard lifted his glass to make a toast. "Let's toast to a decent middle ground, if there is one. May we become the gay Golden Girls!"

"Just look around here...you got a little bit of everything in here. You got the preppies, the Harley Davison riders, some of this and some of that...I was watching that woman over there go from stool to stool, hanging all over those guys. I don't think it's a matter of if she's going home with anyone, just which one."

"And your point is what, Sebastian?"

"Michal, my point is simply that by now everyone knows that the bogey man is out there. They know that there's something out there that good old penicillin can't touch...I seriously doubt if but a handful of the those in here uses a condom."

"Sebastian, what do you think should be done? How much more preaching is needed to get the message across?" I asked. "But then again, when you go to a gay bar, you can always find a container of rubbers. Do you honestly think that some of the tricks stop long enough to grab a few on their way out the door?"

"I would have never said anything to Gregory, but he actually scared me...Knowing that being intimate with someone caused him to die really frightened me...I still see those images in my mind...the way he wasted to nothing...this beautiful man was ugly...I just can't get over it." Sebastian's tears rolled down his face.

"Man, it wasn't because he had been intimate with someone else...that damned disease killed him."

PANELS

"But Richard, where did he get the damned virus? He got it from his lover! He got it from someone he loved and trusted. Gregory is ashes and that son of a bitch still lives."

"Sebastian, not every relationship is like their relationship was...I know guys that have been together for years and nothing has happened to them...Don't get me wrong, I was shocked as hell when I found out that he had died from the bug...Not our Gregory, I thought....But that wasn't the case; it caught him."

"Michal is right, Sebastian. Sleeping with a lover didn't kill Gregory but sleeping with a whore did...I'm actually thankful that I didn't see him while he was dying. This way, I can always remember him the way he was, before AIDS took over his life...You, unfortunately, saw him dying...but regardless, don't let it overcome you."

"At the time of his death, we didn't know anything about AIDS. We didn't know how you could get the virus. Yeah, we heard about it but we also heard just as many rumors." I paused. "Even now, we are still learning."

"I know that I haven't been myself lately. That's an understatement. At night, I lay awake afraid of closing my eyes...Images of Gregory's emaciated body parade around in my mind...Remember the character in Poe's 'Pit and the Pendulum'? My own heart seems to beat louder and louder and louder. I just know it will explode one day...The very thought of the virus anywhere around me stifles my every breath."

While the days numbered and progressed into years, my relationship with the circle began to strain. It appeared that we were individually divorcing ourselves from the circle. In hindsight, perhaps it was easier for us to avoid each other rather than be there for the next death. Nonetheless, as if we were crackling dry pieces of tumbleweed blowing across the desert, we started going our separate ways.

For continuing education in my field, I completed a practicum in working with the inner city adolescents. I was assigned an internship working with poverty stricken children. The children came mostly from poor Black and Hispanic homes. I must confess, initially I was probably more cautious than I would have been if the children were white. But, over time, I was able to overcome whatever prejudices I had. Sure, some of the children were in their natural habitat and were quite territorial but they were just warm blooded all American kids.

PHIL MICHAL THOMAS

The administrator was a young black woman that all the children called 'Miss. Nancye.' She was a beautiful woman, not as old as I. She had a gentle heart. She always wore a smile across her cherubic face.

Miss Nancye was raised within a few city blocks of the day program. She was one of them. The neighborhood accepted her and actually idolized her. Over the short time that I worked under her supervision, I quickly learned to love and respect her. She knew just when to be stern but not angry. She knew how to reach out and hug a crying scared child. Miss Nancye also knew how to reach out to us scared adults.

Miss Nancye taught me that there were no boundaries for positive love where a child is concerned. Through her sincere vision, I was able to realize the beauty of the naïve. I soon found comfort in their innocence. Nobody messed with Miss Nancye's kids—nobody.

While I tried my hand at tutoring, Seth and Richard teamed up in the music arena. Jazz became their main repertoire spiced with a little country on the side. Richard's honey laced baritone voice often accompanied Seth's graceful tickling of the ivories. They performed regularly at various nightclubs whenever their work schedules permitted. Their audiences grew from Elliston Place to Printers Alley and back. Cleo eventually joined them. Her soft mellifluous voice brought balance. Watching them perform gave me certain awe. Their ballads often made me rethink my own past especially when they would sing "Where've You Been" or anything by Kathy Mattea, Oleta Adams, Reba McIntyre, or Dionne Warwick..

Aside from sharing the stage, Seth began attending church with Richard. I would have loved being at Seth's parents' home when he told them that their nice Orthodox Jewish child was attending a Christian church where a woman was the pastor!

Satan must have had one hell of an icy storm since Bradley was able to meet Jeffery. Jeffery was much older than Bradley, which was much to our surprise. Actually the whole situation was a great surprise to all of us. No one imagined Bradley ever settling down. No, not this man that maintained his socio-sexual agenda of keeping his sensual skills above average. In other words, Bradley was quite promiscuous and had worn it proudly until this moment. Maybe people can change.

To say that Bradley and Jeffery were quite smitten with each other was an understatement. They appeared to really adore each other. Jeffery, with his well-defined gray streaked hair, sported a physique of a younger body builder. His Scandinavian body was in better shape than mine and he was fifty! If

PANELS

Bradley was able to find someone, I know there's someone out there for me.

Bradley began to retreat from the circle to a great extent. Bradley rented his condominium out and moved in with Jeffery. They became inseparable. When you saw one, you saw the other. I'm sure the bars were in mourning at the loss of one of their most generous benefactors.

Miracles continued, Sebastian had an emotional makeover. He no longer walked around with his head in the sand. He was so damned perky he got on my nerves. It was if he had taken a new lease on his life, but he wouldn't bulge at what had happened to him. He was a different soul. No, actually it was the old Sebastian that came back to us.

Our dear diva was busily working her fingers through heads of hair and extensions in the daylight hours while she danced her feet off later that night on stage. David attempted to dissolve the unusually slow slump in his salon's clients. He copied hairstyles from various European magazines and with some minor changes; he transformed his clients into unbelievable creations.

His alter ego, Tiffany Lynn, continued to strive to become the Diva of all stages of illusions. Lately, when I did see her perform, I noticed how beautiful she had become. It was as if it was the same fabled fairy godmother had left Cinderella and waved her wand across Tiffany. Everything changed about her; she no longer did trashy songs of lush and desire.

Over the next five years, our directions took us away from the madness of the past. Our lives became complacent and to some extent respectful. My only complaint was that our bond had changed; we rarely saw each other now. I was to the point of resigning myself to this new way of life for us when the earth turned.

One evening after an exhaustive day, I collapsed head first on my sofa. The television soon became a faint ignored whisper as I drifted off to sleep. Without a concern, the phone broke my solace.

"Hello stranger! Long time no hears." The voice on the other end of the phone said.

"Who is this?" I mumbled from my interrupted sleep. I tried to focus on the clock's illuminating numbers. It wasn't even eight o'clock.

"Man, it ain't been that long...I'll call you later."

"No...wait a minute! Who is this?"

"Michal, it's me, Richard."

"Richard! Hey man, how are you?"

"Okay, Michal...Look, I'm really sorry for waking you...I just knew you would still be up."

"It's okay, I'll get over it...what's going on?"

"Well, I haven't heard from you in days, so I thought I'd break down and give ya a call."

"Don't I feel honored! So what's going on with you nowadays? You and Seth still cutting the rug with your jazz?"

"Yeah, it keeps me busy, with work and all, you know the drill...So, what's going on with you? How's your love life?"

"Richard, remember who you are talking to...I can't even scare up a date. What about yours? Are you and Seth an item yet?"

"I don't know what you are talking about."

"Alright, Richard. Go ahead and play dumb. I know the tea on y'all." I rose "I'm sure he's tickling more than just those piano keys."

"Whatever...I mean, I do like Seth a whole lot. But, man, I don't want to do anything to jeopardize what he and I have. He's a real cool dude...anyway, friends don't sleep with friends."

"Richard, in case you didn't know, half the gang have slept with each other already."

"Are you referring to yourself? Did you sleep with the others?"

"Maybe, maybe not. I'm not one of those with the perfect bod."

Before I could finish my words, the phone beeped. There was another call coming in. "Hold on a second. Someone's calling." I fumbled around on the receiver until I depressed the button.

"Omigod, Michal, I'm glad you are at home. I was afraid I was gonna get that damned machine of yours...I need your help!" Cleo was frantic and out of breath. "Tiffany is going off on me!"

"Wait a second...where are you?"

"I'm inside his salon. I'm in a closet where he can't get to me. Michal, ain't a soul here. No other staff...nobody is here. Not a soul except for this fool and me. He done lost his fool mind. Talking crazy as hell of seeing snakes all over the floor...Can you come get me?" Her voice was pleading.

"I'm on the way." The phone went dead. As I was shoving my feet into my shoes, the phone rang.

"Did you forget me?" It was Richard.

"Sorry about that, man, but Ms. Diva of the Universe has gone off on Cleo!"

"Not our girl Cleo! Surely you've got to be kidding."

"I wish I was...David has gone ballistic. I'm on my way to the salon now to get her."

PANELS

"I'll meet you there." Richard's phone went dead.

While driving north on Clarksville Highway to Enchanted Hills, I began to wonder about what had just transpired. Was Cleo's life really in danger? Where were the affluent African American women that he so charmed to become his clients? He was always swamped with curls and twirls. He had transformed many naturals into his glamorous creations. So where were they now?

Within what seemed like minutes, I was standing outside the salon's doors. I tried to peer inside the beveled glass but didn't see anything but darkness.

"Thank God you came!" Cleo was standing outside near her car. "He scared the hell out of me...damned fool!"

"Where is he now?"

"I guess he's still inside talking to those damned non-existing snakes."

"What happened? What made him go off?"

"How the hell do I know! He just did!" Cleo looked angry and bewildered. "I just came here to get my CoCo Chanel evening gown I lent that fool to wear at the pageant...well, David was all alone in the salon with the lights off. Michal, it is daytime. Just look, not a soul around here...I only went inside because I heard David yelling at someone...but when I got inside, nobody was there, just him standing in the middle of the room screaming about seeing serpents crawling on the floor...Michal, there wasn't nothing on the floor...Like a fool, I went and sat down on one of the chairs. The dumbass turned and started calling me everything but the child of God. He called me all kinds of bitches and said he had to destroy me because I was evil."

"What was going on with him? Was he doing acid and tripping out?"

"Who knows what he was high on...he turned at me and stared at me like I was next week steak dinner."

By now, Richard had joined us. He looked as puzzled as I.

"Obviously, you wasn't packing your revolver. If you had been, then David would be one less queer in drag...what did you finally do? How did you get away?" Richard held her in his arms trying to console her trembling soul.

"I eased out of the chair, watching his every move towards me...I was sweating bullets. I thought my heart was going to beat a hole in my ribs."

"So, how did you get out?"

"Michal, my guardian angel sent the postman a knocking. When the mailman opened that door, I bolted out there like a bat out of hell." Cleo gasped for more air. "But I tried going out the back door and got stuck in the closet. I waited until I didn't hear nothing and flew out here."

"So the diva queen finally flipped his own wig...a girl can only take so much curling irons to the roots." I laughed.

"Yeah, but our Cleo almost became a victim.." Richard stared back at the salon's doors. "I'm just glad you are safe."

"Let's get the hell out of here before that crazed fool come barreling out that door...I ain't ready for no round two!" Cleo fumbled with her keys trying to open her car door.

"Hey man, why don't you help Cleo get the hell out of Dodge." Richard turned and faced the building. "I'm going inside to see what the hell is going on." Before I could object, he waved us away and walked inside. "God, I hope he knows what he is doing. That fool is crazy in there." Cleo started her ignition.

"David may act like he's crazy but he has enough sense not to go off on Mama Richard. When Mama Richard finished dusting his ass around in there, the sparkle off the chrome would blind ya...but I will follow you to make sure you are safe...You sure you want to drive? You still shaking?"

"Oh, I'll be alright...but I could use a damn good malt right now."

Eventually, my favorite illusionist Tiffany Lynn no longer performed with any regularity. She had established an unfavorable reputation among the bar owners of being incredibly bizarre and out of control. Rumors said she was stoned on crack and booze.

David began to live as Tiffany full time. I knew something was wrong when I first heard about this change. Living in drag had always been against his doctrine. David used to say that it was difficult to give the illusion of a female impersonator if you stayed in drag all the time. Something was seriously wrong.

Tiffany Lynn now wore the bouquet of stale alcohol. His pores reeked of liquor while his overall appearance weathered. The once graceful movements ceased as she now stumbled through her numbers. I was embarrassed for her and maybe for myself. I wanted to help David but I was afraid I didn't know what to do. No one else, except for Richard and Bradley, wanted to help me find out what was wrong with David. He was still our friend, regardless.

Tiffany Lynn's climaxing night of final destruction came on the night of the Miss Gay Athens Pageant. The most coveted female impersonator pageant of Middle America was being held in the Jackson Hall at the

PANELS

Tennessee Performing Arts Center. The nationally known gracious queen of the divas Della Reeves was scheduled to perform alongside of two recording artists. Contestants from across America attended to compete for this diamond-studded crown of glory.

Walking towards TPAC, I saw several stretched limousines lined the streets. Crowds of people dressed in their after six attire strolled in merriment escaping through the revolving doors to fantasy. Inside, cash bars served the multitude. Wine glasses clinked and laughter captivated the grand hall. The spectators wore a gamut of styles from chic to freak.

Inside the theatre, the massive backdrop was painted with scenes of people draped in white togas pouring water into urns outside Greek temples. The Parthenon appeared to have the main focus. Two well-toned boys in togas were standing guard to the entrance to the temple of Athena. Petals of white roses littered the path around the stage area.

"There you are! Look at you, gonna catch a man tonight!" Cleo screamed across the foyer. She wore a gorgeous butter cream-colored sequin gown with gold laced spidery high heels. Around her neck was her favorite Cartier diamond tiered necklace. "You look so sexy in that tux. Too bad you're gay and I'm married."

"Well look at you! Don't you look beautiful as always," I said. "Don't tell me you got old Eddie boy to come with you tonight?"

"Yeah…Be for real…you know he ain't going to risk anyone seeing him in a pleasure dome like this. He's at home making love to his scotch."

"And he allowed you to come here all alone, looking like this?"

"Don't go there…he doesn't have to allow me to do anything. I'm my own woman."

"Oh, lest I forget, right?"

"Michal, I could die for some of these flawless threads…I haven't seen so much bugle beads and sequins under one roof in my life…You know, some of the girls look real and some look sorta…"

"Like dogs, go ahead and say it. You know that some of those queens are looking boo wrong…you know, real scallywags! Baby, if the designers saw these tired out of shape sissies wearing their dresses, they come here and slap the queens silly for destroying their fashions. Some things just can't be worn with a blue light special figure!"

"Honey, you are so evil. I love you anyway…If I'm right, Seth and Richard are coming. I don't know about Sebastian or Bradley."

"Bradley coming here…for this? He's too much of a man to appreciate another man in high heels."

"Oh yeah, I forgot about Mr. Macho Slut himself...Michal, did you see him wink at me?" Cleo appeared startled at a stranger leering at her.

"That old troll probably thinks you are in drag.... Go ahead and show him some leg. Give him a thrill."

"Michal, now you will protect me, won't ya?"

"Scouts honor!"

"Boy Scouts or Girl Scouts?" Cleo laughed.

"They will just let anyone in this place, won't they?" Richard strolled across the room.

"Oh look, Cleo, it's the Ebony and Ivory twins." I raised my wine.

"I can't believe you actually got off some money for a drink...not in here!" Seth glanced over at Richard. "Let me guess, the bartender was hot!"

"Yeah, but I cooled off mighty fast when he asked me for the fiver for that taste of stale wine."

"Michal, you are such a tightass...lighten up some and live a little."

"Don't remind me...in fact, I really can't believe I'm in this place tonight."

"But you are, Blanche, you are in this dump!" Seth smirked. "Cleo, darling, you look absolutely marvelous! You already got my vote!"

"Did you guys hear that our girl is in the pageant?" Seth smirked.

"Who?" I asked.

"I know you ain't talking about Tiffany. She's too wasted." Cleo adjusted her jacket. "Anyway, whose gonna sponsor her drunk ass?"

"Somebody did, 'cause she's in it." Seth smiled.

"You know, I wouldn't put it pass Bradley to sponsor her. He ain't right no way." I drained my glass.

"Yeah right, I believe that when I see it." Cleo frowned.

"This was always a dream come true for her...winning this grand diva name. Who knows, she may have gotten her act together enough to compete," Richard said.

"I don't care. I'm still pissed at her for going off on me and then scaring the hell out of me. I'm the one that should have went off on her for keeping my Chanel so long!"

"I think she has been exorcised since then." I brushed her hair from the inside of Cleo's neck. "Her demons are gone bye bye...But then again, maybe her talent is turning her head completely around."

"Well, guys, the lights just blinked...shall we take our seats?" Cleo

PANELS

grabbed me. With arms entwined, we walked into the massive redecorated auditorium as the symphony began the prelude. The others quickly followed.

The shrill high-pitched voices of merriment clashed with the sounds of the orchestra tuning up. Conversations echoed throughout the massive auditorium. From my angle, there were no empty seats. A sea of black tuxedos and sequin gowns covered the floor.

The enormous mural on the backdrop was painted to depict the "School of Athens" by Raphael, who portrayed statues of Apollo on the top left, and Athena on the top right inside a Temple. From stage to ceiling, the olive branches hung. Owls were placed about the room in honor of Athena. The smell of incense permeated the previously perfumed air.

"Just leave it up to a queen to try to decorate this place like a museum." Seth looked around the room.

"I think they wanted us to believe we are in the real Athens…Look at the flawless marble pieces…you know, I could use a new floor for my foyer," Cleo said.

"This actually looks like it's going to be a first class act." I leaned forward in my seat. " Even the little boys on stage have chiseled features."

"I can't believe that Bradley is missing all of this." Richard stood to take his jacket off. "Nashville has become NashVegas!"

"Have you ever seen so many diva wannabes in one place?" Sebastian snorted.

"Oh, I really don't want to use the 'C' word…but some of these girls really look cheap. Their faces has more mortar in those cracks than Brooklyn Bridge." Seth joked.

"Wait until the lights are dimmed, they all look better then…is that mothballs I smell?"

"Michal, you are sooo mean…actually I thought it was formaldehyde."

"You definitely would know what that smell like, I mean, isn't that what Eddie is pickled in?"

"Seth, you of all people! I just don't know why I deal with you fools."

"'Cause you love us…and you don't love him. Honey, speak the truth and you shall be free!"

"Maybe I really do love him. What do you think about that?"

"Maybe I'm gonna turn Republican, marry, and have a station wagon full of yard ape brats!"

"Omigod, can you imagine Michal with a wife and some yard apes?" Seth asked.

"Honey, if that was to happen, baby, I can only imagine the trauma." Richard snapped back.

"May the goddess Athena fall on your head the next time you go inside the Parthenon." I waved my hand as if casting a curse.

"Then I could honestly say that I was laid at the park!"

"It certainly won't be the first time!"

"Michal, my bitter heart, I do beg your pardon...You ain't never heard of me laying up at the park with anybody...you must have me confused with yourself."

"I'm so glad we all love each other. It just makes me tingle all over!"

"Love! Cleo, I don't love these strange things...I merely keep them company until something better comes along."

"That's okay, Michal. I do love you. In fact, one day, I hope to grow up to be as beautiful as you think you are!" Richard grinned. Both he and Seth did a high five.

"Whatever flips your skirts...now, be quiet, the show's about to begin." I leaned back in my seat as the orchestra began to play of piece from the Orphic Hymns. The piece celebrated Athena's virtues. The lights went dim and the curtains rose amidst the silence of the crowd.

Several performers graced the stage. Evening gowns were quickly shed for skintight sequin costumes. Dancers accompanied most of the performers in well-rehearsed choreographed routines. It was definitely all that jazz.

"Like I always say; you ain't seen nothing till you see the queens compete in a pageant." Richard grinned.

"Yeah, the divas really come to life." Seth paused. "I'm not talking bad about the old girl, but do you think she stands a chance tonight?"

"Don't worry, she ain't gonna come a short stepping tonight. She has wanted this title for years. Are you even sure she's here?" I asked.

"Michal is right. Our girl Tif is probably back stage selecting her crowning number." Seth looked around the room. "I'm just surprised that Bradley isn't here to cheer her on. He knows better than we do what this night means to her."

"I love him to death but you know he's where he wants to be...cruising for the next lay." Cleo shifted in her chair.

Suddenly the room darkened. A song began to play. It was *Angel*, a slow number by Angela Winbush. The spotlight hit the small opening of the curtain. As the vocal began, the curtain opened around Tiffany. The music played but she did not move. She appeared confused. Finally, she took a step

PANELS

forward and again froze. Even at the distance, I saw her trembling.

"Did you forget the number, you tired old piece!" someone yelled from the audience.

"You ain't supposed to retire on stage…"

"Move ya decrepit old ass or git off!" another one screamed.

"Omigod, she looks like hell!" Cleo shrieked.

"Don't tell me she's drunk…not tonight. What the hell was she thinking?"

"That's just it, she's not thinking…Damn it, why couldn't she get her head together…of all nights, and this was not the night to throw a drunk!" Seth cupped his face as if he was disgraced.

"Wait! Isn't that my Chanel she's wearing?" Cleo rose slightly to get a closer look.

"Baby, that gown is just hanging on her…She looks so bony…didn't she pad tonight?" Sebastian asked.

"I don't think I can watch this…it breaks my heart seeing her like this." Seth shook his head in disbelief.

"I agree with Seth. I want to pull her backstage and spare her this embarrassment."

"Richard, honey, just what do you plan to do, go up on stage and escort her off? She would make a fool out of you."

"I don't care, Michal. Maybe you have forgotten that she is one of us. I haven't. If I make a fool of myself, so be it. I could care less what these bunch of pretentious fags think of me…Stay where you are if you want, but I'm going to her!"

"Oh shit! Richard, she just tripped down the steps…I'm going with you." Seth rose from his seat.

"Well, I be damned…Bradley is on stage helping her to get up!" Cleo pointed.

Tiffany Lynn, obviously bewildered and stunned, abruptly sat on the edge of the stage glaring bitterly into the audience seething. From the left wing, I could see the judges lowering their heads. Some of the judges whispered to their neighbor while some laughed. Finally, the stage lights dimmed, the music ceased, and Bradley rushed her from stage. Immediately, we left our seats and went backstage.

A large room was partitioned into smaller areas with materials draped for privacy. Suitcases and wardrobe trunks littered the walls and floor. Stage runners darted in and around other contestants lining up for their moment. As we moved through the maze of dragdom, our presence appeared unnoticed.

I heard Bradley arguing with Tiffany. Their raised voices competed with the orchestra. As we entered the room, Tiffany turned on her venom on us.

"What the hell do y'all want? Ain't nobody call y'all tired asses!" Tiffany's voice appeared sluggish. Her face extremely weathered and tired. Her face had a blank stare that showed nothingness. Tiffany stumbled around on a broken heel.

"Girl, something is definitely wrong with this picture...We are here to help you so quit ya bitching." Richard walked closer to her.

"We love you and we are concerned about ya." Seth said while reaching out his hand. "What's going on?"

"I don't need y'all damned asses. Get out of here before I slice you mothers..."

"Tif, chill out baby. This is Bradley you're talking to. You and me tight, you know that, don't ya, girl?"

"I don't give a damn who y'all are, get out!" Tiffany screamed and she lunged forward with her erect switchblade.

"That bitch is still crazy!" Cleo ran from the room.

Tiffany brandished the switchblade as if she was slicing the air. She was a madman. In the midst of the turbulence, Seth ran from the room for help. Bradley and I tried to subdue Tiffany. Tiffany whirled around, partially blinded by the crooked wig, and cut Bradley across his shoulder.

"Damn it to hell, Tif, you cut me!" Bradley grabbed his bleeding wound. I snatched a piece of fabric from a table and wrapped it around the cut but it was bleeding too much too fast. I stood back and watched as Tiffany shredded all of the gowns of the other contestants in her reach.

Immediately, the doors flung opened. Four muscular guards stormed her. They eventually interrupted this tirade of hell only after one of the guards was cut on his right hand. After gaining control, the men proceeded to beat her into a state of bloody unconsciousness.

Over a period, the impact of that night gradually dissipated around us. It was no longer the talk of the town. One fact remained true: the officers arrested David and charged him with several counts of destruction of property, aggravated assault, and attempted murder with a weapon.

I can still remember seeing him trying to stand before the night commissioner. David was barely able to stand in position. He fell against the glass as if resting. The guard pushed him away from the clear wall. He was still partially dressed in woman's clothing. His eyes were swollen and smeared with mascara. He turned and looked at us, or least I thought he saw

PANELS

us. David had a blank stare. Nothing! We watched our friend being led away in handcuffs and leg irons.

I will never forget that particular Monday morning. Traffic was easy. The sun was shining brightly although there was a forecast for rain. I arrived to work earlier than usual. I was on my third cup of coffee when she came in.

Evelyn was distributing cases of possible new clients that had been previously assessed by our initial bridge team. We knew the drill: make contact immediately and begin the services.

"Good morning, Mr. Michal. I hope you had a restful weekend!" Evelyn's voice was as spirited as ever. "Don't worry, I'm only going to give you three new cases…I haven't forgotten your caseload."

"I appreciate that…How was your weekend?"

"You mean there was a weekend? I wouldn't know, I have been on call since Friday."

"Well I'll be damned!"

"What? What's your malfunction now?"

"Evelyn, I'm sorry but I can't take this case."

"And why not, may I ask?"

"This guy 'David.' I know him personally."

"And? What's your point? What are you trying to say, Mr. Michal?"

"Evelyn, he's kinda like an old friend of mine…He may not want to talk to me."

"What better reason for you to have his case…Listen, I have read his intake psychological…There is something really wrong with this picture…He needs someone that will take the time to process with him…not someone that has to go learn what they think he's all about…You can do it, I have faith in you." Evelyn patted my shoulder and left.

For several minutes, I just sat there and read and reread his file. I began to feel guilty. I had always discounted my friend's behaviors as being those of a drunken maniac. Through these pages, I started seeing a different person. Someone I guess I really didn't know. David was someone that actually relied on emotions. He wasn't that cold hearted soul that cared less for others. He was actually a frightened soul struggling to survive. Glancing closer at the printed words caused my breath to catch. A sharp piercing pain went through my chest as I read his medical profile. I didn't know. I had no idea that he was so sick.

I questioned myself on how I would approach him. Was he still angry at me? Bottom line was, would he talk to me?

I fought the impulse to pick up the phone and call Richard. Lately, Richard and Bradley were the only ones that remained in contact with David. What would I say to Richard? How could I justify even bringing up David's name to Richard? At the same time, I knew that Richard could help me reach David on whatever plateau David existed.

David was no longer just a friend but now a client. There was this small wish I had that perhaps David would refuse my services and then, only then, would he be reassigned to someone else.

My guts pushed further into my chest cavity. I closed my eyes and winced at the deadening numbness as I reread the medical section. Oh no! Not again—Not AIDS!

Later that night, I paced the floor. I became obsessed. Each time I glanced at his file, the lump in my throat lodged deeper. I needed to talk to someone. Anyone!

I sat and stared out the window as the sun descended; I sipped on scotch and water. It was mostly scotch. The liquid burned my throat. I laid back and closed my eyes and tried to listen to the radio. When I thought I was relaxed, images of David rushed my mind. I drained my glass and reached for the phone.

"Hello Michal!"

"Hey Richard, you and that damned caller id! How am I supposed to creep up on you and whisper sweet obscenities?"

"Whatever! I was just thinking about you."

"Were you busy?" I could feel my heartbeat vibrate the glass as it rested on my chest.

"Naw, just chillin' to some Jazz…What's up?"

"Nothing really…just haven't heard from you guys…"

"So, were you freaked out or something?" Richard's voice was so calm and yet assuring.

"What are you talking about? Freak out over what?" I sat up on my bed. I started gasping for air. My hand tightened around the glass. "What are you talking about?"

"You know, about you case managing David."

"What are you talking about?" I jumped off my bed. Beads of sweat formed around my brow.

"Relax baby, David spilled the beans." Richard paused. "Are you sure you can deal with him? You realize he's like reading a book full of instruction with most of the pages missing."

PANELS

"He ain't mad?"

"Naw, the dude's over it…He says he can't wait to see ya!"

"That's what I'm afraid of…Listen, I need to see him but I don't know what to say…He probably thinks we all deserted him that night he got arrested…."

"Michal, you really need to take a major chill pill…I said he's okay now…A little drugged up, but still himself."

"How much do you know?"

"Everything…trust me…I know what you are getting at…I was with him when he found out."

"But…"

"Stop worrying, Michal. You know he's a fighter…He ain't about to let that AIDS crap get him…in fact, he actually took it better than I did…I totally freaked out!" Richard laughed. "You would have thought it was me and not him when the doctor told us."

"Remind me to leave you at home in case I have a crisis."

"If your computer crashes, call me. If you emotionally crash, ya ass better dial 911." Richard laughed. "Seriously, he really misses the gang."

"When are you going to see him again?"

"Michal sweetie, when do you want to go?"

"Well, I do need to see him as soon as possible…what about tomorrow around three?"

"I can do that…yeah, I can…Do you want to meet at Central State or do you want to ride together? Either way is fine with me."

"Let's ride together…I may need some moral support from you."

"It's cool! But, Michal, seriously…chill out…he don't hate you or nothing…"

"Richard, you have been a damned good friend."

"Trust me, I have my moments…I'm no angel, but you already know that…I just feel that we are all we got…Our little group is a family no matter how dysfunctional we are…We got to stay together."

"Richard, did it surprise you when you found out?"

"You mean about him being sick? Naw, I kinda already suspected as much."

"Why didn't you tell me?" My pity turned to anger.

"Be for real! I didn't have any proof. And that ain't something that you just blurt out without facts especially concerning David…I knew that something wasn't quite right when I went to see him before the pageant…I was blown away at the garbage all over the place. I mean, real slimly garbage. It smelled up his whole house…You know that's not like him. He always kept a spotless crib…Baby, roaches were taking over the place…I had to clear a path just to walk to his bedroom…his thuggish brother was sitting in the front room getting his crack on…"

"Were you afraid?"

"Afraid of that low life thug? Hell no, I would have capped his ass in a heartbeat…Anyway, I stood in his bedroom doorway. Michal, he looked like hell that night and he was talking about going to do a show later that same night at the Chute. I wanted to cry at seeing my bro like that."

"Did he talk to you?"

"Yeah…but it was a weird ass conversation…I mean, we talked about dying, burial, his hatred for his mama, and talk out in the streets about him having sickle cell anemia…Now, I ain't no doctor, but I knew he didn't have no sickle cell shit…I don't know why I said it but I said something about welcoming death and that I wasn't afraid of dying."

"What did he say when you said that?"

"Something about me needing to fight whatever offends or threatens me…he said he would have if he thought his life was about to be over…then he said it."

"Said what? What did he say?" I poured myself another scotch, this time without the water.

"Something about certain queens out on the streets yelling at johns that he has the big 'A'…Honey, before I could say a word, David said it was all lies and that because he was suffering from sickle cell that it was no one business…but get this, David started bitching about no one wanted to help him because he was black."

"Excuse me! No one wanted to help him because he's black!"

"Michal, you ain't heard all of it…David had this little pity pat party going on. Everybody had done him wrong…People only wanted him when they could get something from him…He just went off!"

"All of this was going on before the pageant? So he was having problems long before then. You and I are not white. Has he become anti-white?"

"Naw, not really. He still loves him some Bradley."

"Yeah, two peas in a pod!"

"You know it…between those two, they have had all of Nashville!"

"What do you think we can do for David? I mean, what does he need the most?"

PANELS

"If I knew that, then I would have your job, wouldn't I?...I really don't know what he needs nor even what he wants...all I can do is listen to him. Even as he rambles on talking about nothing, I'll listen."

"Well, if he's not ready to deal with reality, that is all we can do is to listen."

"I don't know, Michal...somehow I think he is ready to change some things...I just hope it's not too late."

"One thing I learned years ago is that you can't make anyone do anything they don't want to do...You might as well dig a hole and stick your head in it for all the good you gonna do."

"Then, I guess we will see tomorrow, won't we?"

"Yeah, we will." I hung the phone back onto its cradle. I took the last swig straight from the bottle. The ringing in my ears roared as my head started to spin.

The sky was clear and the warm air breathed softly across the land. As I walked from the parking area to the main office, I passed a few patients resting on benches. Some of the patients asked me for a cigarette. I shrugged them off. As if undisturbed, they just turned and approached the next person walking in their direction.

I was signing in at the reception area of Central State Psychiatric Hospital when Dr. Sanders walked in. Dr. Richard Sanders, with those gorgeous deep darkening blue eyes and smile of an angel, was standing behind me.

I had known him professionally for many years. He was the medical director at the agency where I work. I had grown extremely fond of him to the point I had a crush on him. I couldn't have him as my psychiatrist since I couldn't look beyond his dreamy eyes. I was secretly in love with him.

Dr. Sanders drummed into our heads the rights of the mentally ill. He fought for his consumers and often went beyond the call of duty to ensure a positive quality of life. He also expected his staff to do the same.

The hairs on the back of my neck felt warm. I felt quite giddy. I was engulfed in my fantasy of him when he spoke my name. The joyous sensation turned tarnished. Oh yeah! I suddenly remembered that I had failed this god.

"I'll take it that we are here for the same consumer?"

"Uh...yes, sir."

"Walk with me and tell me what you learned from your previous encounter."

"Actually, sir, this is my first visit seeing him."

" Michal, I'm quite disappointed in your irresponsible actions." Dr.

Sanders grimaced. "Hasn't he been here over a week?"

"Yes, sir...I've been planning on seeing him before now, but..."

"But you figured if he was to mentally decompose further, he was at the right place, is that it?"

"No, sir..." My battlement was breached.

"So, what is it? What caused you to forget about him?"

"Sir, I didn't forget...I was waiting for another person to come with me."

"Someone from the agency? Why? Is this supposed to be a collaborative effort?"

"No, sir...the person doesn't work with us...He's actually a friend...you see, David is a close friend to both of us." I lowered my head to avoid his eyes.

"Did you tell Evelyn about this when you was first assigned this case?"

"Yes, sir. She thought that me being his friend would help me to understand his dilemmas more so than someone new to case management...something about lost time just to start to process."

"Well, I'm glad you finally decided to connect with him before he turned a year older...I'll get back with you on this matter...now, it's time to see Mr. Flynn."

"Yes, sir." I walked behind him towards the locked doors of H pod. My head still lowered.

"Hello, Dr, Sanders. How are you today?" An attending psychiatric nurse greeted him while totally ignored my presence.

"We're here to see Mr. Flynn." Dr. Sanders signed very unmoved.

"Well, the last time I saw him, he was in the group room a few moments ago...I will go and find him for you." The nurse hurried away.

"Just look at this place...people sitting around idle...no structured activities...how is this therapeutic except for the lazy ass staff watching television?" Dr. Sanders pointed at a cluster around the nursing station. "This is why we need to remove our consumers from this hell hole...they can get worse at home on their own. They don't need this help."

"I'm sorry I'm late, Michal." Richard rushed to my side. "Traffic was murder!"

Richard appeared short of breath. The gleam in his eyes reassured me I was doing the right thing.

"Dr. Sanders, this is the friend that I was telling you about..." I felt somewhat relieved but still slightly embarrassed.

"Well, when Mr. Flynn joins us, we will have enough to play bridge, won't we?" Dr. Sanders grunted. "If Mr. Flynn gives us a release, I will speak

PANELS

with you further regarding your friend. If that is alright with you?"

"Sure, no problem." Richard smiled.

As if a stage curtain opened, David made his entrance. "Hey Ms. Thang, girl! I have died and gone to gay heaven…Y'all got some nice looking specimen coming to see little old me…Darlings, I would haul you to my crib but there's some nasty thang in there drooling all over the place…baby, you better believe me when I say that girl crazier than me! She's like all the *I love Lucy* and the *Three Stooges* reruns all wrap into one soul!" David continued to twirl around us. He was wearing a thin blue cotton bedspread around his shoulders as if it was chiffon.

"I won't ask why you are wearing that." Richard lifted the material from the floor.

"Oh this, this little piece of art! Honey, this is high fashion in here…it's to die for…in fact, some of them crazies can't have this priceless gown. The damned fools tries to hang themselves…honey, you got to get me out of this place before I start to think this is all I got." David danced around us.

"Let's go to the classroom where we can have some privacy." Dr. Sanders nonchalantly moved away toward the empty room.

"Baby, the way you look…honey, I'll go anywhere…Let's ditch these nobodies and make a run for it." David winked.

"Are you ready to leave this place? Are you really ready to go home?" Dr. Sanders asked.

"Does a bear dump in the woods? Hell yeah, I want to get out of this place. I ain't a damned loony." David stopped cold in his tracks. He sized up Dr. Sanders with a glee in his eyes. "Richard honey, who's this flawless piece of meat?"

"He's the man…he's the doctor that gonna get your fool ass out of here."

"Well, I will be damned!" David flirted. "You are so cute. Can I come and live with you? You need a wife or a husband? Honey, I can be both!"

"Hello, David," I said from behind.

"Oh hi…I see you finally got off your grand horse and come to see me…Were you afraid to come alone? You thought I was gonna do something to ya? Is that why ya got back up to protect your sorry ass?" David started twirling again and waved the cloth against my face. His eyes were cold and remote.

"Regardless of how long it took him, now is the time to go forward…what are you ready to do to get out of here?" Dr. Sanders interrupted.

"Anything…anything it will take for me to return to my real world. You just tell me what to do and I will do it." I noticed how sullen David's face was.

"Well, if we are finished with idle chit chat, perhaps we can proceed." Dr. Sanders cocked his eyes upon us.

"Now, I don't mind y'all helping me but I don't want all my business out in the street. That ain't right…you know, people still scared of this shit…Too many people already knows too much now."

"Are you referring to having AIDS?" Dr. Sanders glanced across the table. His voice was nonchalant and not moved.

"I ain't got no damn AIDS!" David reared back. "Ms Thang, if you must know…I'm only positive." His tune was almost patronizing.

"I'm afraid your T-Cells proves otherwise…I won't lie to you and say that it doesn't matter what you think. It does matter. It matters because you are going to have to deal with reality head on and not with avoidance, that is, if you want to live…If you don't want to live, tell me and I will leave. I don't have time for foolishness." Dr. Sanders glared over the rim of his half glasses.

"Just who the hell are you?" David stared. His voice quivered. "I didn't ask for your funky ass…so, go and leave. I don't need your help…See, Richard, ain't that some shit? This is exactly what I been talking about, ain't nobody out there gonna do a damn thing for me!" David turned to Richard.

"David, damn it! Listen to the man. He knows what he's talking about…Stop acting like some punk and work with us." Richard's voice was stern.

"Oh, I see! Now you have gone and turned white on me. Richard, you of all people I thought would know where I'm coming from…Naw, you gotta be some Uncle Tom. I guess if you sleep with enough of them you start to act like them."

"Whatever…if I didn't like your tired self, I wouldn't be here…and neither would they…you just need to open your eyes and see the light before it's too late." Richard rose to leave. "Gimme a call me when you get some sense in your fool head!"

"Hey doc, maybe you need to talk to him…I think he got some major issues." David nervously laughed.

"Why, because he genuinely cares for someone that doesn't give a damn about himself?" Dr. Sanders continued with his head lowered in David's file.

"What the hell makes you so sure that I don't care about myself? Am I supposed to fall to my knees and thank the old master for coming to my rescue? I may be sick right now but I know what I'm saying. I'm not as crazy as you think I am."

PANELS

"Well Michal, I would assume that our work here is done...your friend says he's not crazy, although he is the one in pajamas wearing a blanket on his head on this locked psychiatric ward." Dr. Sanders stood and gathered his items. "So, why are we still here?"

"Hey man...wait a minute!" David grabbed Dr. Sanders' arm. "You can't leave me in this place. I'll die!"

"I have no control of whatever happens to you, you do...and when you are ready to deal with reality, then, and only then, will we work with you...Look around you, look at yourself...Is this how you want to spend the rest of your life?"

"Man, please, give me another chance," David cried. "I just don't know about this...all my life, I have had to fight something or the other. I'm not used to strangers being nice to me without wanting something back in return...Please, that's all I ask of you, please give me another chance."

"Do you think he is worth another shot, Michal?" Dr. Sanders winked in my direction..

"I don't know...it depends on just how serious he is, I guess." I tried not to smile. We had him in our grasp although he was still slippery.

"Michal! You know me. You know I ain't like this. Gimme a break. Do I hafta beg, you know I will," David pleaded.

"Okay then, lets get with it." Dr. Sanders tapped on the empty chair beside him. David hurriedly sat. The session began. As David spoke, I saw tears mounting. Without missing a beat, he reached over the table, grabbed my hand, and held onto my hand. With a slight smile on his face, I felt that he was no longer afraid.

Later that night, I had dinner with some of the guys at the West End Cooker. Cleo was at home playing the Donna Reed role but in a dying marriage. Bradley was somewhere in between sheets with his latest prey. David was still on a locked unit playing all three faces of Eve.

I knew I was in a strange mood. I really didn't want to be around others but I didn't want to be alone either. I longed for some form of normalcy. Although they were my friends, I felt very much like a stranger. Absent was the usual jovial banter. Silence took its place.

I watched Richard toss his food about his plate. He cut the food into small morsels but never ate the food. Seth said Richard was unusually quiet during the drive over. Sebastian appeared captivated in his own misery and ignored others' distress signals. Seth and I struggled with small talk. Obviously, we all wanted to be far away from reality and ourselves. Finally hoping to break the monotony, Seth suggested that we walk through the park before we parted for the evening.

We ran across West End dodging traffic in eerie silence. The only sound was the car engines that whirled around us. Even now, I realized just how uncanny the scene was. The mood was somber—actually gruesome.

In the distance on our left, the Parthenon, home of Pallas Athena, stood gloriously as ever as the white spotlights cascaded upwardly on its granite exterior. Lake Wautauga was directly in front of us on the right side of the park. It was nine o'clock at night. The air was warm. Car brake lights glowed sporadically as if imitating mating calls. The moon was full and very bright. We had two hours before the park closed.

As we walked closer to the mouth of the lake, we heard laughter echoing across the water. Figures in the dark walked in pairs alongside the bank. Crickets replaced the sleeping ducks that nestled on the island in the middle of the lake.

"Let's walk over by the lake." Seth broke the silence.

"Anyone wants to skinny dip?" I blurted out my ill attempt at humor.

"Yeah, you go ahead and I'll join you," Sebastian said. "I'm sure duck shit can do wonders for your complexion."

"Just look at the traffic…the flirting lover boys of the night." I said while ignoring his remark. "Remember when we used to cruise around the lake. Going in circles…"

"Yeah, I remember y'all wasting my gas trying to catch a glimpse of fantasy." Sebastian paused. "Cruising is what probably got David where he is now."

"Oh, are we playing Ms. Prude now? I vaguely remember you passing out your number a few times to trade," I snapped.

"Isn't it unfair to say that David got what he deserved?" Seth stared at Sebastian.

"All I'm saying is that you got to be careful these days. Blowing all caution to the wind is foolish," Sebastian retorted. "He's paying the price for being a whore."

"How dare you act so damn pious! You are nothing more than a sanctimonious bastard." I jumped in his face. "You are a bitter queen!"

"Oh, so I'm the enemy now!…Is it because I'm angrier than you? Ever since Gregory died of that damned disease, we all became aware of that bogeyman that lurks in the shadows waiting." Sebastian's body became rigid. "Hell, all I want to do is to keep living. And if it means not being intimate with

PANELS

anyone, so be it."

"Oh, it is so nice to find someone that truly understands." I paused. "I guess it's just easy to walk away from those you once loved."

"Damn it! Quit ya bitching! Why are we fighting each other? Are we our own enemy?" Richard cried. "Why can't y'all look beyond yourselves? Grow up and stop being so damned selfish."

"Hey, what's with the tears, man?" Sebastian grabbed Richard's shoulder. Richard pulled away and turned his back to us.

"He's worried about David," Seth said as he rubbed Richard's back. Richard turned around and faced Seth. The look they both shared told me it was something else. I learned later exactly what *that something* was. Tonight, we were not as friends but as unwanted strangers in the midst.

"I already told David that no matter what, we will be there for him." Seth proclaimed.

"Well, I don't know about *all of us* being there…you know that Cleo is still miffed at him for scaring the daylights out of her…but, you're right, he has to want us back in his life." Sebastian balked. He walked over to the broken two-seated glider and sat down. His shoes scuffed the earth as the swing moved.

"She will come around. She always does." I said. "But, where the hell is Bradley?"

"Stop worrying…we are here," Sebastian said. "He's family, remember!"

"What does that mean exactly? I have family too but they can't stand the ground I walk on." Richard threw a rock into the lake. "Family don't mean shit!"

"Whoa, Nelly…! What brought this on?" I asked. "Richard, you of all people know what we mean to each other. Man, you have always said that we are a family. What gives?"

"That was yesterday…" Richard muttered.

"I've never realized just how beautiful the moon reflection was on water!" Seth interrupted the flow as he stared at the lake. "The water looks like black ice. So shiny and yet so mystic. Waiting to yield some dark secret."

Richard walked over to the swing and sat beside Sebastian. Richard pointed at the Parthenon. He appeared to have taken a deep breath which he exhaled slowly.

"When the Parthenon was dedicated, the King Constantine of Greece was invited to the celebration. He had lost his throne to the Fascists. So much for the fabled 'Cradle of Democracy' theory…" Richard paused for a moment.

His voice still quivered from the crying. "You know, we also risk the threat of no longer being free or even having pride in who we are…" Richard's tongue unrolled with uncertainty as he stole glances at each one of us. "AIDS scares off friends."

"What kinda person would any of us be if we walked away from David?…Gregory didn't let us into his life until it was too late…I'm still angry at him for watching him die…You can't even imagine the hell it was to see someone you love die before your eyes…" Sebastian pushed the swing with his heel. His face remained lowered.

"Yeah, we would have been there…but he didn't call us, he called you, remember?" I said.

"What damn difference does it make who got what call? Why does that matter? Would he have lived longer if someone else had gotten his call?" Richard stared at me. His eyes filled with pain.

"Actually, Gregory wasn't the one who called me, another guy did…You remember that Duncan fellow…Hell, I don't know why Gregory didn't call any of us but he just didn't…." Sebastian raised his voice. "Next time someone calls, I'll tell them to call you first. Is that what you want?"

"Don't be foolish. You know that's not what I'm saying."

"So Michal, what are you saying…David told Richard about himself and I don't hear any flack over that or does David matter in the same respect?" Sebastian asked. "Why are you so pissed off at who was told first? Why should it matter?"

"It doesn't matter…who cares who knew first. David matters a great deal to me, which is why I'm having a really hard time with what is going on with him…or any others like him. Unlike yourself, I can't just turn off my emotions and only look at life through clinical glasses." Richard paced in a circle. Finally, he walked over and stood beside Seth.

"Richard, my dear friend…are you trying to say that I'm cold and callous? That I have no feelings…which one is it?" Sebastian stopped the swing.

"Sebastian, I did not mean to imply that about you at all…I just meant that I can't handle seeing people in pain. You and Michal work with people all day long in some form of a crisis. I could not do it. " Richard sounded almost apologetic.

"Relax, Sebastian. No one is blaming you." Seth skipped a few pebbles across the water. "That was really a difficult task on anyone. Actually, I'm glad it wasn't me."

"Seth is probably right…that was a raw deal you got." Richard wiped his eye.

PANELS

"Guys, just listen to us...Listen to us tear ourselves down or question our motives. Why? Why are we doing this to ourselves? We have done nothing to be ashamed of."

"You're right! Michal, we have remained tight. Through all our hell, we are still here for each other." Seth smiled. "No one will ever change that!"

"Remember, guys, we are all fragments of one soul." Richard laughed.

"Including Bradley and David!" Sebastian raised his hand to the sky.

"Of course, what would we do without our saintly brothers of the night?" I asked.

"Guys, just suppose that Gregory and David weren't the only two in the group that fought AIDS. Tell me, could each and everyone of you honestly sit here and say that you would still be there regardless?..." Richard paused as Seth took his hand. After a nod from Seth, he proceeded. "Suppose it was one of us right here right now...suppose it was me?...are you gonna be there for me?" Richard asked in a whisper.

Sebastian immediately stopped swinging and looked over at Richard. I stood completely still while wishing the words to be untrue. I watched Seth pull Richard into his arms. The moonlight reflected off their tears.

The full moon's likeness descended across the intensifying ripples of Lake Wautauga as night drew on with a hush.

The year was 1990. The battle against AIDS was fine-tuning and in rapid transition but not quick enough. Since the discovery in 1981, the Center for Disease Control reported more than 307,000 AIDS cases. A bill to force pharmaceuticals to lower the cost of AIDS drugs was vetoed by President Bush. AIDS hit the film festivals and told stories that included the minorities. AIDS was no longer just for the "pretty preppie white boys." Ryan White died. Queer Nation was born.

Over the next few months, my life appeared to realign itself to the universe. I no longer felt stranded on the edge of the world. Life was back on the routine cycle. There was a major change; we were seeing each other with less frequency. In after thought, I wondered if we were avoiding the reality around us.

Richard and Seth were still inseparable, although they still denied any coupling of the slightest intimacy. Sebastian appeared to have taken a new lease on life and moved away from his island of depression. I no longer dodged him since the changes made him tolerable. Cleo labored at making her marriage work. Even though I thought her work was in vain, I continued to be supportive

After two months, David was released from Central State. I was walking to the main building when he came running towards me, flailing his arms while constantly pushing his duffle bag back on his shoulder. His clothes hung on him like sheets on a clothes line. At first I thought he had lost weight but remembered he had always worn his clothes several sizes to large. He was smiling.

"Girl, I thought you was never coming!" David walked past me to the car. "I've been waiting since last night."

"But, you wasn't discharged until this morning." I had to think.

"And...what's your point?" David tossed his bag in the back seat and jumped in the passenger seat. "Get me away from this place!"

"Are you hungry?" I fastened my seat belt. "I thought we would grab a bite."

"Honey, just as long as the food ain't on no damn plastic inserts and cold." David pulled down the sun visor and stared into the mirror. For a moment, he said nothing. "Baby, ain't enough foundation and make up in the world to bring the lovely Tiffany back."

"Something tells me that she be out again real soon." I smiled.

"Naw, the old girl has taken a long exotic retirement." David flipped the visor up. He turned and looked at me. "I thought we were going to get some grub."

Between intervals of ordering and getting our food, we discussed his return to the world. Surprisingly, he was quite optimistic. The days in confinement returned his body weight. Anti-viral medications were given in addition to his psychiatric doses. He had accepted the changes in his life. In fact, David recaptured ownership of his life. He vowed to never touch liquor nor crack again.

" I'm gonna show you and that cute little Doctor Sanders that I'm gonna make it." David laughed. "This is one queen that gonna put a whupin on that bug like you ain't never seen before." He smiled as he swallowed a mouthful of his burger.

"I really think you mean it." I stared at the man before me. He was no longer a stranger but my old friend.

"Michal, you just don't know...chile, I feel I have been blessed with a new lease on life." He looked around the half filled diner. "I'm so glad to be out of there."

PANELS

"I'm glad you're out too. No ill feelings?"

"Naw, I ain't got no time for that foolishness. I'm ready to go home."

Within a week, David began attending twelve steps meetings and HIV/AIDS support groups religiously. Through Nashville Cares, he joined the First Person Tour that went to schools and various other places to speak on the impact of AIDS. The old David had returned home, the caring one.

Bradley, on the other hand, was still Bradley. His wildness never ceased. He and Jeffery separated but remained friends. Seth and Bradley appeared more distant than ever. No one would have ever imagined them being brothers. As different as fire and rain.

The stillness of the night can often breed bewilderment and doubt. I was in deep sleep when the phone rang.

"Hello..." I muttered from my grogginess.

"Hi sweet cheeks! Whatcha doing?"

"I was sleeping...who is this?"

"It's me, Bradley...I figured I'd call you since your fingers are broken and unable to dial me...How's it hanging?"

"Bradley, do you realize it is three in the morning?"

"Is that all...I thought it was later than that...Anyway, I needed to talk to someone so I called you. Isn't that exciting? I haven't seen you in eon years!"

"I can barely hear you...where are you calling me from? All that noise in the background. Are you in a bar?'

"Now you know ain't no bar opened this time of the morning. You know Nashville rolls up the sidewalk at the stroke of two...Naw, I'm at Las Bradley's Hacienda...wait up a sec while I turn down Ms. Aretha...okay, that's better. What have you been up to?"

"Bradley, I'm sure that we could carry this conversation at better time than the wee hours of the morning."

"Look, if you don't want to be bothered just tell me. I will be the least of your worry."

"Bradley, that is not what I meant and you know that. I was merely suggesting that we talk later, that's all."

"Well, apologies excepted. I guess. Anyway, now that you are wide awake, I want to invite you out this Saturday to the Cab."

"Why? What's going on there?"

"That's a surprise. I can't tell you now...Look man, sorry but I had to reach you before it was too late. You are such a busy man these days; I was afraid you had already planned something foofy."

"No, I didn't have anything planned except to just chill out." I glanced over at the clock and winced. "Is it really important?"

"Hell yeah, it's important...Just promise me that you will show up." Bradley appeared to almost be pleading. "Can you do that for me?"

"I will try."

"Groovy! That's all I ask." Bradley paused. "The rest of the gang will be there...Don't forget...and if you do, you're gonna have one mean queen coming after you!" There was laughter and then the phone went dead.

Later that day, I was still dragging. I dared not sit still. I knew if I did, I would probably go to sleep. Have you ever notice that whenever you are so tired and full of sleep, that the world around you is extremely hyperactive? The minute hand on my biological clock seemed stuck!

"Was it good!" Sebastian grinned.

"Was what good?"

"Ah, play dumb, will ya!...You look absolutely like crap."

"Thanks for the compliment...I feel like that too."

"So, what happened?"

"Our prodigal brother Bradley paid me a late visit early this morning...by phone."

"Whew, he still remembered your number...Knowing Bradley, was the moon hanging or was the sun breaking thru?"

"I think the bars had just closed."

"Oh, I see...why didn't you tell him to call you at a more decent time?"

"Oh, don't think I didn't try...but he gave me so much grief at not wanting to talk to him, I felt I had to."

"So, what did he want?"

"He wanted to make sure I knew to go to the Cab this Saturday. He was so cryptic about it. He did say that the rest of the gang would be there."

"Yeah, I got a similar message...I figured I'd go and see what's happening. I ain't got nothing to do anyway. It's not like my social calendar is filled with hot sweaty bodies."

"What! You mean you don't have a date?" I smirked.

"I'm afraid so, in fact, my life is sorta like yours." Sebastian cut his eye at me. "So, I guess I will see you there as well."

"It depends on whether or not I hear from Matthew Broderick!"

"Blanche, like I said...I will see you there."

As I arrived at the Cabaret, I noticed the marquee: an AIDS benefit. Plastered were names of performers from the past and the present scheduled to perform for the "Cabaret Reunion."

AIDS was causing financial hardships for many individuals. Medical insurance was not a priority to many of us during the pre-AIDS days. Many of us had jobs that merely paid the bills of the day. Life had been free and without burdens. Many of us lived for the night. So when AIDS crossed our paths, we were caught literally with our pants down. Many couldn't afford to see doctors let alone pay for the medication. We became the new poor of the decade.

Occasionally, gay bars had benefit shows. Creative themes were designed to not only provide awareness but also put a little fun in the venture. What better excuse to dress in drag. Tip money was used to pay rent, buy food, buy medications, etc. It was the gay welfare. We took care of our own while we could.

Inside the crowded bar, the mood appeared increased in jovial celebration as laughter escalated and resounded off the ceiling. Familiar faces I have not seen in ages were there. As I continued to look, reality overwhelmed me. I realized the absence of many.

Couples joined in laughter and spirits in the knee deep mixed crowd. It was a costumed ball from reality. Just for this night, there is passion in the air.

Finally, my eyes caught them. Cleo, Seth, Bradley, Richard, and Sebastian were seated at table only inches from the stage. Beside Sebastian was an available chair. This night was the first night we had all been together for several months.

"So you did make it after all!" Bradley kissed my cheek.

"I take it that Mr. Matthew didn't call you?" Sebastian nudged me.

"Who's this Matthew?" Cleo appeared curious.

"He's Michal's new lover, except Mr. Matthew doesn't know it...only in Michal's warped mind." Sebastian smiled as he pat me on my back.

"Anyway...It's so great seeing y'all here tonight. I really miss our times together...Too bad that David isn't here to join us," I said as I ordered a beer from a waitress.

"Well, actually...*he* is here." Bradley smiled.

"Oh...should I get another chair?" I asked. "Should he be here? Is he all right? I can move over and make more room."

"No Michal, just take a chill pill and enjoy the show." Bradley reached over and squeezed my hand.

The evening events gradually began with the presentational opening of two elderly lovers giving their brief personal accounts of the actual night that the Stonewall Inn was invaded by New York's finest. One of the individuals himself was battling with AIDS. I noticed how he had walked slow across the stage with his lover by his side. His speech slurred as he told the packed house of his past. He closed with words that quieted much of the noise; he spoke of how he had fought for his rights. Now, he was battling a mêlée that he hoped no one else would. The foe was AIDS.

Later, after several acts left the stage, the house lights went dark. Quietness prevailed. Then there was light. From the ceiling directly over the lowered dance floor, red laser lights beamed and danced across the stage and the audience as soft piano music played in the distance.

A masculine voice softly penetrated the darkness's solace. I tried to understand the words. Something was said about someone sharing the struggle with others battling AIDS. Something about being thankful for having friends when they are needed the most. My attention returned to our table. I watched as Cleo reached over and grabbed Seth and Richard's hands. Whenever the strobe lights crossed her face, I saw tears.

The voice ceased as the music evolved into 'That's What Friends Are For." Several performers took their places on stage on cue singing their parts. People lined around the stage and gave tips, brief hugs and kisses. Tears mounted in my eyes. I found myself singing the lyrics with the others at the table.

I noticed that Seth appeared emotional. His body shook as he quietly cried. Everyone appeared touched, even Bradley. The words to the song hit home with a reality I had become accustomed to.

After the performers had finished, the emcee waited for the clamor to settle down before she brought out the next act to the stage. Suddenly, a vaguely familiar song was being played. A rush went over me as I watched a very familiar face graced the stage from the right wing. It was Tiffany Lynn.

Tiffany Lynn was far more beautiful than I had ever seen her. The white Severin sleeveless dress in rayon Venetian lace captured a soul of an angel. The appearance of rich simplicity with the pristine column of ivory lace covered her body slightly below the neck. She was simply radiant!

In the past, her unforgiving sultry numbers always amused me but tonight I was in total awe as I watched her sing a ballad titled "Make It Like It Was." Her graceful movements of her hands and body strengthened each note.

People stood in several rows to tip her. Her hands filled with dollars until someone brought a basket and placed at her feet. Then, she looked directly at us. Tiffany reached out to us. Cleo was the first to reach her. Seconds later,

PANELS

we were all huddled together even after the music had finished.

Eventually, the night ended. The house lights turned on and fantasies disappeared. The masquerade was over and reality became the mainstay. People shuffled around us exiting into the early morning air. I was drunk with pride. Once again, our friend Tiffany was back on top of the world.

"Anybody for coffee?" Cleo gathered her purse.

"Yeah...a cup of brew to watch the sun rise. I'm game," I said.

"Like the old times...isn't it?" Seth smiled as he rubbed Richard's neck.

"I'm getting too old for this vampire life. Why can't we have our glitter earlier?"

"Richard, my dear, do you really want to see some of these darlings in the day light...Remember we only come out at night!" Bradley smirked. "Anyway, old Tiff has already left the house."

"No! We want her to join us." Cleo pushed Bradley towards the dressing room. "It won't be the same without her."

"Baby doll, are you deaf? I told you she left already on the red eye...She said she will see us tomorrow. She was too exhausted to stay lovely all night," Bradley said.

"Did you see all those duckies she made tonight? Girl ain't got to worry about her rent money this month." Richard laughed.

"You know, I am so happy she bounced back. She looked great tonight." I started walking out the door.

"Correction, Ms. Thang, she was flawless...simply faboo!" Bradley snapped his fingers in the air.

"Whatever! It just goes to show you that if she can turn her life around after all that shit she had to go through, then anybody can." Cleo swayed past us.

" Tiff's like a Timex, you know, she takes a licking but still keeps on ticking. Ain't nothing gonna get her down."

"Bradley, honey, that means that there's hope for you yet!" Richard patted him on his back.

I still remember the sickening feeling in my stomach of the news. David was found dead at his home the next day. He was on the floor near the front window. Sebastian and Richard had tried reaching David by telephone. When they arrived at his house, the police were already there.

David had mentioned that he needed to talk to us about something very important to him. I guess we will never know what he had to say to us.

According to the forensic report, David had been stabbed numerous times about the face and neck. Fragments of broken steel protruded from his head. His face was horribly disfigured and mangled. He was partially still in drag clothing. Recent filled prescription bottles littered the floor around his body. All containers were empty including the vials of demoral and morphine. His addicted brother was nowhere to be found.

I found out later from another performer that David was extremely sick on the night of the benefit. Bianca Paige told me later that David spoke of wanting to give something back to the community, something that he was given: unconditional love.

We buried him a few days later after his body was released. Bradley paid for the casket. He was appalled at the thought of him buried in a simple pine box furnished by the city. Cleo gave the morticians her Coco Chanel gown to dress him in.

The casket was kept closed. There were two pictures, one as Tiffany and the other as David, placed on pedestals. Amidst a few others, our circle were in attendance. After all, we were his family.

According to the small partially hidden newspaper piece, "David Flynn, age thirty-two, was killed by an unknown assailant at his North Nashville home in an apparent foiled robbery attempt. There were no leads."

Outraged, I flung the paper across the room. How dare the authorities discount his death. We all knew damn well who his assailant was. Did his life have less value because he was queer? To others, David was merely a crime statistic, but to us, he was one of us.

I still remember all too well that day we watched our friend being lowered into the cold dry ground. No one there except for us and the cemetery laborers impatiently with their shovels in hand. Waiting like vultures ready to attack the mound of dirt.

All of us, Richard, Bradley, Seth, Sebastian, and I followed behind the bronze coffin to the open grave. Cleo walked behind us. She was trying to find some passage from her bible.

"I'm sorry, guys…I just can't find anything that's right to read. I don't know what to say…"Cleo appeared frustrated through her tears.

"What about reading the Lord 's Prayer?" Richard cocked his head.

"Yeah, I'm sure he would like that one…you know he was kinda religious, at times." Seth nodded.

"What! No drag numbers? No grand finales to leave us with?" Bradley smirked.

No one responded. Instead, we began in unison to recite the prayer. After

PANELS

the casket was lowered, the laborers proceeded to shovel. Something really got to me as I heard the sound of the first piles of the earth fall upon David. My breathing became labored and short. I could feel my heart race, beating hard against my chest. Sweat formed across my brows and upper lip. I wanted them to stop. I did nothing except to stand there and cry.

Even as I walked away from his grave, I knew he would not be the last. I hated myself for thinking that way.

Less than a week later, Cleo called me. Her voice was as spirited as ever. I had just arrived at home from the office. I dropped my brief and kicked my shoes off my tired swollen feet. I listened as she gave me the details.

"You know I really think Bradley is bummed out more than he's willing to say. I mean, we are all hurting…but you know how close they both were. Now he has lost his partner in crime." Cleo paused to sip her wine.

"Yeah, the dynamic duo is no longer terrorizing the innocent."

"He called me this morning. Guess what he wants to do?"

"I only work with feeble minds, I don't second guess them. What, pray tell, is he going to do now?"

"He wants us to make a panel for David," Cleo said with confidence.

"Our Bradley! Are you telling me he wants to do something for someone else? Cleo, surely you jest."

"No, he was serious…so are you game?"

"Sure, count me in."

"I knew you would…we are meeting over at his place on Saturday around noon, bring some material and some wild ideas."

"Do you know where I can get a tiara, bugle beads, and plenty of rhinestones?" I sunk in my chair.

"Now you're talking…see ya there. Love ya!" The phone went dead.

Nashville, during the autumn months, becomes a kaleidoscope of natural beauty. The foliage turned crispy green. The loose leaves from the various trees emulated male peacocks that flirted with newfound love. The calmness of the moist earth harnessed the bitter wind that made each leaf crackle as it fell.

Fall was my favorite season. I could close my eyes and feel the billowing wind. I became a child again with a pure heart. I imagined flying a kite in treacherous flight patterns high above the hills. Sweaters escaped from their cedar prison to protect me from the damp coolness. I was alone watching the flaming embers of the fireplace roar as kernels pop. Rain quickly arrived as summer's heat bid farewell. Seasons left as abrupt as some lives. I eventually learned what it was that Richard was trying to tell us in the park. Deep down, I still wished that all of the words had remained cryptic and without translation. Life doesn't work that way; it doesn't give you a choice.

It was a cool brisk day that Sunday afternoon. There was a knock at my door. Standing on the other side of my peephole were Seth and Richard. Seth held a bag of ice and glasses while Richard held onto a bottle of Jack.

"What do I owe this superb honor to?" I waved them inside as cold damp air rushed in.

"We just happened to be out and about. So we thought we'd drop by…we brought another good friend to join us." Seth smiled. Richard raised the liquor bottle.

"I think I may have met him before…Why don't you guys come on in and let's get reacquainted." I closed the door.

"Are we interrupting? Do you have a stud stashed under the bed?" Richard walked towards the kitchen.

"I wish…no, no one is here. Just my little bed bugs." I grabbed the coke from the refrigerator.

"Oh, I'm scared of you. Remind me to never sleep over here…speaking of which, how is your love life?" Seth dropped the bag of ice on the counter.

"How does one speak of something so nonexistent?" I paused as I glanced at them. "However, I'm sure I can't get the same answer out of you two, now can I?"

"My dear Michal, I am indeed shocked! I haven't the faintest idea of what you are referring to." Richard feigned surprise.

"Oh no! Who let the cat out of the bag?" Seth giggled.

"I know you guys didn't think you could hide something like that from the rest of us. So how long have you guys been kicking it?"

"My goodness, Michal. You are not too keen on subtle hints, are you?" Richard poured a round of Jack and coke.

" Life's too short to walk the maze. Hell, I say, jump the bush!" I took a swig of my cocktail. "So, how long?"

"Well, actually, we are not sleeping together, at least not that way." Richard sat across from me.

"You mean, no sex, right?" I was bold.

"Yeah, kinda like that." Seth came and sat beside Richard.

"Please educate me, I see two guys here that are obviously hot for each

PANELS

other, sleeping together, but no sex. What gives? Are you waiting for a ring?"

"Richard is afraid of us being intimate.."

"Richard, now I know you're not virgin nor are you squeamish about sex...I heard the stories about you. So what gives?" I raised my glass in his direction.

"Should I tell him? What do you think?" Richard glanced over at Seth. Seth nodded and swirled his liquor. "Fasten your seat belt, you may be in for a bumpy ride...I'm positive."

"No shit! No, I mean, I'm sorry...when did you find out? How long have you known?" Without thinking, I took a big gulp of my drink. The liquor burned.

"You remember a few years ago when some of us walked around Centennial Park after eating at the Cooker? Do you remember me asking you guys if you would be there for someone else in our circle if they were positive?" Richard walked towards the balcony window and stared out.

"Omigod, I didn't think you meant yourself. Forgive me for saying this, but I actually thought you were talking about Bradley. I would have never thought about you...Of course, I will be there for you. Man, I love you. You have been like a brother to me...You mean you have kept this all bottled up inside of you all this time? Who else knows?" I wanted to go to him.

"Besides Seth and Cleo, just you...now, do you see why we can't sleep together. I love Seth way too much to kill him."

"Michal, I have tried to tell him that we could take precautions but he refuses to even want to try." Seth had moved to the kitchen for more ice.

"Richard..."

"Save it, Michal. How do I know those little raincoats really protect? I couldn't live thinking I gave it to him." Richard sat back on the sofa. I saw tears in his eyes.

"What made you go to find out?"

"I saw Daniel's name in the paper."

"Daniel, your ex?"

"Yeah...it was his obituary. So, I called his best friend Shannon. Let's just say she confirmed my fears."

"Richard, I'm so sorry...How are you handling it?" I poured more Jack.

"I take it day by day. My church has been very supportive. They don't cringe when I walk by. No whispering behind my back. They still hug me...However, I try not to plan anything long termed." Richard laughed.

"Are you sick?" I was taken aback at the thought.

"Actually, I'm not. I'm what you call asymptomatic. Meaning I don't have any of the wonderful opportunitistic infections...my viral load is still undetectable right now and my T-Cell count is around 2500. So, I guess I'm still hiding within the land of the living uninfected."

"How long have you known, Seth?" I turned to face him.

"Michal, I was with him when he went back for his results." Seth reached over and massaged Richard's arm. "And I'm going to be right there with him until..."

The year was 1996. Within six years after David's death, Richard became symptomatic. He was taking a mound of medication. Often his legs gave away while walking. He complained of having a tingling sensation and sharp pain throughout his body. He was diagnosed with neuropathy.

One Saturday morning, I met at Richard's for lunch. Seth was in the kitchen scrambling eggs. The quaint apartment smelled of Lysol and fried foods. Medicine bottles captured space near the toaster. I glanced without wanting to at the prescriptions.

"I thought if I was just sitting at my desk that I could still work." Richard winced. He woke me from my trance. "But, my body wouldn't listen."

"What about the Americans with disability act? Won't they make your boss accommodate you?" I wanted to know. I felt his eyes on me but I kept my eyes away.

"Lately, the only way they have been accommodating anyone was to show them the door." Richard started rubbing his raised leg that rested on a side chair. His veins appeared swollen and clearly defined. His legs reminded me as a child of seeing my grandmother's exposed varicose veins with the blood waiting to burst.

"But Richard, you can fight that. Man! That's nothing but flat out discrimination."

"Michal, my naïve dear child, yeah I can fight it...Whatever...in fact, just the other day another dude was fired while on restrictions...Hell, he only had temporary limitations...imagine what they would do to someone having AIDS...Face it, Michal, I'm history."

"Man, that's a raw deal! You really don't have any job security? I thought there were laws to prevent that from happening. I still think you should fight it!"

"Michal, I'm just too tired to fight. I simply don't have the energy. Oh, don't get me wrong, I'm scared...I'm scared because I really don't know what would happen to me if I lost my job...I have been on my own for years. I can't go back home. You know, if they didn't accept me for being gay then what do you think would happen if I showed up at their door with AIDS?"

"Michal, that's not something he has to worry about...He will always have a place here with me." Seth came around from the kitchen and hugged him.

Richard eventually lost his job because of his failing health. The tingling sensation had moved to his fingers making them numb. He couldn't type anymore. His medications gave him bouts of diarrhea and cramping. He wasn't flat out fired for his health. He was merely downsized. Funny, how only those on restrictions were downsized.

He gradually did move in with Seth at Seth's request. Richard had confided in me once that he feared losing his own identity by moving in with Seth. Deep inside, he resented anyone having any control of his life. Seth, he said, tried to assure him that he would be treated equal and not as some pathetic invalid. The proposed transition was only to last until his disability checks rolled in.

Seth became extremely articulated, hopeful, and aggressively extroverted in his will for Richard to live. No longer the introverted timid person afraid of facing the truth. Ironically, for his swan song, Seth had contracted Bradley's contagious knack for assertiveness. Seth told me once that he knew that Richard would be the one to fight the virus and win. Seth was definitely Richard's eager confidant and soul mate. Their constant tireless companionship appeared to prove positively beneficial.

One rather warm autumn evening, several of us went to the Belcourt to see the movie *Long Time Companion*. I had only heard bits and pieces about this movie. Cleo and Richard had suggested this particular flick, ranting and raving about how progressive this movie was and how it expressed such a sensitive matter as AIDS. Without questioning, I joined my friends.

I sat still through the entire movie afraid that if I moved, I would flood a river of tears. I gripped the cloth arm of my seat so tightly that my knuckles hurt. I wasn't prepared for this much reality, not at this time in my life. I tried to convince myself that it was only a fictional flick. Who was I trying to fool?

Afterwards, we walked across busy Hillsboro to Fido's for espresso and Danish. We remained quite solemn even as we dashed and darted in front of passing cars. Sebastian arrived first and held the door opened for us. The room was sparsely filled with yuppies and students tapping on their laptops. We gave our orders to the face-jeweled girl and spied the room for a spot. Near the window, we found two small tables. Seth was the first to break the silence.

"I've been reading lately about alternative healing processes…even for those fighting things like cancer and even AIDS." He leaned forward.

"Crying must have some healing quality in itself…I mean, I don't think I have cried so much at a movie as I have tonight." Cleo cupped her face in her hands. "Oh god, I need something stronger than this espresso." Her mascara slightly smeared.

"Did anyone notice how some of those people kinda resembled us?" Richard leaned back against the window. His wooden chair balanced on its back legs while his legs rested on a chair.

"I sorta lost it when the lover was telling his dying mate that it was okay to let go. That was really compassionate love." Sebastian poured more sugar in his coffee.

"The only thing I didn't like about the movie was that it made gays appear so materialistic and basic whoremongers…not everybody has a flat on Fire Island," I said.

"Yeah, and we don't always do drugs, at least not all of us." Seth shuffled in his chair.

"Speaking of which…has anyone seen Bradley lately?" Cleo looked over the brim of her mug around the room.

"Seth is right…I mean the movie was right on target on some things. There was the mass hysteria that surrounded the fear of AIDS. I can remember people I knew that freaked out over hearing of someone being sick." Richard shifted his weight.

"Remember the days when anyone was skinny was thought to be sick and we assumed the worst?" Sebastian grinned. "Honey, talking about a decrease of crash diets!"

"Yeah, a lot of us started putting the pounds on. Even you, Michal. You got a little pudgy there yourself for a while." Seth punched at my side.

"It's all good…in fact, my stock went up. People looked at me and knew I was healthy." I smiled.

"A dangerous myth…now we know that weight doesn't equate to someone necessarily being negative or safe." Richard stood up.

"What do you need?" Seth rose. "I'll get it for you."

PANELS

"Naw, I'm okay. I need to stretch my legs anyway." Richard pushed him back down. He went for more espresso. Discrete stolen glances were made of his staggering.

"Oh God, I can only hope he isn't in too much pain," Cleo whispered.

"Have you guys ever heard of Louise Hay? She has this philosophy that it is dangerous for any of us to have internal negativistic poison. That this impacts our healing process." Seth changed the subject. "Help me out, Sebastian and Michal, do I have it right?"

"By George, I think you do have it...Seriously, there has been some scientific evidence to suggest relieving one's mind of the bull and only concentrate on the positive can lengthen one's life." I stirred a half filled mug. The natural sugar grains scratched the sides.

"True, but one must also surf around the garbage and decided what is important and what is not. I mean, denying some fatal illness won't make it go away, but how you approach it matters a great deal," Sebastian added.

"Oh Lord, we all gonna need care plans now." Cleo laughed.

"Well, it's certainly worth a try. You know, something I think that has helped Richard deal with this ordeal is his faith and his church...I don't care how weak or sick he is, he always wants to go to his church." Seth moved over as Richard returned to his seat.

"Speaking of church, did you guys notice that the only time church was mentioned was during somebody's memorial?" Richard sipped his hot brew.

"Well, that's understandable...not many of us have a church to feel welcomed in...We are looked on as something evil and worse than the lepers...Don't let me in your church, because if you do, then all of the congregation will turn homosexual. Puff!" Sebastian waved his hand in the air as if casting a spell.

"That's why I like Edgehill...everyone is treated the same." Richard smiled.

"Isn't that the church that has the reconciling flag on the wall?" Cleo asked.

"Yeah, that's the one...my passage back to my God."

"I have gone with him several times and no one freaked out." Seth rubbed Richard's back.

"What! I know you are mistaken. Not our little Jewish child up in somebody's Christian church. Seth, what would your father say?" Sebastian reared back in his chair.

"What's to say?" Seth answered.

"Hmm...knowing the other dear child is so wayward, your father probably glad you are going somewhere that doesn't involve a bar." I had a smirk on my face.

"Careful, he might hear you belittling him." Cleo grinned.

"Yeah right, this place sells coffee and not booze. I'm sure that child is miles away at some liquor watering hole. Speaking of the devil, has anyone seen the prodigal son lately? What about you, Seth?" I asked.

"He calls sometimes...but he never really stops by anymore. He told us that we were too depressing to be around. We didn't know how to have fun anymore."

"Actually, if the truth be known, I think he is scared to be around me...you see, I remind him of the bogeyman." Richard glanced hard into Seth's face.

"Let's not worry about that right now. He will come around in time. He always does." Seth returned his stare.

"You know what? You guys remind me of a gay version of *Designing Women*." Cleo laughed. We all laughed. It felt good to laugh.

Several days later, I met Seth for lunch at Noshville. I parked on the street. The brisk wind caught my breath. I saw him waving from inside the window booth. I glanced at my watch. Surely I wasn't that late. Okay, maybe a few minutes.

"Welcome to my side of the world." Seth motioned for me to sit. He fished at a pickle from the small porcelain bowl filled to the rim with others.

"I actually like kosher food...except for the salty fish." I smiled across from him.

"I believe you are referring to the lox, gifilte fish isn't really salty..." Seth stirred his iced tea. "You have to acquire a taste for lox."

"You may be right...have you ordered yet?" I glanced at the menu. "I'm starving!"

As if on cue, the waitress appeared with glasses of water with lemon wedges. She raised a smile as she poised her pen for our order.

"I know how you love salads, I would highly suggest you try the 'Nosh' salad?" Seth spoke confidently. " I usually end up taking half of it home."

"Sounds like a deal to me." I closed my menu and handed it to the waitress. "I will have the 'Nosh' salad, as recommended by my friend. Blue cheese with thick feta."

Seth made his selection and she left.

"So...how are things with you and Richard?"

"I'm in love with him...Michal. I know it sounds crazy, but I love the way

PANELS

he makes me feel."

"So I take it that you made home base, right?"

"Naw, I'm still on first." Seth laughed. "It's not about sex with him; it's actually more than that…for once, I have learned that you can love someone without sex being involved.…"

"Being that I haven't had any lately, I tend to agree with you," I joked. "You're really serious, aren't you?"

Seth paused before he answered. The waitress had returned with an abundance of two meaty salads that would have easily fed a family of four.

"Omigod, now this is really a salad!" My eyes rose.

"I told you…now, are you man enough to devour it?"

"Make sure you save room for a piece of delicious cheese cake." The waitress patted my shoulder and left.

"Now let's get back to Romeo and Romeo…you are really serious, aren't you?"

"Yeah…like the other night while it was storming, the raindrops hitting my window pane woke me. I got out of my bed and went to his room. I stood in his door way. Watching while he slept…Richard began to stir around and I saw him open his eyes. I asked him if he wanted anything and he nodded. I approached his bed and he patted beside him…Richard was sweating. His face was soaking wet. I reached over and grabbed a wash cloth and wiped his face…Richard looked so sheepish when he asked me if his bed was wet…it wasn't…not saying a word, I laid beside him…I slid beneath his arms. He kissed my neck." Seth paused.

At that very moment, I became distracted as an aged white man strolled by the window. His face was sullen and distraught. The man had eyes that were black and glaring. Our eyes caught until I heard Seth swirling the sugar into his tea glass.

"I thought you said no sex…"

"Michal, intimacy doesn't always have to be clouded with sex. There can be passion in just holding someone or being held by that special person that you love…"

"Seth, baby, you got it bad…just how long have you felt like this about him? Was it always like this and you was afraid to say anything to him or to us?"

"Michal, believe it or not, it wasn't until that night we all went to the Chute for line dancing…They played that song by Kathy Mattea, you know the one, "My Last Word"…No one wanted to dance with me. There I was, standing there bobbing my head to the beat when he came over and asked me to dance...He held me tight and we moved so well together. Have you ever listened to the lyrics to that song? I did that night...I actually closed my eyes and let him guide me all over the floor...I felt safe in his arms...something just went through me."

"Is that why you hated Daniel so much? I always wondered what he had ever done to you."

"He ain't done nothing to me...Daniel was beneath him...Daniel never believed in Richard's dreams. He was a user." Seth stabbed his corn beef with his fork. "I wish to God that he had never ever met Richard."

"Do you think that Richard feels the same way? What does he say about you?"

"He told me that he was scared of messing up the close friendship we have. You know how he believes that friends shouldn't sleep together."

"Yeah, I do. That's why I was sorta blown away when I first heard of you two. Sure, we have always teased you both about being more than just friends...What's really important is...are you happy?"

"Michal, that's putting it mildly...sometimes when I'm around him, I feel like some silly giddy school girl...and when I'm away from him, I feel lost."

"Aren't you afraid of falling in love with him because of his...?" I caught myself. All I could see in front of me was that old beggar in his filth. I could smell the stench of death ruminating from his veins. Then I saw the face of Richard. *Has Seth lost his mind? Is this his death wish?*

"Because of AIDS? Is that what you was going to say? I won't lie, I'm more than afraid. I'm bitter and I'm angry. I'm angry because for once in my life I have found someone that I want to share my life with...For once, I know that I can cry out in the night and he will be there for me." Seth used his napkin to wipe the tears from his eyes.

"I'm glad for you both...I really am. I have always loved you guys, and it helps me to know that he will never be alone...Is there anything I can do?"

"Yeah, be there for me when his time comes," He grabbed my wrist. "Can you promise me that?"

The season of spring came in like an old soul on crutches. Flowers dared to bloom. Coolness of the days and nights lingered past the usual time of departure. Winter's wind fought to stay. Richard became sicker.

"Did you hear about Seth?" Sebastian came in my office and sat down.

"What has he done now?" I closed my planner and looked at Sebastian. Somehow I felt I knew what he was going to tell me. I could see the pain in his face.

PANELS

"He's in the hospital...He has a upper respiratory infection...Did you know he was positive?"

"Oh hell, no! Don't tell me that...I thought he and Richard weren't doing anything!" I fell back in my seat dazed.

"He didn't get infected by Richard..."

"But, Sebastian...how else could he have gotten it? He's the only one that Seth has been with...How did it happen?"

"Michal, you know as well as I that that little virus is a funny thing...it can lay in for years before it rears its ugly head...believe me, I was as shocked as you are. Seth of all people. Bradley, yes! Forgive me, Lord, for saying that but you know what I mean." Sebastian stood to leave. "He's at St. Thomas."

After he left, I pulled out that letter and read it over and over. The words never changed. What was happening to us? Why was it happening to us? I closed my eyes and prayed. Will this madness ever end?

I stopped briefly to visit with Seth. I found most of the gang already there. We all laughed and joked about the superficial things while obliviously fearing reality. We all behaved as if we were living in the past. Amidst the settings of the actual room, it really felt good being with my friends.

Seth really didn't look the same to me. He appeared thin and pale. His speech was slurred, almost like a whisper. I tried to avoid looking directly in his eyes. His damned eyes held too much truth, more than I was willing to accept.

All of a sudden, I felt warm. Although the room was quite cool, I could feel beads of sweat forming on my forehead. My mouth was dry. I needed to leave, and leave soon.

Looking around the room, I saw my friends trying to smile. Cleo stood on the left side of his bed. Richard stood on the right side brushing Seth's thinning hair from his face. It was something about their glances towards each other that gave me comfort.

Bradley stood with his back to us as if he was searching out the window for his comfort. He was quiet, unlike his normal obnoxious self. His cockiness was absent. In fact, he said very little to Seth or anyone else for that matter.

Sebastian sat in a nearby rocking recliner. He appeared to be studying the entire room. I knew his look. Our conversations were as if none of this madness was really happening. No one was sick. Everything was just like the old days, right?

"Hate to bother you, guys, but it's time for your evening meds." A nurse said as she entered. Without missing a beat, she grabbed Seth's arm for his vital signs. She popped on his bed tray a small plastic cup filled with various pills.

"I can remember when popping pills was cool," Bradley said. He had suddenly turned from the window and returned to the living. But as quick as he turned to us, he turned back around facing the window.

"Well, I'm sure we can find you some of these beauties." Seth pointed to the cup.

"That's perfectly alright, Ms. Thang…what pills I want is definitely not in that cup." Bradley leered.

"You know, I've always thought you used drugs…No body can be that whacked without being on something." Cleo laughed.

"Oh, you must have me confused with your husband or one of your breeder friends," Bradley snapped.

"Looks like someone has touched a very sensitive nerve here…Retreat with your claws, Bradleymeister, everyone knows you used to trip on uppers and downers," Sebastian said.

"Used to, hell, I'm sure he's still skipping down the yellow brick road looking for the little munchkins," Seth joked.

"It helps me to deal with y'all tired asses…anyway, ain't a one of you in here walking the lily white road to sainthood…" Bradley recoiled. "So don't do me; I ain't the one."

"Please excuse him. He doesn't get out too often…we usually keep him under lock and key." Sebastian told the nurse. Although I did notice the nurse strain a smile, I also noticed that she quickly picked up her pace and left.

"We all can't fit in the closet, if you know what I mean, Michal and Sebastian, and I'm sure you do."

"Bradley, dear, we still love you…even when you are a royal pain in the ass." Cleo smirked.

Bradley mumbled something that I didn't understand and left abruptly amidst the catcalls from us. He didn't even say goodbye to Seth.

"Omigod, now we have really done it! We won't see our beloved Bradley before the next eclipse," Seth said with a grin.

"Hey, Michal, I wished you wouldn't talk so damn such," Sebastian said.

"Yeah, Michal, what's with the silence?" Cleo asked.

"Oh, it's nothing…just a lot on my mind. I keep telling myself that things will get better," I said.

"You know, Michal has got to be one of the most positive person I know,

PANELS

with the exception of Seth of course. Michal is always saying it will get better...But, Michal, when will things get better?" Richard smiled.

"It's cool! I kinda like having someone around me that still sees the good, someone that is still optimistic even when all hell breaks loose." Cleo rubbed my back.

"I have to agree with Cleo...it really helps me to fight this damn disease...Who knows, I may even beat it!" Seth grinned.

"Who knows...you just may," I said. My voice betrayed me. I still avoided any direct eye contact. I still felt faint and weak at my knees. I needed some fresh air. I was feeling closed in and my air was thinning out. I quickly went to the bed and rubbed Seth's toes. I told him that I would see him later. I left without waiting for a reply from anyone.

Frantically, I walked straight into a maze of sterile corridors. Everywhere I turned, I smelled that cleansing antiseptic odor. The glare of the waxed floors mixed with the white walls blinded me. I felt my heart beat like crazy. Finally, I found the door that led to the parking area. I flung the door wide open so hard it made a frightening thud against the concrete wall.

"Michal, hold up one minute!" I turned and saw Sebastian. "You mind telling me what the hell is going on with you?"

Now, I faced Sebastian head on. I closed my eyes. I was hoping he would somehow disappear before I opened my eyes. Go away from me, I wanted to scream.

"What in God's name is going on with you?"

"Nothing...I don't know what you are talking about," I lied.

"Michal, don't try to bull me...I know you all too well, hell we all do. So, are you going to tell me or are we going to play the million question game?" Sebastian walked closer to me. "Either way, I'm not leaving until you tell me something."

"Sebastian, you know you kill me with your overly righteous self. You always want to play some damned martyr; ready and willing to band aid all the wrong doings of the world...You sit so smug and look down on us like we are some damned helpless lot that doesn't know their head from their ass." I was angry but not really with him. He was just in the line of fire.

"What the hell are you talking about? Are you tripping on some drugs or what? You are making as much sense as that frigging wall." Sebastian's tone of voice showed a rigid anger.

"Why don't you just leave me the hell alone! I don't need your damned pity." By now, tears were streaming down my face. I so wanted to take back every last word but I didn't know how.

Sebastian grabbed me. He held onto me as I fought to be free. His grip was far too strong. He hugged me tightly. My body began to shake before I went limp into his massive arms. I cried on his shoulders. He gently stroked my face.

"Michal, I love you, you know that? We all love you. You are a part of us and there's nothing that can change that," Sebastian whispered. " Michal, we have been to hell and beyond together, and we will continue together."

"I just feel like a damned fool. I knew better, damn it, I knew better!"

"I'm here…you have my undivided attention…" Sebastian paused. He appeared so calm and reassuring. I felt my walls crumbling…perhaps I could trust him.

"Do I also have your undivided love as well?"

"Michal, need you ask?" Sebastian released me from his hold.

"You know, there's no one in our circle that I wouldn't do anything for…even for Bradley."

"Yeah, I know, and we all feel the same for you." He was looking directly at me as if waiting. Waiting for me to explode!

"I was looking at Seth and wondering just how sick he was…I couldn't bear looking in his eyes…It hurt me too bad to see him possibly dying…his thin crumpled body underneath that sheet scared the hell out of me…I'm afraid, Sebastian, I'm really afraid."

"That's normal to feel that way, you know that."

"You don't understand, Sebastian. I'm not afraid of Seth…I'm afraid of being like Seth."

"I think I may have missed something here."

"I think I may have been infected."

Sebastian takes a deep breath. "I'm here…talk to me."

"Remember when I went to the seminar in San Francisco last year?"

"Wait a minute…I thought you said that you did nothing with anyone while you was there."

"I lied." I lowered my head.

"So…what happened?"

"I had gone out for a few drinks. It was my last night. I went to the Brass Elephant near Castro Street…The place was somewhat crowded…Bodies all around, some in suits and some in leather and jeans…Typical mixed scene…I was standing in line waiting for the bartender when he approached me…His steel blue eyes mesmerized me…Of all the people in the bar, he picked me out."

PANELS

"Yeah, new meat!" Sebastian said. "I'm sorry, go on."

"Anyway, and you might be right...I almost forgot what I was ordering so he ordered something for me...He was sort of a take charge man...I felt like a clumsy school girl after being caught in the boys locker room...we danced...we danced...we talked seemingly for hours and then I went to his home."

"So, I presume that you both got to know each other in the biblical sense?"

"I think so...but, to be honest, I really don't know if we did or not...I mean...the whole night seemed so blurry."

"You don't think he used ecstasy drug on you, do you? Tell me you did use a raincoat, didn't you?"

"Naw, at least I don't remember...maybe we did use one of his...I really can't remember...Hell, I don't even remember how we even got to his place...I later found mine still in my pocket the next day."

"Michal, just because he's from San Francisco doesn't necessarily mean that he was infected. Not everyone in California has the virus."

"True, and I was praying to God that he wasn't one of them...then, yesterday my whole world came to a screeching halt...I received this letter from him." I handed Sebastian the crumpled letter I carried in my coat pocket.

Sebastian leaned against the car and read the letter. The mere expression on his face alarmed me. I wanted to snatch the letter from his hands and act as if it didn't exist, that it was all a cruel hoax. But it was too late. The horses had all left the barn.

"Go ahead...say it." I reached for the letter.

"Say what?" he asked.

"You know...what a stupid ass I was."

"This is not the time...are you going to get tested?"

"Yeah, real soon."

"Regardless of the outcome, please know that I am here." Sebastian held me close in his arms. "God help us."

Everyone has a particular friend that appears to be an outlaw in life, the attention seeker, the challenger to society without guilt or remorse, someone that constantly required attention, never down staged. No matter what, they were always the beautiful ones. Bradley was indeed our token from the world of perfection.

For as long as I can remember, Bradley and I have shared countless moments from the others. Gaining his trust wasn't easy. Whenever he experienced the possible mirroring effect, he told me. He said he felt trapped and struggling for the essence of his own sustaining air of courage. The walls closed in on him too rapidly as he fought to be free. He once told me that he felt that we would never understand his feelings.

One evening, Bradley and I met at the Sunset Grill for drinks and a meal. An artsy chic diner for the young and the beautiful. The restaurant was full of patrons straight from the Abercromie & Fitch catalogue. The high shriek voices with teasing laughter were abounding. I was waiting for the table when he arrived.

"Sorry I'm late." Bradley hugged me. "Been waiting very long? Parking was a pain."

"Actually, I just got here myself." I pointed towards the dining area. "I thought we could also grab a bite as we drink."

"I forgot this place was so active during the week. We can go some place else if you like."

"This is fine." I heard my name paged and we followed the hostess to our table. A non-descript waiter took our order and hurried away. He appeared nervous and avoided eye contact.

"I think I had him." He was nonchalant. Just a trick.

"Bradley, is there anyone in Nashville you haven't had?"

"A few…you know I don't do troll and scaly wags. I save those for you, my dear."

"You are way too kind. But, I think I will pass for now."

"I hear you, man. In fact, I am so aware of the tension between the others and me. Seth even told me that he blamed himself for telling me he was HIV positive. He thinks I stay away from every body because I find them miserable."

"Is that so far from the truth?" I sat back in my chair. Bradley paused while the waiter placed the cocktails on the table and stood at attention for our food order. Moments later, he darted away.

"At times, no. Then other times I find their lives horrible. Cleo locked into a dead end marriage where love never existed. Sebastian and Richard act like two decrepit old men on Social Security. Man, they are always so damn serious about every little trivial thing. Seth and I are as different as salt and pepper. At times, I really don't know him. My girl Tiffany lost her poor soul to leave the land of dragdom. And you, my friend, you act as if your life has ended…We used to party all night, every night. Remember?"

"Yeah, but times have changed. My body can no longer adjust to one hour of snoozing and twenty-three hours of boozing. We are getting old."

PANELS

"One thing that I learned from Gregory's death was that I needed to live my life until my eyes close for the last time. Then I will rest."

"Does that mean you can't live your life and still be around the gang?"

"Michal my dear man, I can always live my life and I will always live my life. I can still come around the others. Whether you believe this or not, there is not a single person in our little close knit family that I despise. You and everyone else mean the world to me. Yeah, I may not always show it but I love y'all"

"Speaking of Gregory, I did notice that you did take a back row seat with us. How come?" I toyed around with my food waiting for an answer.

"Gregory scared the hell out of me, that's why. Sure, I had heard of AIDS but it was always somebody else dying that I didn't know or people from a distant land. Gregory brought it home!"

"Not everyone has AIDS."

"Yeah, not everyone. But look at our own. Tiff didn't die from it but he had it. Seth got the bug and even Richard. Now tell me how the hell that was possible. I see more action than the both of them together."

"It only takes one exposure."

"Now, how fair is that? How fair is life to crucify someone before they can even find out what life is really about?" Bradley's eyes turned glazy "Seth hasn't harmed a soul."

"I don't have an answer…I doubt if anyone does. But intimacy doesn't have to involve just sex.

"But I'm addicted to sex. I could care less about being intimate. Remember one of my old rules was to find them and another rule was to forget them."

"But you can still be intimate with your friends without expecting sex."

"I'm quite aware that the intimate contact should not be confused with actual sexual relations," Bradley said.

"It is important that you do realize the difference. The acts of touching, massaging, holding, and caressing are vitally important in positive growth. Basically psychological factors affected physical conditions," I said.

"When you speak, you make everything sound so damn clinical. Talk to me in street terms that I can understand," Bradley asked. "I can't tell you enough how I despise all those damn modifications that are so strongly encouraged. Having to stop in the middle of wild sex just to put on a condom is a total downer. Trying to remember what is safe destroys all of the spontaneity of the moment."

"I'm surprised, but glad, to hear that you are being safe. Maybe there's hope for you yet." I grinned.

"I'm horny, not a complete fool. I've been lucky so far. What about you? Have you been tested yet?"

"As a matter of fact, I've recently been tested."

"And…"

"Good question. I don't know anything yet. What about you? Have you been tested?"

"Sweetheart, I've been tested like clock work every six months and the little bastard hasn't shown up yet, thank God for small miracles." Bradley reached over and knocked on a piece of the wooden table.

"So, you are playing safer and decreasing your partners. That's good."

"Well daddy, I'm glad you approve but I said nothing about limiting anything. I still love men in the worst way and still seek a good piece daily if I can. Don't get me wrong, I no longer cruise the parks or the lakes, too many damn trolls running around. How about you, my dear? Are you getting any?" Bradley smiled that trademark enticing smile.

"I'm saving myself for my wedding day," I joked.

"Why did AIDS have to come and destroy our lives? Where did it come from? My whole life has been nothing but risks. Some I wanted and some life dealt me. I have never ran away scared of anything in my life…but this virus hangs on my shoulders, tormenting me…" Bradley paused. There was still much pain in Bradley's eyes in accepting how having AIDS had affected his life in general. "I mean, after both David and Gregory got sick, my life hasn't been the same…I love you guys, you know that…but it's too painful for me being around. All our lives have changed…Nothing is fun anymore…With the fact lingering that the end of many of our friends' lives were drawing so near, I find myself wanting to stay away. I can't face it anymore…" Bradley cupped his face in his hands.

"I can only hope that you don't venture too far away."

"Michal, tell me something…and be honest with me. How do you deal with it? How do you handle seeing people you love being eaten alive with AIDS? How do you wake up in the morning knowing that you might one day become a walking dead yourself?"

"It's certainly not easy…I just try to be supportive and listen to them…I won't lie, it scares the hell out of me…but I refuse to let it overcome me."

"Please tell me, then, how I can do just that. Tell me what I need to do to make sure it doesn't overcome me as well. Tell me that all those countless

PANELS

nights that I toss in bed, unable to sleep, afraid of the bogey man…Afraid of being alone and yet afraid of being with someone for fear they may be infected."

"I wish it was that easy. I wish I could say that I have control over my own emotions but that would be lying. I just take it day by day."

"I know you guys think I'm some kind of a hard ass non-caring son of a bitch for the way I deal with Seth…Y'all just don't understand what I'm going through…It's easy for y'all to judge me…none of y'all have a brother that's dying…None of y'all have to stand and watch someone you was raised with being destroyed…watch and can't do a damned thing about it…if I knew this would have happened, I think I would have let him kill himself years ago…at least, he wouldn't have to go through this shit!"

"Michal, I really don't know if I should be telling you this. I mean, I like you as a friend but I really don't know if I can really trust you with what I'm about to say."

"This really sounds deep. Maybe I should order a stronger cocktail." I tried to joke but he was obviously not kidding.

"Please, I'm not in the mood…If you don't want to be bothered, just tell me."

"I'm sorry…please forgive me."

"The world has always been a stage to me. Constantly acting roles that wasn't really me but what I thought others wanted me to be…I know that there's something wrong with me." With a stern expression on his tense face, he stared into my eyes. The moment became cold. "I'm fighting demons and I might be losing…Months before Gregory's memorial, I noticed a tightness in my chest. While in bed, I could hear a faint rattle after I breathe out. I'm getting tired easier than before. Maybe I'm just getting older and my life is catching up with me."

As he spoke, I became uncomfortable. Why did I already know where this was leading? As if anticipated by me, he went on to say that it began with night sweats, which left his bed drenched with wetness. His temperature soared. He decided that he was just sweating alcohol through his pores and promised himself that he would cut back. He began to hate the hellish headaches.

"I crossed some drugs off, but had to keep my poppers and my coke. Don't act surprised! Yeah, I'm a bonafide coke head. David knew but he ain't telling no one at this point…Now you know."

During another one of our talks, he informed me that he kept a personal daily journal. Bradley's thoughts showed a person with an unfulfilled life who desperately wanted to cling to another without really knowing how. He hated being around anyone sick or depressed because he couldn't justify or tolerate mood changes, their pain, frustration, hurt, sadness, or their pending deaths.

Later, I read in his journal a bit of a revelation. His initial reflection over his own diagnosis proved surprisingly indifferent to his life. He blamed himself for not taking better precautions. He soon welcomed death as a release from his world of uncertainty. Maybe in death, he would have a final focus, a sense of direction.

His continued addictions served only as a smoke screen, hiding his private emotional mutilation. His impulsive sexual drive temporarily made him feel better about himself. It had a rather calming effect. Bradley refused to buy into theory that he was perhaps suffering from depression, which was an inherited illness until he also remembered his maternal history of alcoholism. In one of his entries, he wrote of what he had titled as the soggy biscuit theory.

"Once, somewhere, I read in one of those mind books, where this particular therapist described behaviors similar to mine as relating it to a 'Soggy Biscuit Theory.' She wrote in her article that even the most negative attention was far better than no attention. She mentioned a small child wanting but not necessarily needing another biscuit during breakfast. There was only one left on the plate. The biscuit had been on the bottom underneath all the others and had become extremely soggy with the cooking juices and sauces from the various foods that rested on the top of the pile. Although the child was clearly full and really didn't need the biscuit, the child craved the biscuit anyway.

"The child eventually got the biscuit and was satisfied not necessarily with the condition of the biscuit but with getting the biscuit. What a brat, but somehow I feel that the therapist was talking about me. Often I have wanted things and even people not necessarily because I really wanted them but because I thought that they would somehow satisfy my own esteem. I would find my true inadequacies through them. They never could fulfill my desire.

"I do not expect anyone to ever understand my ways. I'm not even sure I understand them myself. Am I flippant or what? Anyway, I realized that I hadn't been functioning emotionally responsible after finding out my cruel fate but I don't really give a damn at this point. It's not as if others don't know that thing is out there.

PANELS

"I have never forced anyone to have sex with me. Why should I feel morbidly remorseful? Sex seemed easier now than it ever was before the threat of AIDS. Why should I take the reins and prove the sane one? Why should I be the voice of reason? Many people think that I am a total ass hole incapable of loving anyone other than myself. That is not totally true. There were many people around me that I really loved but I feared dreadfully that they too might eventually leave me as my mother had left me. David has already left me. I hate him for it. I refuse to think of him anymore. Richard is very sick and dying. He was sicker than I wanted to realize. I don't want to go around him anymore. He smells foul and strongly of death. He scares me. My own brother is moving against me. How could he destroy what we had developed between the two of us. Does he not remember that I love him?

"The weeds in my yard are growing high. I no longer have the strength nor the desire to clean the growth away. I feel a strangeness growing inside me; I'm too weak to stop it. Maybe it's for the best. I have never been happy or even content with my life and maybe this is my way out. I wish no harm, but they should also know better in this day and time to not always drop their pants for the quick good feel.

"Long after my demise, people may realize just how unstable I was in my life. They may even realize how I fought feelings of rejection and of disillusion. Even as the stages grew inside me, I refused to stop picking up tricks.

"I knew that it was wrong, but God help me, I couldn't bear people possibly walking away from me. I needed them at my side constantly. I needed to be told how beautiful I was. I could never be alone. I hate to admit that I don't even remember their faces just their bodies that raced savagely against mine. Don't ask me their names; it is more blurred than their faces.

"Like the song implies, I definitely found comfort in the arms of strangers...I don't want to live the remainder of my days as Richard has nor die an ugly death like Gregory nor go stone mad as David had. I hate them. God only knows just how much I truly despise them...Why did Gregory have to start this damn chain reaction? Why couldn't life be as it once was? Why should I be at all surprised at anything disappointing about life, hasn't life served me nothing but a silver platter of bullshit?"

Three years after our talk, Bradley was tested for the virus. I know because I was with him. As the physician spoke with Bradley about the procedure, the tears swelled in his eyes. Bradley reached out and shook the doctor's hand attempting to stop the medical spiel. Looking straight into the doctor's eyes, Bradley informed him that he knew how AIDS affected the body. He knew all to well because someone close to him had previously died with KS. He assured the man in white not to worry about him because he would not die from KS. Bradley smiled and left. We walked in silence.

Bradley sat motionless in his car. The sun glared brightly off the other vehicles. His silent tears impaired his vision. Bradley drove to the city's cemetery. Although I was a bit surprised, he appeared extremely calm and collected.

Parking his car near the opened rusty black wrought iron gates with the pointed steeples, his action was done extremely mechanically and probably without thought.

He did not immediately move from his car. He sat and reflected over his troubled life.

"I just want someone to hold me and never let go…Hold me as tight as possible…I want you to be able to reassure me that I will be alright…I want you to forget ever seeing me cry." Bradley stared into space.

"I only wish that I could do all that you ask…and more." I grabbed his hand and squeezed it.

"All I can remember was the hurt in my folks' eyes when they found out about Seth…I can't do this to them…not again!…I remembered their raised voices and tears over one of their children dying…I remember the absence of laughter in our home…they must never know about this…No, they will not know about this! It ain't right to expect my folks to even think about the possibility of losing two sons at once." He cried. He didn't try to keep them back at that point.

As we sat in the park, life continued without our consent. The sun lowered its rays across the granite monuments casting various shadows on the earth and us. Somehow, I sensed Bradley made his decision. He went after the weeds of his life. What that consisted of, I did not know. We hugged each other and parted. *Please, Lord, remember your flock even those that stray*, I prayed.

I doubt if Bradley was aware of Seth being admitted to St. Thomas Hospital with a bout of pneumonia because Bradley himself left town for several days. He told all of us that he had to leave town to complete an accounting assignment for one of his clients. Later, after reading his journal, I learned differently.

PANELS

We learned afterward that Bradley drove ninety miles east to a distant land that society as a whole had not discovered. Clothing was optional at this particular kingdom. Basic rules of the land that applied to all which were maintaining peaceful harmony and not disrupting other's flowing concentration of positive energy. The land and the reality belonged to the radical faeries located far from the norms in the sanctuary called Short Mountain.

The land wasn't a stranger to me. I had been there numerous times. The sanctuary was nestled in the midst of the mountaintop with steep hills blending with sparse developed areas. Paths circled the treacherous rocky terrain.

There were no paved streets. The main house was the focal point where social meetings or dinners were held. Art and craft items lined the wooden railings and rafters on the porch. Nearby, were canned natural jams, jellies, and fruits. Various items were available for sale or to barter. No one was ever turned away for lack of money.

Short Mountain's creed was devised to maintain the Sanctuary as a safe haven for lesbians and gay men, a place where people learned to trust their environment and experience the joys of cooperative and harmonious group living in an alternative community. There were no one leader but all were leaders. The people created a list of behaviors considered inappropriate for existing in the rural setting such as discounting emotions, to comforting others physically without first asking for other's permission. The guidelines secured the concept that individuals were extremely significant and their thought patterns just as important as others. It was a place for equality for all.

Bradley wrote that he walked over to Goat Child as Goat Child sat on a grassy knoll breathing ancient Celtic melodies into his battered Irish flute. Introduced by the moniker of the "Goat Child," the stranger explains how he had readily accustomed himself to the untouched land, finding the opportunity to express what he termed his radical wit. Bradley's initial urge was to sexually attract the hunk of a man into running off into the woods for a moment of hot passion. Instead, he was afraid to approach him or anyone else. Bradley's symptoms were slowly becoming visually apparent. He tired easily. He needed rest more than usual. He still did not possess the courage to tell anyone about his fate. He was determined he would battle his war alone without pity.

Goat Child raised his head slightly while he continued holding the flute to his lips, their eyes met. Bradley looked away. He imagined that the man had known everything about him, even his silent fears. Tears formed in his eyes as he continued to sit facing the musician. He was totally unaware of others that sat around him. Someone was talking to him but his emotions blocked him from comprehending the words. He thought they all knew his inner pain. The moment became nightmarish and anguished. Bradley felt outwitted. He felt that his face was flustering warm. He felt as if he was suffocating with those around him laughing at him. He knew that they saw the blemishes about his face. Confused and scared, he ran from the circle into the dense woods as the flutist played to those remaining in the circle.

The Mountain brought nature to the inner darkness of the mind. The tranquility of being accepted no matter how extreme the torment. Included in the vast array of occupants were a dog and a goat. The Mountain proved a true shrine and haven to those battling with AIDS.

The grounds were quiet and life was still as Bradley emerged from his solitude within the darkened woods. His eyes swollen with tears. He needed someone to talk to about his anxious fears, but did not know where to go or who to turn to. As he wandered among the exterior of the community, he noticed a few others around him that had similar blemishes about their bodies. He noticed a few wrapped in blankets on the unusually hot night. He saw pain in their eyes but also their doubtful will to survive.

Suddenly Bradley found himself face to face with a man covered with cloudy snow-white hair. His equally white beard extended past his neck. Bradley found immediate relief in his caring eyes. He wanted to touch the cloud of whiteness to assure his reality. The angel first asked permission before he opened himself to speak to Bradley. After being given the nod, the man, identified simply as Gabb, slowly placed his left hand sympathetically across Bradley's shoulder, and told Bradley to feel free to allow his hurt to leave his faltering soul.

Gabb spoke directly but softly into his trembling eyes. Bradley's knees buckled underneath his weight. He fell, mentally exhausted, into Gabb's massive but gentle arms.

"I won't ask you to tell me what is bothering you. I won't invade your privacy, your inner thoughts, unless you permit me the privilege. May I suggest a bit of unsolicited advice? Look back into your heart at your responses and consider the balances of both your pain and of your joys as representatives of concepts that you have already chose to lead your life. Ask yourself if the paths that you have chosen have any value in your life today. Has your life given in to negativity? Has your life been altered because of the pain or of the joys? Look deep inside yourself. Search for the determination to refuse to be damned. As you move through your private world, observe what exact foundations you have created in your image. Watch the sunrise and the sunset. Breathe in the real tranquility of nature's grace. Notice how the perfect circles form as you skip pebbles across the waters. Are the circles really perfect or is that an illusion? Is it reality to be perfect? Question the concept of a perfect life that we as man attempt to strive for, the calming harmony. Does it really exist? Find the love that you earnestly desire within the inner boundaries of your soul. Allow the hate to dissipate as vapors in a raging heated storm."

Allow me to introduce myself. My name is Cleo. I'm the real woman of the circle. Even though the men were gay, I was in love with each of them. They made me feel quite special. Like a queen with knights in shining amour waiting with raised shields fighting for my honor. With them, I learned what a woman was. A woman was not a doormat waiting to be crushed by the next foot but a gift of grace. A woman was beautiful, strong and delicate. A woman was a person.

After the first few years of my marriage, whatever compromising structures we may have had soon dissipated. The vast difference in our ages proved much more than either of us wanted. Edward, my husband, was much older than I. The relationship gradually deteriorated; we were strangers unfortunately sharing the same domain.

Edward was an alcoholic. His excessive drinking came with an increased act of aggression towards me. His anger evolved from the verbal mistreatment to actual physical assault. As his age increased, his sexual ability greatly decreased. Edward became passionately impotent and blamed me for no longer being able to arouse him. He constantly told me just how worthless I was. With the smell of the harsh liquor on his breath, he screamed a sea of profanities my way. He graduated to slapping me. During his violent drunken state, he would laugh until he passed out.

In order to hide our disintegrating marriage, I tried to paint a deceptive picture of an affectionate couple, embracing close while whispering into his ears. Alone, we separated and barely spoke. Edward's initial love and devotion dissolved due to his love for bourbon while my real companions became my crutch.

Although I obviously failed, I kept much of my marriage from even my closest friends. I didn't want any of them to really know how I had failed in my marriage. However, I soon became aware that Seth and Michal were aware of the tension and lies.

"Baby doll, I know that there's too many good men for you out there that can bring some measure of joy back into your life. I can tell even in your voice that Eddie boy is giving you grief. Why do you put up with it?" Seth asked.

"Don't be silly. Everything here is going okay. I mean, there's no relationship that is perfect. We just have our problems like any other couple. It may flair up today but gone tomorrow. Nothing that I can't deal with," I laughed back.

"Cleo, this is Seth you're talking to. Believe me, I know from experience that you can't kid a kidder. Why don't you leave that bastard before it's too late," Seth chided.

"No, why don't we just change the subject. I'm with you right now and no one else matters now. I mean no one else." I wanted to change the subject. I looked away. I was nervous.

"I'm staring at a beautiful woman that has set up housekeeping in the land of denial." Seth pointed at me.

I was dumbfounded. What could I say? I had been a dutiful wife to Edward for the past fourteen years. The marriage, still childless, was quickly dying of boredom. To escape, I created my own world. I often fantasized about being the passionate sultry singer with an inseparable following. I captured the center of attention as adoring roses showered me. As with Seth, I tried to escape into my own world of imagination. It was my only release from the reality of bondage. Someone was threatening to steal my dreams.

My thoughts had no bearing on his reality. I wanted to run back to my peasant family in the village of Santillana del Mar. I wanted to run back to the conforming arms of my mother. I so wanted to leave him but I was afraid of his wrath. For many years, I had survived the mental anguish and the physical beatings laced with the on-going threats of me being deported back to my homeland for being an undesirable wife to Edward. I feared the stigma, so I endured the hell.

The intimate few friends of mine were the circle. Edward groaned in acknowledgment of their presence and hurriedly left from the room in disgust.

I once told Michal and Seth of another fantasy. Within my mind, I became mesmerized by thoughts of a lover touching me gently as he stroked my soft hair. His palms touching my face, sensually caressing. I was rendered

PANELS

powerless as his hands slowly circled my bodice. My body gave way to the unfamiliar sensations I felt down below my waist. My imaginary lover trailed his hands while feeling the smallness of my waist as he stroked his way from the curves of my svelte hips up my back. His tongue played twisting against my ears as he barely nibbled on each lobe. I was ready to be taken.

Edward spent one early Thanksgiving with us. Actually, it was one of the first years our gang was together. It definitely wasn't a Hallmark moment. He sat in a dark corner nursing his warm bourbon, while he watched some of the guys dance around in the kitchen. The tops of the small lampshades were covered with scarves. The scarves cast shadows of various medieval figures that danced to the blaring music. David clumsily clacked around in my four-inch heels as he begged in his shrill-pitched voice for people to kiss his Miss Piggy doll. She was his idol in life. A gift from Sebastian and Seth.

Laughter interspersed with the sound of the electric can opener starting our feast. Canned creamed corn slightly seasoned with flour and pepper sizzled in the frying pan.

Quart bottles of beer and strawberry wine replaced the traditional egg nog. Boxed fried chicken replaced the turkey. Edward continued to sit in the darkened corner inside the tattered chair. His eyes flared at me. He occasionally yelled something in our direction as he poured his bourbon. None of us responded except for Bradley casually raising his third finger. Finally, he left. With his departure, someone cranked up the music louder as the door slammed behind him.

One rather warm autumn evening, after we went to see a movie, Seth invited me for drink. We went to the Boundry. Seth wanted the world to disappear so that he could repair my damaged heart. As we sat outside on the enclosed patio, Seth said that he wondered if he really knew the lonely person across the table from him. I looked around the room. Surely, he wasn't referring to me. Unfortunately, Seth had noticed my unsteadiness throughout the film especially during the violent fight scenes between a husband and wife. He had also noticed that I kept my head lowered and away from him. Often in the past, we held hands, but not this time. Seth wanted to close the distance between us. My hand trembled around the fragile stem of the wine glass. He placed his hand across the top of my free hand and looked deeply into my swelling eyes.

"Enough of the drivel. Such senseless empty words only to fill the air.

How long are you going to try to keep hiding your hurt? I mean, how long are you going to keep pretending everything is wonderful when inside your heart, you are screaming to be free?"

"I don't know what you are talking about," I said, avoiding his eyes. I brushed my denim skirt downward as if annoyed by some presence on the clothing.

"Cleo, I love you enough to say this to you. Cut the shit and be real with me. You don't have to hide a damn thing from me. I've never judged you, nor will I ever. I hate to see you constantly being beaten by that old son of a bitch you live with. "

"Wait a damn minute. Just because we saw that shit on that movie doesn't mean my life is like that."

"Look in my eyes and tell me that Ed doesn't kick your ass."

"I don't have to take this from you. Of all people, I would have never thought you would rib me about it." My voice angrily rose. I awkwardly rose from the table knocking the glasses over and ran towards the door. The disturbance caused other patrons to turn and look. Seth quickly ran to my side and held my quivering body. I tried to fight his touch. Then I just lost it. I cried softly as he gradually released his arms from around me.

"I've been to hell and back trying to hide the obvious…I feel so ashamed at anyone knowing the truth." I whispered as I sat down.

"But, you forget, I'm not just anyone. I'm Seth. I've watched you for months trying to hide his beatings. Several times I've wanted to kill the bastard with my bare hands. You don't deserve that shit; you're much better than that. When I first saw that movie, I saw you as Tina. At first I never could comprehend why she or anyone stayed in that hell until I realized that women are raised to endure this macho shit. You can walk away like Tina did."

"Yeah right, except Tina was born here. I wasn't. Edward constantly threatens me with having me deported for being an undesirable alien. Me, the bended knee wife at his beck and call. "

"That's total bullshit on both your parts. His threats are as idle as his limp dick. You can't be deported because of some trumped up shit as being a bad wife. Enough of this nonsense. We must find you relief from this, unless of course, you like to have the hell beat out of you?"

"Not hardly. Why couldn't you both have been straight?" I tried to smile through my tears. I let out a deep sigh.

"Why couldn't you have been a man, sweetheart?" Seth smiled back. The

PANELS

movie had proved to be a catalyst for me. I was strengthened with the knowledge that Seth believed in me including my weakness.

Over the next three months, I worked on myself. I transformed internally and the gang played the supportive role. Without anyone's knowledge, I enrolled in counseling sessions for battered women through Nashville's YWCA. My determination for my own independence and fair treatment grew with each individual account I heard from other survivors. Sickness mounted within the very pit of my stomach each time I winced at their stories of their near death experiences from their abusive mates. I cried with strange relief, realizing that others shared my pain and that no one condemned me for being a bad person. I learned to love myself as a whole person.

Through my struggle for equality, I fought back. I no longer hid behind screens of deception. I refused Edward the privilege to denounce my womanhood. I freed myself from living the life of lies, dishonesty, egotism, and manipulation, unless it was at my command.

Now, whenever Edward balked, I threatened him with public character assassination. I now challenged him on all of his idle bluffs. I openly advocated feminist concepts within my home. Edward ceased requesting my presence at formal conservative functions, fearing that I would embarrass him. My perceptive attitude quickly progressed as AIDS continued penetrating my life and those that I loved.

Without the knowledge of anyone, I participated in a weekend training seminar sponsored by Nashville CARES.

While I sat quietly, I listened to others who had experienced similar hurt and confused turmoil brought on by the impact of AIDS. I listened as a panel of both volunteers and people actually living with AIDS spoke about their heartfelt experiences and rewards. Their pain and tribulations gave little relief to me as I reflected over my own internal grief.

My ignorance of the subject turned to anger as I realized the overt insensitivity of the current government and the world in general. I wanted to make others realize just how insurmountable AIDS was to the general society. I wanted others to further realize that their bigotry towards those with AIDS was wrong. No one should blame any specific group with spreading the virus. Gays didn't create AIDS.

Having been raised Catholic, I have a natural inclination to lower my head in the presence of a nun. However, one of the monumental impressions that were left on my mind during the seminar dealt with a catholic nun who spoke on death and dying issues. Sister Beatrice related her own experience dealing with her own grief. Dressed not in the usual habit, but instead in conservative clothing of a navy blue knee length skirt with matching jacket. Sister Beatrice spoke with firmness in her convictions. I regressed to my childhood persona of Juliana for the moment, remembering the nuns that lived in her village. I felt a peculiar familiarity. I smiled as I carefully reached up and carefully stroked the crucifix I wore around my neck.

Sister Beatrice explained to her listeners how one could feel closer to their God.

"Traditionally, people have been told and fiercely warned never to question God's decisions. To question the Almighty showed much disrespect, and those who were foolish enough to do so would surely receive the wrath of God. No one should ever place themselves on the same level as God, but is it really wrong to question him?" Sister Beatrice paused as she surveyed the faces around her. All eyes were on her waiting for her next revelation.

"Let's think about our own actions and involvements when we're in a intimate loving relationship. Whenever there are problems, we don't want to confront the situation at hand? Don't we become angry because we love the other person so much that we demand to know what has gone wrong in the relationship? Think of the connection you may have with your God as a relationship. A close intimate relationship where you can share all of your darkest fears without any remorse or guilt. A relationship where you feel comfortable enough to allow your defensive barriers to tumble down and still feel secured. It's out of love that you question your creator. By allowing yourself this choice, you have fully acknowledged closeness to your God that is definitely love. Get angry, yell at the top of your lungs, scream, and then cry to your best friend. He will understand. Death has never been easy on anyone. Denial is not a reasonable preventative measure; it's not even a cure for what ails you. Denial is merely procrastination in the worst form. The longer people hold on to their pain, the more unbearable it becomes. Accept the loss, allow yourself to cry and whatever other emotions you need. The loss you have experienced is only a physical loss. The memory will forever last inside, where it really matters, in your heart."

Sister Beatrice ended her words and smiled. As she finished, several participants quietly wiped their moist eyes while others nodded in silent agreement.

PANELS

Over the course of my volunteer hours at Nashville CARES, I befriended a lesbian couple during the seminar. Ruth Kydex was a registered nurse and her partner Patricia Majors was a second year law student. Together, they had adopted an infant boy, named Justin, born with the AIDS anti-bodies. I longed to hold the precious child that rested peacefully in Ruth's arms. He was so adorable.

Patricia glowed as she described the antics of her new child. She beamed as she suggested that Justin might develop his own anti-bodies. Ruth stated that the significance in his given name was that, as long as he lived and bonded with them, his name would always be Justin. But, should he die a needless death because apathy on behalf of bureaucratic red tape, his name would become injustice.

Winter threatened to take territorial rights rather quickly. Darkness came about the earth earlier ending the day. Others predicted that the winter would be colder than previous years. Life had slowed to a crawl. A cooler temperature has a tendency to lower anger and mellow the moods. At least it was true for my clients. Crises lessened.

"Michal, can you leave?" Sebastian stood at the threshold of my office. He appeared troubled. His face was white.

"What's up?" I glanced at my calendar.

"Kari just called." He paused and took a deep breath. "Richard is in Vanderbilt Hospital."

"I'm there!" I grabbed my keys and went with Sebastian.

The drive over was extremely subdued and long. No one spoke a word. I'm not quite sure if it was the glaring sun that struck the glass covered buildings that blinded Sebastian as he drove or the tears I saw forming around his eyes

Kari had told Sebastian and I which room number although we knew the floor all too well. As we walked from the elevator, we passed the familiar Formica white nursing station that extended length ways down the sterilized corridor while white clad physicians and nurses stood engrossed in various charts. No one appeared to have given our presence any notice.

Outside the designated room, we paused shortly before I knocked lightly on the door. I took a deep breath and pushed the door open. Abruptly, Richard shouted at us to stop and place one of the blue facial masks on our face that rested on the outside railing of his room. I despised wearing the facial covering.

We soon learned that Richard was having several tests to determine his exact illness. The reason for the masks was due to the doctors not completely ruling out Richard having tuberculosis. Chest X-rays and skin tests were not sufficient to actually distinguish between tuberculosis and mycobacterium avium complex. MAC was a horrible fungal infection usually seen only in birds. Richard proceeded to tell us that his immune system was severely suppressed. He felt confident that he had MAC instead of TB.

The results returned several days later stating that he had MAC outside his lungs as well as in the GI tract. The MAC in his lungs was found after a series of blood cultures. Richard had undergone a series of bone marrow biopsies. Both Cleo and Kari were present, with Sebastian and myself, when Dr. Raffanti explained the diagnosis. Richard had asked us to stay.

Kari squeezed her brother's bony hand as she winced at the foreign words. He was immediately prescribed medications. Some of his medications had to be eliminated due to the serious side effects as well as the levels of toxicity.

Kari told me the next day that on that previous night, Kari rested in the chair beside his bed. Richard attempted to rise from his bed when the bed creaked.

"I guess he thought I was asleep...I was squinting my eyes and saw him glancing at me. I got up and helped him. He was so weak and hot. He was burning up!"

"I'm surprised he didn't tell you to go away."

"Michal, if he could have, you know he would have told me in a heart beat to sit back down...The doctors say they are doing everything possible, but I don't know if I believe them."

"Kari, there are times when we need divine intervention."

"Michal, honey, say no more. I've been praying day in to day out. The good Lord ain't never let me down and I know he ain't gonna start now."

Kari told me how Richard was covered in his own sweat. He fell back against his bed, too weak to rise. Slowly, he pulled his body into a loose ball as he tried to relieve himself from the cramping in his stomach. As he pulled up the drenched sheets to shield his trembling body, a book of poetry fell to the floor. Kari abruptly stood at her chair and looked at her brother. Without saying a word, she wiped his forehead softly.

She proceeded to change his linen. As she worked, Kari hummed some ditty unfamiliar to Richard. She slipped her thin manicured fingers into the powder filled exam gloves as she prepared to bathe her brother. There was no talking between the two except for her to instruct him on which way to turn.

PANELS

Somehow if there were no communication during those times then the moments of embarrassment never actually took place.

Unfortunately, even with all of the precautions taken by all of us to decrease the risk of bacteria, Richard gradually became worse. Richard developed symptoms of severe wasting. He lost weight rapidly and the ability for his body to absorb food or the nutrients decreased. His physicians prescribed additional medications. Richard was taking mega doses of liquid nutritional supplements. The treatments only slowed down the illness' path of destruction.

Richard began to pull away from his sister and us. He became extremely combative. He wanted to be alone. Some of us reacted with bewilderment and anger. Richard wanted the curtains pulled closed at all times, not wanting to see the daybreak or the daylight, which reminded him of the life outside his sterile prison. He slept or at least pretended to be asleep while we tried to talk to him. He began to store his pills within the lining of his parched mouth, refusing to swallow, and would later discard the medicines as soon as he was left alone. Richard, later, told me that he had refused to look at himself in mirrors or any object that would have cast a reflection of the stranger before him.

"Do you ever notice my presence anymore? Do you ever take the time to see beyond yourself?" Seth said.

"You don't have to be here, I never asked you to come."

"You are too damn stubborn to admit you need anyone around. If I waited for you to call me, then I'd be shit out of luck."

"What's your point? If you want to fight, then go find someone else to fight. I'm too tired for the shit."

"That's your problem in a nut shell. You have lost your fight. You're no longer that Richard that I once knew who refused to walk away in defeat. You're nothing now but a pile of scared shit."

"In case you haven't noticed, my life is about to end any day."

"So, you're going to just give up that fucking easy. What about the days you have left? Has our friendship meant nothing to you? I know that I can't imagine what you're going through, but I do care. This is not like you to take this damn pity trip. Damn it, you ain't dead yet." Seth stopped. He turned away to keep Richard from seeing the tears.

Some days, Richard tried to hit Seth. Once, while I was present, Seth pushed him back against his bed and Richard stopped screaming. Countless times, Richard threatened Seth, which Seth teasingly welcomed. Seth told him to get well so that he could kick Seth's ass as promised. Seth said he wanted Richard to realize that he hadn't died yet.

Once during one of their conflicts, Seth told Richard that he knew exactly what Richard was attempting to do. Richard ignored Seth's theory regarding his creation of barriers. Seth promised him that it would take more than rude bitchiness to make him stop caring about him. Before Richard could rebuke his words, Seth swiveled around and told him that he needed to get off his high horse of pity and live whatever life he still had.

Richard turned away from Seth's eyes. In sudden frenzied frustrated anger, Seth jerked Richard around and shook him violently before he ran from the room in tears.

Several days went by without Richard seeing Seth. As others came to attend to his essential needs, not one of us said anything about Seth.

Finally, as he was being spoon fed by me, Richard turned his head slightly away, tried to clear his throat, barely speaking above a whisper, and asked me where Seth was. I fell back in my chair and stared at Richard. Richard's eyes were warm and soft. He placed his hand carefully on the top of my hand. I swallowed hard, taking a deep breath.

"Seth is in the hospital. He has pneumonia. But he is doing okay; in fact, he should be home in a couple of days. Seth often asks about you," I ended my sentence with a sincere smile.

"Who else is here with you," Richard whispered. " Please tell them to come in."

I went immediately to beckon others into the cramped room where Richard tearfully told us that he was very sorry for the way he had acted towards us. Richard explained to us that he hadn't wanted to hurt anyone but felt that if we walked away bitter then he wouldn't have felt so guilty about dying and leaving his friends behind. As his voice weakened, Richard whispered that he wanted Seth to know how he loved Seth. I told him that I would make sure he got the message. Richard said he loved Seth very much especially for not allowing him to give up. He didn't know what life had for him but he knew that he wanted to be with us if only we would have him back.

Cleo cried as she told him that she was just glad he was off his damn throne and back down to earth with the real people that loved him. Kari threatened to inflict the worse pain imaginable should he ever act that way again. A tear fell from her face onto his as she reached down to give him a slight hug.

PANELS

Seeing him fast becoming tired, we soon left the room as he fell into a deep sleep.

The next morning as Richard stirred from his fitful sleep, he opened his eyes and found Seth and I standing over him smiling. Seth appeared somewhat haggard. Richard extended his hand towards Seth as Seth gingerly caressed the bony hand across his face.

"I understand that we both came back home," Seth said as he lowered his head to kiss Richard on his cheek, "I love you. Do you know that?"

"Yeah, but not as much as I love you," Richard said.

Richard gradually left his dark confinements and with the aid of his close friends, especially Seth, reentered his old world. At first the light was harsh to his sensitive eyes. Richard's outlook began to change as he finally accepted each moment of life with delight and chose to live life. He knew he was dying but his priorities improved.

Seth and Richard spent much of their waking hours together merely talking and laughing. Using a borrowed wheel chair, one of us often took Seth and Richard to Centennial Park or to Edwin Warner Park where the three strolled casually void of any concept of neither time nor space. Sometimes Cleo packed picnic lunches, which they ate while spread across the three blankets covering the hard ground.

By this time, Kari had to leave her brother. Kari had to report to the Indiana National Guard for active combat in the Gulf War. Kari promised Richard that she would write him every week. The letters poured in almost daily from the various places in the Middle East. We took turn reading him his letters. The letters usually left him with mixed emotions.

Richard and Seth began talking about their living wills. Sebastian and I arranged for a lawyer to draft legal documents for our two friends after they had requested the service. Neither Seth nor Richard had wanted anyone to change their final instructions, and wanted to insure it by putting their wishes in writing.

I contacted a lawyer friend who was also a lesbian. Abby Ian clearly understood the men's decision and wrote accordingly. She, too, was aware how absent families reappeared at the hour of death to reclaim the dying. Both men themselves witnessed the other's signatures on the living wills along with Sebastian, Cleo, and me signing.

Richard fought his own diagnosis with laughter. Amidst the pain discretely now hidden in the depths of his eyes, he maintained a renewed stronger smile. Richard became far more concerned with others around him and refused to live in the sea of pity anymore. He shared the last few days with his new partner that he had always loved very much. There wasn't much difference in their marriage. People, regardless of their sexual preferences, become crucially involved in the lives of their mates. No one could invalidate their existence or their struggling relationship.

Richard openly received members from Edgehill Church as they arrived to give him commune on Sunday afternoons. An African American woman named Christine looked deep into his eyes as she placed the piece of bread on his lips. Her voice was deep but reverent. Richard felt forgiven by God.

Richard's health faltered quickly. He developed additional opportunistic infections. He was constantly monitored due to the toxicity levels. Various medications were either deleted or added, trying to circumvent any further negative reactions caused by the medications. Richard continued being optimistic instead of pessimistic.

Edgehill Church sponsored an AIDS support group that Richard participated in. He volunteered when his health permitted. He spoke to various groups on the impact of AIDS in his life. He wrote letters to various newspapers and to numerous elected officials asking for an increase in financial assistance to those battling with AIDS.

While in the hospital, Richard often entered the rooms of other AIDS patients to talk to them. He noticed a few patients in rooms close to his room that appeared to never receive any visitors.

When Richard was warned not to visit the rooms of other patients due to both of them being highly susceptible to other viruses, he understood. He realized the hidden dangers of possible infections. Instead of visiting, Richard either wrote short notes or asked some of his supportive troupe to occasionally check on those who appeared to be deserted by their own family and former friends.

After Seth was released from the hospital, he remained with Richard. Often Seth slept over on the small metal cot placed near Richard on the floor. Richard started having frequent nightmares always waking with his body shaking tremendously as Seth held him. Seth rocked Richard back to sleep and stayed on the side of his bed softly wiping his brow with a cool damp cloth. Seth never left him until he believed he was out of danger. Nurses entered the room constantly, administer medications, and check his vital signs, chart their findings, and left quietly as not to disturb the tranquility that

PANELS

existed between the two friends. No one interrupted the lovers' privacy.

Seth was sitting in the side chair beside Richard when Cleo and I walked in the room. We watched as both slept. Richard's breathing appeared greatly labored and unsteady. Seth's contorted body shifted into a gradual ball with his head lowered into his knees. Someone had placed a light blue blanket across his still body. Cleo turned back to Richard and leaned over and kissed Richard's forehead. Cleo was no longer shocked at the sight of his gaunt form. She also had grown accustomed to seeing the various tubing and needles penetrating his skin. Cleo glanced at Seth and sat between her two friends on the bed. Seth was sweating heavily. His breathing appeared labored. Cleo reached over and touched Seth softly on his arm and felt the heat. Seth's temperature was extremely high.

Seth suffered another bout of pneumonia. He was re-admitted to the hospital. At this point, Richard was too weak to leave from his bed. He was fed directly through to his stomach using inserted tubing.

Seth had fought pneumonia twice before this episode and told us that it was only a brief set back and for us not to worry. Seth realized that his infections were further destroying his immune system. He told us that he would not give up his battle too easily. Cleo laughed as she told him that he was too mean to die.

Bradley briefly stopped by to see him, usually at their parents' request, to check on him whenever they couldn't be there themselves. He stood quietly at the foot of Seth's bed. Once, while no one was in the room except for Seth, Bradley, and I, Bradley reached nervously for his brother's hand and squeezed it ever so lightly. Seth saw the tears that clouded Bradley's eyes. Seth told me that he longed to soothe Bradley's fears and tell him that he understood.

Finally, as Bradley stood facing the closed window, he cried softly. He turned and looked at his brother and whispered in his sincerest tone that if it was possible for him to take that gun from Seth's hands, he would, if only he knew how.

"The reason I fought with you that time you had that gun to your head..." Bradley tearfully continued, "was because I had already lost someone I loved dearly to the hands of death and could not bear the thought of losing anyone else to death again." Seth reached out with his hand to Bradley. Bradley, no longer fearful, leaned over and hugged his brother.

The sky was empty and the land was still. There was a bright fiery red sun that warmed the earth. The wind wasn't blowing when Death took another life. Seth and I were returning after Seth had another series of chest X-rays. He was in an unusually jovial mood, engaged in conversation with his attending orderly and me..

Seth had not actually seen Richard in two days. He knew that he couldn't go inside Richard's room on his way back to his room but still wanted to go by the room just to at least wave and say hello from a distance. Andy Pippin, the orderly, just arrived for his shift. He knew how close friends Seth and Richard were. Andy did not see anything wrong with merely pushing Seth briefly by Richard's room.

As Andy pushed him towards the room, we were involved in deep conversation and were laughing as we neared the corner to Richard's room. The charge nurse rushed away from the nursing station, attempting to stop us. While the orderly was busily trying to explain what he was doing, Seth looked curiously around the nurse into the room at the empty bed. I closed my eyes not wanting to realize the obvious. Seth rolled his chair closer to the room. The nurse placed a sympathetic hand on his quivering shoulder as he sat quietly inside the threshold of the now barren room. His lover forgot to say goodbye.

As he had wished, Richard's body was cremated, with his ashes sealed in a crystal urn that Richard selected for his remains. Kari arrived minutes before his service at Edgehill was to begin. No other family member was present from Indiana.

The church was filled with not only his closest friends but also with numerous congregational members. There were many faces that I had previously seen in the waiting room, praying and singing spirituals softly. For many days, a host of church members came to visit him. Many came bearing food for us as we waited. Richard was right, they didn't forget him.

The infamous banner hung from the ceiling underneath the window behind the altar. I remembered that same image of the lone figure in the kaleidoscopic background with outstretched hands to the sky. I thought to myself, Richard had found a piece of his Heaven right here in this place.

Various individuals took their turn speaking on Richard's behalf. Their words appeared so sincere and loving. Knowing Richard, I'm sure he was blushing. He hated anyone complimenting him on anything. He never knew how to answer. I would simply tell him to say "thank you." He loved working from within the shadows.

My eyes became moist as his pastor spoke about him. His words were simple but quite eloquent. When Pastor Barnes finished, he walked over to

PANELS

Kari and they hugged. The piano started to play an all to familiar spiritual. I remembered Connye from the Sunday Richard had joined the church. Eyes closed and head held high, Connye sang his song.

Why should I feel discouraged? Why should the shadow fall...for his eyes is on the sparrow, and I know he watches me...I sing because I'm happy, I sing because I'm free, for his eyes is on the sparrow and I know he watches me.

I was certainly not alone as I cried. He would have been so happy.

The remaining circle of friends was sitting around Kari. I noticed how she glanced around the room but avoided looking at Richard's portrait and his remains.

She told me later that the flicker from the burning candles reminded her of the burning flesh. Cleo had given her one of her rarely used valiums hoping to calm some of her grief. Her face was swollen from her pain. Kari tried being the perfect little soldier, wishing that Richard could somehow see how strong she could be for him.

During his illness, her tears stayed imprisoned, fearing exposure to her true mask of despair for her brother. Marvin, her fiancé, held her shuddering body.

Beside Kari sat Seth. He no longer cried. Seth stared directly into the face of the portrait and smiled. Cleo wrapped her arm around his shoulder. Bradley was on the end, on the other side of Cleo. He discretely quickly wiped away his tears as he read the small card held in the sweaty palm of his left hand with Richard's full name written along with his birthday and the day of his death. There was a short prayer that read, "May thy soul and the souls of all the faithful departed, through the Mercy of God, Rest in Peace."

Sebastian stood proud at the podium behind the altar. Now it was Sebastian's moment to not say goodbye but to offer his wishes for a safer journey. While he thought of appropriate things to say, he told us of something that his grandmother had once said about death. He never understood the significance of her words until later in his life.

"For twenty plus years, I integrated myself into various lives where people themselves dealt first hand with terminal illness. Each time there was a death and a funeral, I promised myself that that death would have been the last for me. However, I unfortunately found it difficult to turn away. While I have learned a great deal from my own experiences. Not only did I eventually touch a life but also that life touched me. There was a certain heart print left forever of the life...through my friends' journeys, I further learned to freely cry and to laugh. Small wonders become magnificent. No longer are things taken for granted. As painful as it was, I have finally made myself aware and even understood with acceptance the right of the individual's decision to finally let go of the reins." Sebastian spoke of how Richard fought his illness with renewed laughter amidst his pain that he discretely hid behind his eyes. Sebastian, pausing momentarily clearing his eyes, proceeded to describe Richard as being more concerned with others around him refusing to live in pity, although life dealt him an unfair hand to play.

"Richard was able to spend the last days with those who he loved and who loved him. This church was his home. To him, he was able to walk with his Savior again…In all my life, I have never seen such an out pouring of true Christian love as I have tonight. His eyes would light up whenever he spoke of this place. I can see why…His dear sister Kari was not there physically but very much present in his heart; he knew that her love was there to comfort him…There was an old story, which Richard had once told me, and I would like to attempt to tell the same story to you…An elderly lady passed away. Although she had a very large family, she was a very lonely woman and heavily relied on the kindness of strangers for friendship and love. At her funeral, her family packed the pews. Flowers were in great abundance. A young girl walked in carrying a plate of baked sweets that the deceased had been very fond of. The young girl placed the covered dish on the woman's breast. She bent lower and planted a kiss on the woman's forehead and whispered softly that she hoped that the woman enjoyed the food. By this time, the family was quite beside themselves with bellyaching laughter. Finally, one family member approached her. ' You foolish girl, she can't enjoy your food. She's dead.' To this, the young girl replied, ' Sure she can just as soon as she gets up to smell those flowers you sent.'"

Sebastian paused and raised his head. He turned to the portrait and smiled..

"Richard, your life has made the complete cycle. At this time, your friends have gathered to celebrate your time spent with us. You have given us far more than just a friendship. You gave unselfishly of yourself. Although your ashes are here in front of us, your wonderful loving memory is etched deep in our hearts forever."

There was a brief stillness in the air as Seth stumbled past Sebastian at the podium. Taking a deep breath, Seth held his head high as he faced the remnants of his fallen lover. The papers crackled against the microphone as he unraveled the pages of the poem that he wrote for Richard. His eyes were dry but sad.

PANELS

Kari helped us design the panel for Richard. Amidst a rainbow background that extended into the sky, his full name sewn. A few musical symbols sporadically placed around the edges. In the very center of the cloth was a child-like figure holding a heavily brown streaked song sparrow. Below the words read: *I know He watches over me.*

Welcome again to the world as seen through my eyes. Cleo's eyes. Once again, I have experienced yet another death among the gang. Tears are no longer common for me as they once were. I continue to mature emotionally through the events that surround my life. I have confronted evil and his name was Edward.

Several days after Richard's memorial, the remaining participants of the gang dissipated. I guess it would be truthful to say that each of us attempted to gather our own remote thoughts, while we searched desperately within ourselves for directions. The losses were insurmountably difficult but I am surviving.

I missed Richard. He was the big brother I never had. I began to remember the countless conversations he and I shared. Richard was never one to judge but one to always listen. I was actually quite thrilled over his relationship with Seth. It was a special love that I know I would never experience. Richard's love for me was always unconditional.

Edward and I quickly left for New York City. Edward was in the process of closing on a hostile multi-million dollar merger involving control over smaller healthcare satellites. He needed the gentleness of me at his side to offset his assertive actions. I wasn't naïve, realized my purpose, and accepted the trip. This time, I set my own agenda.

To this very day, I still laugh at how Edward tried to educate me of the grand dazzling historical landmarks common of his past. Edward reserved elaborate accommodations at the famed Waldorf Astoria Hotel. It wasn't for me rather for the image he had to uphold.

I will admit that I walked in constant amazement, with my mouth possibly gasping, while I goggled at the study of the twenties classicism with soaring white spaces that were guarded by numerous massive squared pillars. I was further intrigued with the toga-clad allegorical figures. The whirlwind of visual thoughts drew me back home to my homeland of Santillana del Mar.

PHIL MICHAL THOMAS

As we continued walking through the main lobby amidst the black marble columns that appeared to extend into the heavens, I admired the restored mosaic that displayed a babe held closely inside larger arms followed clockwise by various stages of life that ended in a mourning scene. I think I closed my eyes and imagined the visual impressions as being images of my own life. Hope I wasn't being too dramatic.

I think Edward sneered as he suggested that I immediately cease gawking before others noticed my stupidity. This angered me. I abruptly pulled away from his side and firmly told him that I would meet him later in our room. I left him standing staring at me as if he was an incompetent fool.

During my lone travels, I think I found myself back at the entrance to the Peacock Alley Bar, which I noticed earlier. It was discretely positioned off the main lobby. Ignoring the lustful smiles of the aged men, I became engrossed in the bronze clock that stood at the center of the lobby. A bellman told me that the elaborate clock was a souvenir from the original Waldorf. In my wild imagination, I saw the images come to life. Adorned with bristling figures of masculine animals that ranged from bears, bulls, bison, and other icons from turn of the century America, including actual people such as President Ulysses Grant. I believed I recognized another icon to be Queen Victoria.

As I moved around the room, I almost strained my neck to see what had appeared to be the Lady of Freedom that rested magnificently at the clock's very top. I offered my hand gracefully to all of the icons as if accepting the vast royalty.

My eyes suddenly rested on the glamorous Steinway grand piano. On this particular evening, a middle aged man in formal attire played softly as he accompanied a slender black woman singing a well rehearsed musical tribute of melodies written by Cole Porter.

I remembered Seth was an avid fan of tunes written by both Porter and George Gerswin. Seth often commented that the two lyricists had lived years before their time without anyone fully understanding or appreciating their novel talents. The liver spots covering the man's hands brought me stumbling back to Gregory's disease ridden body. I wanted to imagine Seth playing. Careful for others not to see me, I wiped a tear from my eye. Oh how I wished that he were really there for me.

I slipped easily onto the elegant Italian bar stool at the corner of the bar and ordered a glass of wine. Forgetting where I was, I absentmindedly ran my fingers down my laced stockings after I crossed my legs. The wine was extremely dry and rather offensive unlike my usual Chablis. I winced at the distorted reflections through the glass as the liquid inside swirled around.

Feeling the effect of the wine, I started humming along with the music. I wanted one of my friends' massive arms wrapped tightly around me, forever keeping me from further harm. I fought back the urge to cry as the tears mounted. Refusing to compromise, I ordered another glass of the bitter wine.

Glancing at my watch, I noticed the time. I charged my drinks to the room, his room. I walked from the elevator towards the suite; I carefully paced my steps slowly hoping that I would find Edward asleep. However, he was standing with his back turned to me as he faced the open balcony. Obviously by his unsteady demeanor and posture, Edward had been drinking.

Initially, no words were exchanged between us. The mere sight of him made me uneasy and absolutely nauseous. I tried to avoid him, which proved extremely difficult due to the close proximity. Still, I pretended that he wasn't there when suddenly the room turned very cold.

"Finally those damn queers are slowly being cleansed from my life. Hell, those faggot leeches that you refer to as friends have totally ruined my life. They've destroyed everything they have touched with their infected hands including you." He laughed as he threw an ice cube from his liquor filled glass in my direction. I quickly turned to him to object. He slapped me hard across my face. I lost my balance and fell forward. I stumbled. Edward laughed harder as he called me names. I became blindly outraged. I felt fire in my bones. I leaped forward and clawed at his face and throat fiercely. I was determined to quiet him. I possessed nothing but dire hatred for Edward.

As we continued fighting, our legs entangled in the loose pieces of our luggage. Both our bodies crashed to the carpeted floor with a thundering thud. Edward continued with his bantering laughter mocking my emotional weakness. Although I was much smaller than him I had my youth in my rage. I was no longer afraid to fight back. I became the lioness protecting her ailing cubs: my friends.

Edward bled profusely from the direct scratches of my long nails. I quickly crawled away from him while still kicking at his unprotected chest. Edward grabbed me by my thin throat. He continued swinging his massive calloused fist across my face. He purposely tore my dress, which ripped away the attached bodice.

I realized that my jaw was numb and swollen and possibly broken. My lips were cracked from the heavy blows. Blood flowed from my face. At a distance, Edward continued his drunken badgering laughter even after I had escaped and ran from him.

With a racing heart, I quickly locked myself in the adjoining bathroom. I listened to him stumbling around outside the closed door. He continued to laugh and curse me until he eventually slammed the door of the hotel room and left.

I stood trembling. I was partially naked. My body blocked the locked door as I cried quietly. I hated him. I stood in disbelief and stared at the unfamiliar nude stranger that stood before me in the mirror. My face was badly bruised, with dried blood caked within the swollen crevices. My unraveled hair throbbed at the very roots where he had grabbed me. My left eye was partially closed and extremely sensitive. Most of my fingernails were broken, with jagged edges. My usually thin lips were now enlarged with the skin opened. With intense grieving hatred, I smeared lipstick maliciously across the glass surface. I screamed out some of agonizing hurt. Hitting the mirrors with my throbbing fists brought no actual relief to my pain. Breathing deeply as I cried, I closed my eyes. I could feel my heart still racing and echoing loudly. I wanted to imagine myself as far from the moment as possible.

I stayed alone in the secured room. I was quick to bolt the doors carefully before I packed my clothes to return home. I called and told Seth everything about the entire battle. Enraged, Seth wanted to rescue me from my hell and the bastard. His words appeared soothing and non-judgmental towards me. Somehow, I felt relieved knowing he had understood and no longer questioned my decisions about my ill-fated marriage. Seth listened and agreed to meet my plane the following morning.

Attempting to get myself calm, I lay inside the massive tub, trying to relax in the soothing hot sudsy bath. I completely submersed until my injured body was covered. The wet warmness relieved some of my discomfort but without much pleasure as the heat stung my sides where he had scratched me while tearing the dress. Wincing, I fell deeper into the inviting waters.

I hate to admit that I did briefly entertained thoughts of drowning. I wanted that bastard Edward to find my decomposing body. I so wanted him to have that lasting image of me dead. I wanted to torture him for the rest of his miserable life.

I had read once that death by drowning was actually quite calming. Neither pain nor real discomfort, just the sensation of fullness. But, I couldn't go on with it. Why should I be the one to end my life and for what? Two things kept me from fulfilling my thoughts. My religious convictions that condemned suicides and the fact that I didn't want to appear so overly

PANELS

dramatic. Solemnly, I lit numerous candles, placed them around the bathroom, and prayed. I asked the Savior for forgiveness and for divine guidance. I actually felt guilty for despising Edward although I felt no remorse in hitting him while defending the loyal honor of my friends.

Still fearful of his eventual return, I dragged one of the enormous upholstered chairs to rest firmly against the bedroom door. I was actually quite thankful for Edward's hindsight at reserving a suite with the additional bedroom across from the formal sitting room. I began moving his clothing into the other bedroom quickly. I was far too weak to fight a second round.

After I felt safe, I tried to sleep but my body was too troubled. My heart skipped various beats at each noise I heard. I didn't want to think that Edward may try to storm at me again. I got out of bed and checked the tightness of the lodged chair. It didn't bulge. I went back to bed and pulled the pillows around my battered face to soften the blows of reality.

Waking slightly disoriented at first, I opened my eyes to the new day. Absentmindedly I rubbed my face. The pain quickly etched deep into the nerves. I focused back on the night before. I remembered and cursed the mere thought of Edward as I reflected on the fight. My stiff body slowly rose from the bed. I tried to put the memory out of my mind and gathered my wits. I went into the bathroom.

I wanted to scream when I saw that face staring back at me. I winced hatefully at the sight from the mirror. Taking a deep breath and cursing his name once more, I grimaced as I carefully covered my face in make up. He will surely pay for this I swore.

An hour later, clad in oversized sunglasses, with full resentment and rebutted anger, I tipped the door attendant and went shopping armed with Edward's credit cards.

In pure defiance, I purchased items that I knew I would never keep for myself.. The flowing beaded designer gowns would be worn once and then discarded freely for a mere pittance to any one of my dragqueen friends. I went wild with his money. I also purchased two half-carat diamond studded cuff links for Seth and Michal. For Sebastian, I selected a warm blue, soft, pure silk baseball jacket. For Bradley, remembering the interior decor of his emasculated condominium, I found a darling set of translucent capiz shells hand layered into oval placemats made from the Philippines from Berdolf Goodman.

PHIL MICHAL THOMAS

After leaving the last boutique, I remembered the cruel comment from Edward about the emancipation and sheepishly laughed to myself as I asked the West Indian cabbie to take me to the Gay Men's Health Center. It brought much joy to my heart as I wrote out a check for twenty five thousand dollars in Edward's full name for direct services to those living with the fatal virus.

Hours later, I was exhausted from my feat of the day. I returned briefly to the hotel, gathered my bags, and returned home alone into Seth's awaiting arms.

"I take it, that you didn't have a great time in the Big Apple." Michal gathered my luggage. He tried to look at my face but I tried to shield my face from him.

"Oh my God! I will kill that bastard if he ever touches you again!" Seth shrieked.

"Let me just say, that seeing your tired old faces is the best medicine for a wearied old gal!" I hugged Seth. "I will never leave you guys

Our prodigal friend was becoming invisible. His presence had become less and less frequent. When others would ask me if I had either seen Bradley or if I knew what was going on with him, I simply lied. No, I haven't seen Bradley nor did I know what was bothering him. I couldn't betray his trust. For the first time, he had actually reached out to me. So, I remained silent. Yes, I knew where he was.

Even now, I can close my eyes and remember back to that moment. The day was serene with temperatures in the nineties. The sky was a bluish backdrop over the burnt earth. The birds chirped softly in the wind. The sun dissipated the clouds. A slight breeze fought to blow beneath the barren trees.

Reflections of sunlight bounced off the buildings. The buildings encircled a large inner city park, which played host to the only full-scaled replica of the Greek Parthenon.

Inside the massive walls stood the enormous statue of Athena in all of her greatness and wisdom. Although Nashville was much more than the Country Music City, it will forever be remembered as a hillbilly haven.

Layers of green paint covered the splintered wooden tables that were placed sporadically around the pleasing waters. In the center of the park was the Lake Wautauga, with its inner island that gave safe refuge to the birds that used the park as a brief homestead. Couples lost themselves in love's solitude while they paddled along the sides of the pond, totally oblivious to the world around them. In the far horizon, separate clusters of elderly men some with children at their sides cast their baited hooks into the clouded waters.

Close by was the office of Bradley's physician, which he and I had just left. Bradley clutched the papers tightly in his right hand. He walked slowly and mechanically, his breathing labored and troubled. His eyes were blank and distant as he continued to move towards the hill where his car was parked. Then he stopped abruptly and began to cry silently. Torn from within the very depths of his soul, he fell heavily against his car and began to cry uncontrollably.

Bradley pounded his fists against the cold steel of his car. People continued walking past him without appearing to notice.

Emotions overwhelmed him. He screamed out in utter despair. Suddenly, people noticed his wildness. Instead of going to his aid, they hurried away, anxious to get out of his reach. Bradley had finally stepped into someone else's shoes. He no longer felt attractive or alluring. So many times he had wondered what he would do if he were ever told that he was HIV positive. The doctor's report pushed him beyond endurable limits of angry fear, beyond hope. His pain was unimaginable to anyone but himself. Not even real to me. There was only silence between us.

No one attempted to rescue him; bystanders hurried their families quickly out of the mad man's reach. In an instant, Bradley rose from his car and ran blindly up the short inclines that led to the lake. I ran close behind him. Cars swerved or stopped, barely missing us as we frantically ran into their paths, then Bradley stopped at Lake Wautauga.

Tears streamed down his face. Spectators laughed and shouted vile profanities. Bradley ignored the people that watched him crying. No one acknowledged his torment except for an elderly frail man who had sat alone on the gravel bank.

The old man stared at Bradley. In a barely audible whisper, he asked, "Are you out of your fool mind, boy?"

"Get the hell away from me, you old buzzard." Bradley yelled as he turned his back on the senior. A diabolical smile appeared on Bradley's face. He decided to torment his foe. Both men eventually stood face to face. Both stood equally forcefully, holding their ground.

"I hate this damn country. I don't care who hears me. This country is so full of moralistic hypocrites who don't care about other people that I could just scream. But why bother puking my guts up. No one gives a damn," Bradley yelled.

"I can't ignore you while you're condemning this great land. The land of freedom for all. This is God's own pure piece of goodness. Stop your childish behavior," the man said. Bradley saw the shocked expression on the old man's face.

"You can't ignore me? Who the hell are you? What damn business is it of yours anyway? Surely your little senile mentality doesn't truly buy into that patriotic bullshit."

Many more angry words were exchanged with no interference from anyone in the gathering. Bradley violently grabbed the man by his shirt collar and pulled him closer until his face was only inches away. He tried to push his tattered papers down the man's mouth as the man fought against his violent actions. I tried to separate them but Bradley knocked me into the murky lake.

While standing in the knee deep murky water, I saw Bradley pushed him backward causing the old man to stumble over the gravel and fall to the ground. His fragile body fell with a slight thud against the dry earth only inches from the water. I tried to fight the water to get to their side. But it was too late. Discouraging remarks came from the crowd as a few people tried to rescue the old man from the ground. Bradley turned his back on them as he held his paper remnants and flung his arms madly into the crowd.

Obviously angered by his fall, the old man reached for a small limb he spotted and brought it hard across Bradley's face bringing a trickle of blood above his right temple. Bradley appeared slightly stunned as the blood flowed down into his eyes mixing with his tears.

By now, four park rangers ran to us and tried to physically restrain us. I was slammed hard against the cruiser and handcuffed. Bradley attempted to fight the efforts of the rangers until the rangers rustled him to the ground and handcuffed him. Bradley finally succumbed. He stopped and yelled at the rangers trying to tell them not to touch him where he was bleeding that he has AIDS. Outraged, the enforcers cursed him. Bradley raised his head and wailed to the sky as a sharp blow of a nightstick downed him.

I desperately tried to go to him but I was pushed into the back of the cruiser, still soaking wet. On the inside, I cried. Not for myself, but for my friend as he lay face down in the dirt.

Hours later, I was released with no charges filed. Enough witnesses testified that my role wasn't as an adversary. Some of the officers recognized me and gave me questionable stares. Bradley, on the other hand, wasn't as lucky. He was detained on a criminal assault charge and resisting arrest.

Upon their separate return from their ill-fated trip to New York, Cleo and Edward started the tedious process of dissolving their marriage. Cleo's

PANELS

counsel encouraged her to list the mental and physical abuse that she had endured under Edward's control. Pictures taken of her upon her return home were included as evidence further sustaining her claims of domestic violence.

No longer the timid peasant girl, Cleo went after Edward with great vigor. Cleo's first steps were to protect herself from Edward, which included changing all the house locks. Seth, as an added measure, purchased a well-trained female Doberman pinscher that was unfamiliar to Edward

While struggling through the initial stages of the divorce, Cleo began to develop a life of her own. She focused on giving life to some of her forgotten dreams. Initially she struggled to find herself. Her own personality sacrificed to become the obedient, doting wife her culture expected. Seth's presence gave her the strength needed to fight and finally break the chains of her oppression.

Initially, Edward balked at the first planned settlement that gave her the house and twenty percent of his current wealth. Further negotiations quickly cancelled when Edward became publicly belligerent and yelled derogatory slurs at Cleo as he walked from the courtroom. He was not aware that the judge had just entered from her chambers. Judge Mattielyn Wilson listened quietly to his ranting then she stopped him. In her decree, she then awarded Cleo the house and fifty percent of Edward's wealth including his future income. The condition of her remarrying would be the only stipulation that would make the arrangement null and void.

We were all standing in support at her side when the judge gave the award. Edward stormed away only after cursing several generations of Cleo's family wishing the AIDS virus on their bloodthirsty souls. Judge Wilson abruptly raised her eyeglasses towards his counsel that appeared dumbfounded with the entire situation. In her soft voice, she stated that Edward obviously didn't take heed to her words and then advised his counsel to be further advised that she was charging Edward a thousand dollars fine for every generation of Cleo's family still living due to his rude comments and then added eighty hours of community service to be completed within two months at one of the local community awareness programs, specifically Nashville CARES. She concluded that after he had worked the assigned hours at Nashville CARES, then perhaps he would have empathy instead of apathy for those living with AIDS. She vowed that her court officers would definitely monitor his involvement at the agency.

Hours later, in the comfort of her home, Cleo sat inside the bay window sipping a glass of burgundy wine. I was glancing through a magazine when

Seth entered the room. She had been waiting for the moment. To me, it was the image of grace and sophistication with her slender fingers caressing the smooth glass stem, constantly twirling the warm liquid around the opening in a teasing manner. She was wearing a gold brocade suit with beaded embodied pockets and jeweled buttons. Although her matching lined slim skirt was waist less, her sleek figure was still very visually alluring.

Cleo looked into Seth's eyes and again she wistfully smiled. After a few more minutes of idle time consuming chit chat, Seth stood directly over her, placed his bony hands lightly on the tops of both of her hands cautiously as if he was touching fine Spanish china. He looked directly into her moist green eyes. Smiling rather innocently, Cleo stared at the stem of her glass. She took another sip and then spoke of her wishes to him.

Cleo reminded Seth of the previous plans for the three-floor structure that was located in the historic section of Edgefield in East Nashville. She reminded him how both Edward and she had carefully devised blueprints renovating their antebellum home for their individual offices on the ground floor and a small art gallery on the main level. Cleo had wanted to invest in limited art pieces that wasn't readily available anywhere else in Nashville. Edward had suggested that the venture was a viable investment and had fully backed her financially before their separation.

I watched as Cleo walked over to the portable bar and poured another glass of wine. Then she turned to him. Cleo explained that she had called him to ask him to move in with her. She wanted the man that she loved living with her. She told him that he would no longer have to suffer trying to pay his bills and his outrageous lease on his West End apartment. She, in turn, could help him should he ever require medical assistance in the middle of the night.

Seth objected to her arrangements fearing that the burden would be too severe for her. Cleo placed her hand softly against his lips, "I need you here beside me. Please don't say no."

Cleo's Heart
I spent a great deal of time with Ruth and Patricia. Seth teased me often asking if I had crossed over. I only laughed saying that he was the only woman for me. This was the first time I have ever had the closeness of another woman in my life since leaving my family in Spain. I guess my maternal instincts became apparent and the relationship I shared with the lesbian couple proved effective and non-restraining. I wanted to fill the vast void that existed in my

life. Surprisingly, I wanted something more reciprocal, I wanted my own child. I longed to have Seth's child, but knew that that was virtually impossible because of his fatal infection.

In developing my person, I became aware of the similarity of the women's movement and the gay movement. Both considered underground minorities evolved within the shadows of white masculine America. I once felt oppressed under Edward's rule, but eventually was able to break free of the shackles.

During my friendship with Ruth and Patricia, I became actively involved in various women's movements. No longer the indecisive woman that I once was under the directives of my former controller, I learned to excel.

Whether I spent my time rushing to the hospital visiting my friends or attending forums on the equality of women, the presence of Justin soon took center stage. Justin slowly became a large influencing factor in my decision to adopt a child. Ruth helped me with the initial arrangements to start the process. Somehow, I managed to keep this possibility from the guys. I had to know certain of my chances.

I was wheeling Seth down to the pediatric level when we first saw her. All Seth knew was that I was coming to feed an abandoned child. Seth warned me about becoming too dependent on the child. I laughed in response to his concerns saying that Edward had broken me from the habit. Seth patted my hand lightly and gave me a faint smile.

The social worker and the charge nurse were already waiting for us. Across from the nursing station, Justin sat snuggly on Ruth's lap. Justin's face was aglow with his cherubic smile and high-pitched giggle. The social worker smiled a reassuring smile as she asked me to come inside her office before I met the child. Before I could protest, Seth looked up behind him and told me to go. Seth assured me that he would be all right hanging out with Justin and Ruth.

"Now, don't leave. I'll be right back in a flash!" I walked towards the office.

"That woman is full of surprises," I heard Seth say. "Does anyone know what she's up to?"

"Like you said, she's full of surprises." Ruth winked.

"How do you guys feel about being uncles?" I heard Patricia tease as I went inside.

Once inside, I was quickly ushered into the social worker's desk. Her discerning expression made me uncomfortable.

"I really do admire you for wanting to take on this rather difficult feat," Julie, the social worker, said. "Not everyone could actually do this, even on a temporary basis. There's still much fear and ignorance when it concerns babies being born with the virus. Are you really aware of the stigma, of the repercussions, the social damnations or the prejudices that you are opening yourself up to? Many people simply would not look upon this as being of any heroic measure. They would not understand about why you want to do this. How aware are you of AIDS?"

During the interview, Julie disclosed that she had fought a battle against breast cancer. Her cancer was in remission. She had found out first hand how detrimental it was to realize that life might be over in just a matter of time. Julie realized how her close friends had kept their distance due to their fear and ignorance. Julie knew all too well of the rejection and the decline of her social status because she was also dealing with AIDS. She wondered aloud if I realized the unexpected pitfalls of taking care of society's forgotten lot.

"Well, I'm divorced. I have too much time on my hands. I'm not the bridge playing type. My experience of AIDS is also crucially painful for me. You noticed the friend with me, that is the fourth close friend I've had that is living with AIDS. The other three have died...Believe me, I know what I'm in for. I know of the pain and the heartache of loving someone dying. I'll never say that I know just how much pain and suffering that they continue to go through. I will, however, say that I will always be there for them. Oh, I'm the first to admit, I still have much to learn. But, I have a great deal of compassion also. I may not be accepted as a potential foster parent. But if I was considered, I know I can give her unconditional love, if you'll let me." I wiped the perspiration that had formed on the palms of my hands.

"The child stands a 50% chance of survival...Yes, there is no cure for the virus, but the antibodies in an infant stands the test for fighting the virus."

"I read somewhere where with much love and attention that kids can live."

"Are you ready to take on such an emotional chance? Have you learned anything from your friends...?"

"Don't worry about me. I'm a fighter. I wouldn't be here wasting your time if I didn't think I could handle this...Where is my child? I have a home waiting for her."

A hour later as I sat outside with the others in the lobby, a nurse soon brought The newborn and gently laid her in my arms.

"Say hello to my sweet little angel!" I held her gently in the air. "Guys, I'm finally a mamma!" Immediately, the child was inundated with affection and compassion from everyone. The newborn was very small for nine months old. She was my black angel. She was in the developmental stage of a five month old. Her sparkling eyes glittered with innocence. She was a dark angel with a battle to fight that she knew nothing about and didn't deserve. Julie explained how the newborn had not been able to effectively bond with anyone, and may have even given up the will to live. Her parents were both crack addicts with a long history of alcohol abuse. Neither parent had visited the infant after she was diagnosed with not only the AIDS virus but also fetal alcohol syndrome.

Before she was ready to come home with me, I went every day to the hospital during feeding times to hold the newborn and bottle-feed her. Once, while I was holding the fragile child in my arms, a nurse walked into the room. The infant was fretting even after she had consumed the entire contents of her four-ounce bottle. I searched the room until I saw the pacifier on the bassinet in the corner by her bed. I kindly asked the nurse to hand me the pacifier.

Appearing somewhat disgruntled by the request, the nurse reached for several paper towels to place over the pacifier. As she handed it to me, I flew into a rage. I flung the pacifier at the nurse, yelling at her to get out.

Moments later, the nursing supervisor came into the room, attempting to calm me. I demanded that the nurse be removed from the floor because of her apparent insensitivity and lack of concern for the fragile child. I was angry knowing that someone supposedly dedicated to treat sick people would intentionally mistreat someone as precious as someone supposedly dedicated to treat sick people would intentionally mistreat the baby I held in my arms.

Later that evening, I wrote a letter to Julie, "As I rocked and held the newborn, I remembered the significance of the process of bonding within the first years of a person's life. Looking into her eyes, which held only her innocence, our own eyes filled with anger. The newborn reminded me of the large delicate plants in the corridor of her unit, specifically the sheffleras. Scheffleras are extremely sensitive and difficult to grow. The fragile plants can easily be destroyed by constantly being shifted or moved about. Similar to the scheffleras, the newborn was bounced from place to place within various unfamiliar hands. Could you possibly exist within those same limits of uncertainty? Children are the scheffleras of the world. They are delicate fragile souls that should not be acquired without knowledge or sincere love to nurture them."

I renamed my child Theresa Juliana Castleman. Named after Theresa

Chikaba, born in 1676, the daughter of a king off the African West Coast. She was a fighter.

Theresa eventually gained weight and discharged to live with me. I was told that my eyes sparkled whenever I held the wiggling child in my arms. She became an inseparable part of my life. Where I went, my living doll was with me. She gave me unconditional love without knowing any previous history of my misfortunes.

A portrait painted in the image of Theresa, commissioned personally by me by one of my favorite local artist Tony Teek hangs above the desk in my study, forever to immortalize the child's precious existence in this world.

Months slowly passed as Sebastian returned to his self-isolation from the rest of the world except for Cleo, Seth, and I. Maybe I was a thorn in his side because I worked with him.

One morning proved crucial in our lives. He stood outside my office with tears streaming down his face. I quickly went to him and pulled him inside.

I was not prepared for what he had to say. He wiped his eyes, regained his usual poise and whispered. "Bradley is dead."

"What the hell are you talking about? He can't be dead. Not Bradley…" I felt the air knocked out. "Omigod, please say it isn't so."

"Now you know how I felt when I first heard." He sat on the desk corner.

"What happened? Who told you?" By this time, I was crying.

"Cleo…she called me this morning before day light." He paused. "My immediate thought was that Seth died. So, not knowing what exactly happened, I said I've been expecting this to happen…asked how was she holding up…I tried to assure her that Seth was now at peace".

"I thought you said it was Bradley?"

"I did…she kept saying how it was so unreal. And how she couldn't get over it. It really made no damn sense…I mean, why did he do it?" I still thought it was Seth until she finally screamed out it wasn't Seth that was dead but Bradley. I jumped straight up in bed at that point. My eyes were wide open then."

"What the hell happened?" I was irritable. "Who killed him?"

"He killed himself." Sebastian stared out the window. "The phone rang again. This time it was Mr. Thomas-McCleane…He wants to talk to me this afternoon."

"Omigod, it must be really hard on them. Is there anything I can do?"

PANELS

"Michal, I need you to go with me...I can't face his father alone...I don't know what to say." Sebastian looked directly in my eyes for an answer.

"Sure...I'll go...who else knows besides Cleo and us?"

"Seth doesn't know, if that is what you're asking."

As promised, Sebastian and I stood outside the entrance to Bradley's condominium, as Ben walked slowly toward us.. The older man wore a heavy-laden expression of much scattered life across his frail shoulders, his eyes swollen with obvious misery. His gait was slower than usual and unsteady. His face was void of any joy, as gnawing malaise prevailed. With a deeper sigh, the keys to Bradley's home turned and the door opened.

Bradley's dwelling was immaculate as ever. That was his trademark on life. The only thing that appeared out of place was the reasoning around his suicide. The rooms appeared colder than usual. Sebastian felt the walls were mourning for their owner. I felt a rather strong presence of Bradley within the rooms. Perhaps, I wondered, if Bradley was somehow monitoring their movements about the interior. Sebastian imagined hearing Bradley's voice and even his sarcastic laughter. While looking at the rather eccentric decor, my own mind envisioned the host being present with us in physical form. Was this denial?

Ben sat on the black pin-stripped chaise with the crumpled letter written in his son's precise handwriting opened directly before his swelling eyes. As his aged trembling fingers clutched the pages, he read once again the reported last words Bradley left him. "By now, you have realized what my decision was. My decision...my choice...Before you fault me, please read all of my words closely. I will try to hurry. I feel the sensations from the incoming fumes. My thoughts are extremely varied and numerous, but I will try to finish before I go to sleep. I do owe you a reason why...Please remember that I do love my family and my friends very much. Try to forgive me and please try to understand...I see the suffering that AIDS has already brought into our circle of friends and especially my own family...I'm not blaming Seth or anyone else. I loved Seth more than I loved myself. Now it's too late for him to know...

"I have to be in full control of my life. Of my total existence. I cannot bear to further burden anyone with my illness. It wouldn't be fair to those that I love. Think of my choice as an answer to having rode continuingly on the roller coaster of life. I merely decided that it was time for me to get off and finally rest. Believe me, it's for the best. Maybe one day, you'll fully understand...I have cried my last tear...always remember that I loved each and every one of you...Father, you have given me the best that life had to offer. You have given me your love unconditionally...now I need your forgiveness. We'll see each other again, but in another place. Your son, Bradley"

Hours later, as the sun finally raised its blistering head, Benjamin stood in absolute horror, as he watched Bradley's dissipated body lying before his eyes. The horrible disfigured corpse on the stretcher draped with the dingy white sheets could not be his blood. He fought back the tears. Benjamin could not bear to look into his child's distorted face. He refused to see Death. Benjamin refused to realize the image before him was indeed his own boy. *Had ha-Shem forsaken him once again?* he asked the heavens.

Benjamin's facial expression appeared opprobrious, as I read the police report. In total disbelief, he was aware of just how cruel his son had died. A police helicopter was randomly searching for reported marijuana crops off the rural desolate roads fifty miles south of Nashville. The pilot noticed a rather expensive car parked close behind an abandoned weathered tobacco barn. Never seeing the strange car in the past searches, the pilot immediately radioed the local authorities to investigate the situation.

The cirrus white 1992 Saab 9000 convertible motor was still running, as the three patrol cars cautiously circled the area. Slowly, the officers walked toward the car with their service revolvers clearly drawn in the direction of the unfamiliar car.

The lieutenant called out to the car, loudly ordering the passenger out of the car with their hands in the air. An officer who eased up from behind the Saab quickly noticed a flexible hose that ran from the exhaust pipe into the driver's side of the car. Immediately, he replaced his service revolver and tried opening the door. He yelled at the other officers to assist him.

The car doors locked, a couple of officers peered inside the slightly tinted windows and noticed a limp body inside sitting behind the wheel. Finally, someone broke the passenger window. The toxic fumes emitted inside the car escaped out the shattered glass. The fumes were so powerful the officers had to temporarily retreat.

Moments later, after placing their handkerchief over their faces, they quickly pulled the body from the car. They gasped at the condition, while almost dropping him on the barren ground. Two officers suddenly became nauseated and left from the scene.

Due to the extreme heat inside the already secured non-ventilated vehicle, his body was totally limp past the rigor mortis stage. The muscle fibers depleted of adenosine triphosphate. His naturally tanned skin was now cherry red in appearance. The heat caused fragments of his skin to pull away and slip from his body. Residue carefully scraped from the driver's door and various other places off his leather seats. Thin transparent layers came off onto the officers' hands, as they pulled Bradley to the ground. His eyes partially opened with the signs of darkness and dryness where once his mucus membranes totally depleted. His former beauty was now a frightful skeleton.

The medical examiner summoned to the unfortunate discovery. A blood sample taken directly from the heart to define the levels of the carbon monoxide poisoning at the actual site. At that point, ruled as a suicide, and no autopsy was required after the officers retrieved the handwritten pieces of papers from his sustaining fingers. The letter was addressed to his family. Foul play ruled out.

Dr. Elizabeth Gooden, the medical examiner for Davidson County, spoke briefly with a sympathetic mellifluous voice, as she stood facing the troubled expressionless faces. She unfortunately experienced moments of this type of pain before. Elizabeth understood as much as she possibly could while considering the delicate situation. There was never anything she knew to say to soothe the broken hearts and mend the dreams of the living. She gathered her charts quietly and eventually left the father and son alone.

Years later, Seth told me that his father existed on the periphery of his family's misery. Through his past, he regained his own history before the days of the German hell. After the Holocaust, he regained his lost hope and pride. Through his family happiness, he found renewed strength in living again.

Ben was the last child born to a German-Jewish family. The family surname wasn't McCleane but Mosherman. There was nothing vastly unusual about his natural family except their heritage and religion offended Hitler's regime. Ben lived the words of the Mishna, especially the Mishna Brura in keeping with the traditional basic Jewish laws. He maintained his own responsibilities for the mincha and the ma'ariv faithfully. Later during his youth, he changed his birthright name. Benjamin was not denying his ancestry. He feared further retaliatory hatred from the world. Even now, he told me that he wondered if his actions had not offended his God.

By this time, others gathered outside, while the father and I stayed with Bradley within the freezing desolate confinement of the city's morgue. In silence, Benjamin stood in distilled horror over the vision of Bradley lying covered partially with starchy thin white sheets that attempted to shield his son's shrunken body. As denial grew within his heart, he desperately wanted the disfigured cursed carcass to be someone other than his son. Silence shielded the brief reality but did nothing for the pain that throbbed excessively within the very depths of his own scarred soul.

Outside and away from their coldness, arrangements made with the morticians. Bradley always wanted cremation. He often laughed saying he could never imagine anyone hovering over him while in a coffin. He never wanted anyone to remember him in that fashion. Benjamin initially balked at the idea of his own blood burning again inside some cruel filthy furnace. In Bradley's letter he left at his home, he tried to reason the rationale of cremation because he vainly wanted everyone to remember him as he lived instead of whatever remained of him. Although he somehow understood his son's wishes, his survivor's stubbornness tried to prevail, refusing to comply with his son's wishes until the moment he regretfully viewed the altered remains.

Sebastian stood with the remainder of the family. All members were present except for Seth. Silence prevailed in their presence. The atmosphere was completely staid with utter shock and disbelief. In our minds, Bradley was not the one Death prepared them for. However, the obvious choice never mentioned. Benjamin turned to me and extended his hand.

"Will you stay with me?"

"Sir, I will stay with you." I went to his side.

"Thank you…I really appreciate your support."

Back inside the room, Benjamin moved the steel-backed chair beside his cold son and gradually sat down. I watched as he removed Bradley's lifeless left hand from his side and placed it delicately up to his lips. With both of his callused aged hands, Benjamin held the lifeless limb against his own moist cheekbone.

"God, why are you so angry with me? Have I not followed your teachings and your examples?…Every morning I wake wondering what I have done so

PANELS

wrong...I saw the misery, and it saw me...Have I not dreamed my last dream of that time?"

Suddenly, he stopped. He kissed the non-responsive hand. Still, he didn't look directly into his son's uncovered face. Benjamin continued to lament on his past, somehow hoping Bradley was somehow listening. Benjamin was clearly stricken with not only grief but guilt as well. Perhaps if he listened to his children more, maybe things would have been quite different. He wondered if he actually ever told Bradley how much he loved him. Was his tolerance dreadfully wrong? Although he never really approved of his son's sexual preference in life, he learned to accept his son, because he was still his son nevertheless. Curiously, he wondered if God had been displeased with him for the deception to the Laws.

"You, my son, have joined the others who have gone before you. You started your own selfish pilgrimage without my knowledge, and now your quest is definitely completed. As in the past, I once again must say the Kaddish for you in all of the mornings, days, and the evening prayers...Death cheated me several times before in my past...I am very angry about you leaving me...Perhaps you considered this way the best for you...I used to look fondly in your eyes and see the reflections of your mother's gentle face. Her precious smile underneath her stern eyes, the expression of an angel...I never told you just how much you really meant to me; I never knew how...But now it's too damn late...Why must we wait so late just to say how we feel?...My heart is broken for you...But, damn, how dare you turn away from your family...Haven't we been there for you in the past? I know I don't know what you must have gone through emotionally when you first were told. Maybe you thought that there was no hope, but at least you could've given us the chance to say good-bye...I feel very cheated, and I'm not ready to yield you...Come back into my life and live, god damn it...Do you hear me...Oh God, what have I done so wrong to lose a child?...Please have pity on my weakened heart. I know that I can't take the emptiness that surrounds my soul...Somehow, I tell myself that maybe my son is finally at rest with himself. Still, that doesn't ease any of my miserable pain any less..." Benjamin fell against his son and sobbed as his own voice neared anger.

A fallen man, Benjamin soon dropped his head down onto the stretcher that now bears his son's scars. Slowly and only after a momentary pause, Benjamin regained his frail composure and continued his conversation with God and his son.

"You were always filled with much more courage and conviction than I.

PHIL MICHAL THOMAS

I know that you had to have suffered impassively in making your final decision. I love you, and I will always love you…Ironically, your death painstakingly reminds me of the older days…Yes, finally, I do understand and even accept your choice after I realized your only destiny…I still hurt, but I do understand. There were times when I too felt like ending my sordid life of routine misery…Days when I had nothing, I thought, to live for except the dullness that I felt after being trampled upon. I couldn't retaliate. At first, I thought that neither should you have…It's against our Law…I wasn't completely scared of death, although it certainly was constantly beside me. It was the constant flicker of hope that forever stayed with me and, in my heart, the hope that better days laid ahead, days of final freedom and peace…Unlike me, my son, you was never offered any hope. Once again, death had twisted its dagger cutting the flesh of my heart."

Benjamin, wishing for the presence of either the cantor or the rebbe or better yet a maggid to offer him answers, closed his eyes and prayed silently the ma'ariv.

Eloise quietly entered from behind the kneeling figure. She also refused to stare at the body underneath the sheets. She held onto Benjamin, as the attendants wheeled the still body away. Pretending to be stronger at that moment, Eloise embraced her saddened husband, as he cried uncontrollably in her own trembling arms. There was no room for any additional words from either. Having faced a barren corner inside the examining room, Benjamin desperately tried to imagine himself far away from that very moment. Eloise clenched her eyes tightly while still refusing to watch, as the attendants transferred their child's body into the body bag. Both parents' bodies stiffened, as the zippering noise echoed throughout the interior.

Later, others joined us as we walked from the room in total desolate silence.

The sun lowered its magnificent rays on the day of the season that began Passover. I have learned from my previous conversations with Seth and Brad that Passover signified the celebrating freedom of the Exodus from Egypt. The day represented the end of slavery and the end of bondage for Jews. Was mankind actually released from the shackles or merely transformed to another arms of devastating imprisonment? One morning while drinking coffee with me, Sebastian told me that he had taken a closer look at the life around him.

PANELS

"With all this shit in my face, I don't see the good in anything anymore."

"Yeah, I know, it's kinda hard staying focused on the positives...no pun intended...when you are drowning."

"My life really sucks," Sebastian announced.

"I remember when that was a good thing...I'm sorry, I just could not pass that one up...So, what's going on with you?" I asked.

"I really hate sounding like some screwy record. But...I must confess...this damn AIDS has really taken its toll on my life...I no longer find myself physically attractive to others..."

"It definitely makes you think twice about having sex."

"Yeah, sometimes more than twice. I mean, it makes you question yourself as whether or not it's worth getting laid nowadays. So, if I need to, I find myself fantasizing to get off."

"I'm sure that the end brought a pleasurable finish. For you, anyway. But for me, even my fantasies leave me dry," I said. "You can always go cyber."

"You better believe it. Man, there's nothing better than programmed sex." He laughed.

"Actually, if the truth be known, it's sad to realize that sometimes the dream is far better than the real thing...but with my track record, I don't always know what the real thing is anyway."

"So, is that by your choice?"

" Hell no, definitely not mine...their choice!"

"I'm far from hating sex. In fact, I love and want sex...Don't get me wrong; I'm not a whore either."

"Have you totally lost interest? Found yourself in the land of no boners?"

"Totally!"

"Welcome to the club, my brother," I said.

"Seriously, the shit with AIDS is playing hell with my love life which was already limited to nil...and if you repeat this, I will swear that you are a liar, but those damned images of our friends battling has become a damn wall blocking my mind...If I were in the middle of sex, I immediately lost my erection...The mere touch of the other person scared me."

"Sebastian, believe me when I say I do understand where you are coming from...I have been accused too many times of not wanting to commit to a relationship. I was told that I was too selfish, arrogant, and even guilty of loving no one but myself. You know that none of that is true except perhaps the part of me needing to love me...Like yourself, I have seen far too much just how AIDS has screwed people."

"Michal, you know that I'm far from being a prudish person in terms of sex but I also don't want to press my luck too often either. I'm scared to fall in love with anyone. I prefer to do without because of this damned fear…but yet, I need someone in my life. "

"Remember that it is better to love and to not love."

"Michal, that's our problem…we don't really know what love is. Do we?"

"Will we ever know?" I paused. "To love or not to love is the burden."

As time went on, I understood why Sebastian constantly fought the urge to have someone in his life. I spoke with him one night after he had stopped at the Gaslite after work.

"Michal, the bar was barely filled. The jukebox was blasting ballads that made you want to cry. Real depressing…Few guys were cruising heavily for that piece of ass…You know the game, eyes met but quickly dropped away. You know the drill, act like you not to be bothered while drooling at the same time."

Sebastian found an empty stool and ordered a beer. The coolness of the bottle awakened his senses momentarily as he placed a few bills on the counter.

"I tried to relax but felt quite awkward…Almost bored to tears, I glanced around at the faces near me and caught a reciprocating stare from the end of the bar. From the distant, the man appeared totally hot. At least for that moment, I found the guy quite sexy…His eyes seemed calming yet inviting. Feeling my wheaties, I rose to greet the stranger who, by this time, had moved to the stool beside me…After stupid chit chat, phone numbers were exchanged with promises of spending time together."

"And…what happened?"

"I never heard from him."

We laughed at this little episode of lost potential love. I understood all too well of his frustration in trying to find that special someone. I, too, was looking for a special person to share my life with. It will happen eventually, we both agreed…or rather hoped.

Months later, Sebastian and I were sitting around the patio of the Chute when someone, who he had previously noticed in our travels through the bar, was standing directly behind him. I winked at Sebastian as he gave this person a glance. Sebastian shrugged his shoulder.

"Don't look now, but this guy was with someone else earlier and he had already tried to make eye contact with me even then," Sebastian whispered.

"Maybe he likes what he sees!"

"Maybe he's a fickle queen!" Now the blond was only inches behind him and his friend was now engaged in conversing with someone else. The blond closed in and was only inches from Sebastian.

I watched as strange hands reach down and massage his shoulders. Sebastian stared at me with a questioning expression on his face. He glanced upward into the awaiting blue eyes of the blond. Sebastian reached and began to caress the massaging hands.

"I hope me taking certain liberties doesn't annoy you."

"On the contrary, it is very wanted...My name is Sebastian and yours?"

"My name is Jonathan but my friends calls me JB...You mind if I sit?" The stranger now has a name. Sebastian gazed into JB's face as well as his exposed body. Sebastian smiled at the muscled hunk before him. He appeared marveled in JB's beauty.

Eventually, JB and Sebastian began seeing each other for several weeks. JB was a waiter working evenings. Sebastian would see him after work and would spend early morning hours together. Their relationship proved more than just sexual, it served as true companionship.

Sebastian once described how he would lay in JB's arms never wanting to be released. He felt secured and loved. Sebastian allowed JB to make Sebastian feel good about him. He felt that the love was genuine.

JB was living with a roommate that had previously tested positive. According to Sebastian, there existed neither sexual influence nor romance between JB and his roommate Hailey, although, according to JB, Hailey appeared to have a obvious crush for him.

I asked Sebastian once what did the two of them talk about in the quiet wee hours of the morning.

"Nothing major. We spoke of our fears and of our painful past...I listened closely as he spoke of his fear for his roommate living with the horrible virus."

"I take it that he doesn't know of our friends?" I asked.

"Hell no...I silently gasp every time he mentions not wanting Hailey to even touch him...let alone sexually...just because he is positive. He says he could care for Hailey but could never love him. I was becoming quite uncomfortable about our talk, so I decided to change the focus. Boy, wasn't that a mistake."

"Why, did he say something that freaked you out?"

"I guess you can say that...For some reason, I decided to ask him why he was not involved with anyone. Why was he still single."

"Okay, so what was his major malfunction? Why is he flying solo? He's really a woman, right?"

"He said he was single because he likes to drink and drink and drink. Drink himself into complete oblivion." Sebastian shrugged off. "So, I asked him if he drinks to accept himself or if he really enjoyed drinking. He tightens up and spouts back that he was not one of my patients and told me that maybe he does try to hide from himself. He says that no one appears to want to be around him especially his family...Obviously his father isn't too keen on his lifestyle since his father tells him constantly that there is this long hand reaching from the Heavens waiting to help him change."

"If only it would be that easy to change." I laughed.

Eventually, Sebastian appeared to have succumbed to his returned fears. He eventually stopped dating altogether. He became celibate, definitely not his choice but perhaps by the will to survive. He said he hoped he wasn't too late to save himself.

"It seems like all I talk about lately with you is the void in my life...It has taken over my life, being frustrated, that is. My levels of depression have increased."

"Do you no longer feel as if you could build stable relationships with others, or even fill the need for belongings or love?"

"No, I no longer feel secure in close intimate relationships. I tried nonchalantly to distant myself emotionally from my clients and even my friends...even to you, Michal...I know that I'm quick tempered and easily irritated."

"Have you spoken to the man or have you just sit back and diagnosed yourself?"

"Actually, I have made an appointment...but you must never tell anyone...Who would fly on a bird with a broken wing?"

"Man, I can relate...Not to take your storm away, but I feel the same anger, fear, and even some slight lack of hope are also what I'm living with. I think my anger exists because of the restrictive present situation, and fear in not knowing the future."

"Michal, I want to know my future."

PANELS

Two days later, Sebastian sat across from the psychiatrist. With careful consideration, he chose someone on staff that specialized in obsessive-compulsive personality disorders. He told me that he hoped to gain answers to his dilemma.

Dr. Paul Thomas, initially, didn't want to counsel Sebastian professionally, since he feared he was too close to Sebastian in order to provide effective treatment to stabilize the healing process.

"Being a fellow therapist, I need not remind you how your extreme rituals and obsessive thoughts separate you clearly from other anxiety sufferers. Are there any experiences of avoidance and, if so, to what degree?"

"People. Yeah, people! It's like I'm afraid of being physically or even emotionally close to anyone. I no longer fear rejections especially since I fear that they'll somehow will harm me."

"What about the levels of intimacy? Are you now prone to fear intimate relations as well?"

"This conversation is about as intimate as I get nowadays. It's like, I have to be constantly on guard and keenly aware of what others around me may try to do to me. Not really paranoid, but, and I know that this may sound so damn foolish and believe me, I do know better, but I'm actually so scared that I could get AIDS from others just simply touching or holding me."

"So, you avoid people in general?"

"Like the plague. No pun intended." Sebastian smiled nervously, as he paused to take a breath before he continued. "I realize essentially and even relate well to the fact of recurrent obsessions being time consuming and definitely interfering with my daily life, but how do I simply ignore the fact that others from my past are constantly dying around me?"

"Have you been tested?"

"Yeah...several times...So far, nothing...Strictly negative, but I still deal constantly with the haunting fear of my past infecting me."

"Is that your way of maintaining pervasive perfection?"

"To be honest, I want to believe that I can keep AIDS far away from me. Maybe I do go to extremes by over modifying my life, but I feel strongly that it is virtually necessary in order for me to survive."

"What feelings do you have for your friends who have died from AIDS?"

"Honestly...I hate them...I truly despise them. I hate them for leaving me and I hate them for making me see their deaths...I hate them for making me cry into a fighting rage as I strike the thin cold air…alone late at night…I hate them…and myself for bringing the enemy closer."

Sebastian later shared his session with me. Although I did respect and appreciate his honesty, his words bothered me a great deal. Secretly, I felt betrayed. My initial response was to cast him aside and treat him with a long handle spoon. However, I knew, deep down, he merely said out loud what I actually felt.

Maureen, a Portrait of Truth

A person can either change or modify to the environment in order to survive. Those living within an unfavorable environment appear to challenge those who intend to carry out their ideal lives in expected measures. During the unhappy periods of one's life, individuals begin to evaluate and justify the value of living so that they themselves can still carry on with their lives mindfully. There may exist a rude awakening and balancing the sensations of fulfillment.

Sebastian's peripheral school of thought consisted of the teachings of behaviorists. Reality therapy was another mainstay of Sebastian's approach. He was direct and often appeared rather harsh at times. He refused to give false hope.

Alone, a person creates the hell or the Heaven in life. Sebastian was very effective in applying these rules to others but failed miserably in creating the truth within him. Isn't it easier to do as one says instead of as one does?

I believe there was a woman that we both counseled that I would swear he actually idolized. Somehow, she lived the life he desperately would welcome. Her name was Maureen.

As I walked near the reception area, I caught a glimpse at her. Maureen was leaning forward in the reception room chair across from alluring eyes of the other gender as she nonchalantly pulled at her spidery silver laced stockings that slid into her satin evening mules. Her long manicured nails with the sparkling jeweled insets caressed her structured thin legs. Her white hooded coat with the down filled silk was draped gingerly across the neighboring chair.

Diamonds coveted her thin smooth sensual fingers. Maureen had worn her "Dog Collar" belt in crocodile while she loosely gasped the bag also in black crocodile. Her blond locks hung shatteringly over her stirring eyes and cascading gently down her back across her raw silk blouse accentuated with

PANELS

the jeweled collar, cuffs, and matching skirt.

Maureen charmed the rather sterile surroundings with her grace. Her sophisticated smile masked her complex fear. Maureen was an independent that required the assistance from no one except the monetary kindness of strangers. Those that had utilized her rather unique personal services preferred anonymity, which she religiously respected. She offered her clients, both male and female, a safe haven in the world of sexual adventures and fantasies with satisfaction as a rule.

"Well, if it isn't my dear high priest! Hello Pastor Michal…Saving any lost sheep lately?" she asked me.

"Hello, Maureen, did I have an appointment with you today?" I replied.

"Oh, no, not with you, darling…it's with my other man Sebastian but I'm sure we can do a group thing, if you know what I mean." She winked. "In fact, no charge…strictly on the house, my house that is."

"Well hey, baby, count me in!" A male patient with disheveled matted blond hair seated nearby said. He was quite weathered in his appearance: missing teeth, tattered clothing, and soiled greased hands.

"Honey, not in your wildest dreams could you ever hope to afford the likes of me…Him maybe…but certainly not me." She twirled around.

The intruder lowered his head and appeared wounded as he lit his cigarette. A woman beside him, in similar attire, elbowed him in his side as she frowned. Other patients in the small reception area seemed not amused to the incident or rather caught in their own world of drug-induced despair. I smiled and hurriedly walked away. I was afraid that I would embarrass myself if I stayed any longer.

In checking the master schedule, I found that Maureen's appointment was scheduled for ten thirty that morning with Sebastian. I knew from my own sessions with her that she was always prompt and extremely punctual in arriving for her monthly appointments. I feared that she would soon grow restless since his prior session was running a bit over. Time was significantly an essence in the dealings in her interpersonal interactions.

Several months before today, she had confided during one of our sessions that while during a routine pelvic examination, the gynecologist investigated what Maureen had complained of as being a foul unpleasant smelling discharge. Immediately, he ordered a laparoscope's to identify areas of possible abscesses or abnormal growths. Maureen had used the suggested IUDs but was still instructed to stop all sexual activities since the items could increase her chances of developing PID.

PHIL MICHAL THOMAS

Maureen was a fighter. She told me how she left the physician's office knowing that whatever she had, she would battle the afflictions as she had with anything else. Maureen cringed at the mere thought of any further suffering.

I was indeed fascinated by her. I knew that she was a vixen who controlled her own destiny. She had always been in complete charge of her rather troubled life since the day she left her family and their sordid memories back in Maryville, Tennessee, decades earlier. Refusing to comply with her father's and/or brothers' sexual gratification and any other further acts of physical aggressions, her flight from home began.

During our break through session, she tearfully recounted her years of abuse she experienced. She decided to leave too late. Unfortunately, only after a younger sister died from a tubal pregnancy. The seed from their father and the silence of their mother blessed the incest.

With much heartfelt anger in her already determined soul and disdain for her family, she decided no man would ever control her body again. Although I was caught off guard often by her disclosures, I appreciated her directness and her honesty. Maureen appeared quite comfortable with both Sebastian and me. We obviously proved no threats to her. I really think she knew about us although we had never disclosed anything to her.

At my last session with her, she described a recent night where she sat on her milky white lounge chaise sipping slowly from her glass of cognac. Candles were burning and scenting throughout the rooms, as the whisper of the soft classical music filled the already perfumed air. The last appointment just left for the evening. Her body was still moist from the hot cream bath. Her wet tangled hair hung sheepishly across her designer silk white robe.

She said she was mesmerized by the wind instruments of the symphony that played in her immediate background. The cognac swirled around and around inside the delicate crystal goblet. Glances at her leather embroidery appointment book reminded her of tomorrow's tricks for the trade. Suddenly, the phone began to ring, interrupting her seldom serenity. Maureen closed her eyes, allowing her service to take the message of the uninvited disturbance. The voice on the other end was not a client. Her tranquil moment ended abruptly.

Maureen reached for the phone that voided the service. Her mellifluous voice quickly turned stunned, as she listened to the doctor's words. Disbelief, she threw the fragile glass against the wall. It smashed into countless wet pieces. He wanted to see her early that next morning for more tests.

PANELS

Knowing what ails a person doesn't always give the person relief; it does however supply answers, not always with comfort. She felt somewhat relieved and equally scared for herself. Very few times in her life had she wanted someone there just to hold her until the dark clouds rolled past her.

Later, after she raised her trembling body from her marble tub after taking another bath, she walked stiffly into her office. With tears formed in the crevices of her moist eyes, she sat behind her well-polished mahogany desk. She opened a locked compartment and retrieved a sealed plastic envelope. Placing the entire contents of the fine white powder on top of the oval flat mirror with her initials engraved across the front, she used a gold-plated razor blade to separate the valuable grains into lines. Each of the four-inch lines was equal in all aspects. Her tears occasionally fell onto the powder. Her agony smeared the residue across the reflection of her. Carefully, she placed her fingers around the monogrammed sterling silver tubing. She pressed one side of her nostril closed, as the other became a welcoming avenue for her delight. With her other hand, she carefully held back her wandering wet hair as her head descended upon the mirror. The fingers stayed calm and completely steady, even until the actual second of the drug's impact.

At a distance, I watched as Sebastian slightly shook Maureen from her daydreaming. He stood only inches in front of her, as he quietly called her name. Regaining her graceful composure, she gathered her personal items and walked behind him to his office.

Inside his office, Maureen crossed her legs immediately upon taking her seat on the leather sectional. Her eyes fell directly in line with his eyes. Both challenged their grounds relentlessly. Maureen long suspected his sexual preference but clearly had no problem with his identity. She knew he was good although she felt he hadn't realized the fact. Sebastian long gained her trust, which wasn't easily given to anyone. She rarely trusted anyone with anything. Ironically, she considered him an equal ally, a non-threatening confidant. Compromises were never easily accepted without furious questioning on either side.

At this stage of her treatment plan, Sebastian and I had agreed that we would take it to a new level. This particular session dealt with Maureen's responsibilities in either discontinuing her experienced practices or informing her clients of her current HIV positive status.

"Do you ever notice my clothes? Take my blouse, for an example, this is raw silk...Just a mere $950..." Maureen stated defiantly, as she raised forward on the sectional. "Do you realize what you're asking me to do? I think not...Hell, I might as well take a knife and slice my throat right here on this damn imitation leather shit...Why should I tell them?...Everywhere you look nowadays, there's always a damn something or the other in the media about AIDS...So, why should I make the lone pilgrimage to misery?"

"You really don't feel any type of responsibility in warning your client about the possible sexual transmissions? What about their wives and families? What feelings, if any, do you have regarding your clients infecting others?"

"As I said before, why should I tell...Hell, you tell others about the dangers of sexual promiscuity and unprotected sex, do they listen to you? I seriously doubt it...And before you start the guilt trip into the land of my own personal anger...I'm beyond blaming anyone for any of my mistakes in this life. I left that stage of denial when I left Maryville years ago. I may never know just how I got the infection...It doesn't really matter to me anymore...I got it, OK. Knowing doesn't erase anything but gives more guilt...I refuse to give up living the way I have definitely grown accustomed. My quest, unlike yours, is not to try to save mankind...Oh, I'm really not bitter about having the infections nor with what life has already granted me nor the promise of a bitch of a death, I've just come too far to go back to nothing...Which is definitely what I lived with in that shoddy hell hole in East Tennessee...Tell me something, could you stop right this moment having lovers?"

Sebastian told me later that he felt as if he had the wind literally knocked from him. Before he realized it, an inner voice rudely betrayed him and proclaimed he already stopped accepting the physical affections of a lover.

"Well, you certainly deserve a medal of honor...But don't ask me to give up my sustaining life...When you have actually walked in my shoes, experienced the isolation and the alienation of other's affection, feeling like pure white trash, no. Make that lower than white trash only because you have never felt loved nor knew how to love...When you fear getting emotionally too close because you're scared that your weak vulnerable heart would crumble into tiny pieces and blown away without the slightest concern...I see couples walking together so damn close that it actually sickens me...Am I envious? Hell yes, I'm envious...I look into the mirror and wonder why someone hasn't ever loved me...You know, my prescriptions have all ran out...I haven't bothered getting any of them refilled...Why prolong my sentence?...My relief comes entirely from my cognac and my cocaine...Don't worry about me, Sebastian. I will continue to live my life to the fullest until my eyes are closed at God's own request."

PANELS

The words continue to make that resounding thud against my own wall of reality. I listened to the taped session several times wondering what I would do if it was me dealing with uncertain fate. Would I be as courageous as Maureen or would I simply cease fighting? What would I do?

The cool weather was fast approaching as the temperatures dropped into the mid sixties. The leaves had not completely changed to their indigenous colors due mostly to the sporadic seasonal climate changes in the weather. Sparse clothing gave way to the bundles as the sun fought to break from the circling clouds. One day, while we both glanced out the window at work, Sebastian stole the moment to talk. No one else had arrived for the staffing so we were able to have our moment alone. He said how he wanted to renew love back into his life. At least he was aspired to do so until he heard from someone from his past.

In a whispered voice, he told me that on the previous night he had received some not so good news. He had just turned off the bedside table lamp to sleep. His phone began to ring. A cursive thought left his dry parched lips as he glanced at the red illuminating numbers 2:00 a.m. that registered across his alarm clock. He wanted to ignore the invading nuisance. He tried burying himself deep inside his over-sized pillows. No relief. He was still too exhausted from the earlier actions of the day. Still, he tried to unwind and relax. But he had too much troubling his mind and the pressure mounted. Everywhere, it appeared, he turned was sadness. Powerless, he reached for the phone.

The voice on the other end was a familiar sound. It was Aaron, someone that Sebastian had known intimately, at least until he realized that there were no exploding stars in their relationship. There was simply no chemistry between the two.

I had met him while he was seeing Sebastian. Although Aaron was white, Aaron had physical features of being interracial. He had an olive complexion. His hair was a thick grade of shoulder length black hair that he often wore in a ponytail. Aaron's body was muscular and lean. He was an avid lover of body sculpturing. He was definitely an uncommon character of the farm working hand, which was the origin of his existence.

Aaron was born and raised in rural Waverly; Aaron possessed the boyish charm of the mischievous kindred soul, a rebel to his very roots. He was born within the matter of a few months before his parents divorced due to their irreconcilable differences. The only son of blue collar working parents, he later realized his gayness during his youth. He finally accepted the reality of having a troubled relationship with his occasional insane father and alcoholic emotionally displaced mother.

He eventually left his home in search of himself. Neither parent openly objected to their queer son leaving. His mother once told him in a heat of anger that her only son had died in her heart the day he told her he was gay. The father only stared.

Aaron and Sebastian eventually became closer only in friendship instead of the lover's role that Aaron still had his heart set. They would meet occasionally for a social cocktail. Aaron was much younger than Sebastian. He was somewhat immature especially in terms of his directions in life, in Sebastian's opinion.

I first met Aaron at a cocktail party that he and Sebastian attended together. From talking with him over a period of time, I soon realized that Aaron never accepted his own disposition in the gay world unless it was altered within the limited boundaries of the drag world. As he painstakingly developed the persona of his alter ego of Raquel, the personalities drastically changed the timid passive person into a wild, sexual vixen full of blissful confidence.

Sebastian admitted that he could never quite grasp the changes of personalities. He finally withdrew his association completely from maintaining further intimacy with Aaron. At least that's what he wanted Aaron to believe. In actual truth, Aaron wasn't masculine enough to feed Sebastian's hunger for a man. Instead, Sebastian craved the unknown burly type that possessed the very charisma that made Sebastian literally melt to his knees. He needed someone to take him. He wanted the misery of his life manhandled from within every inch of his bones. Nonetheless, Aaron stayed infatuated with Sebastian. He refused to believe that Sebastian could not possibly love him.

Through the years, Sebastian rarely encouraged any form of communication between the two unless it was extremely necessary. He thought his distance would circumvent Aaron's prevalent interests. Instead, Aaron felt his kindness trampled by him. Aaron once scorned Sebastian about being misled by his initial feelings for Aaron. He couldn't understand how Sebastian could so easily turn his affections off as one turned off the water faucet. He felt rejected by Sebastian who clearly refused to have sexual relations. Sebastian embarrassingly tried to explain his dilemma regarding

PANELS

his frightful fear of sex with anyone. Aaron balked angrily. Defiantly but calmly, Sebastian tried to encourage Aaron to look elsewhere for intimate affections since he himself wouldn't be able to satisfy Aaron's desires. Aaron cried. Sebastian found it as a way to manifest his attention further. They would argue and then depart in their angry and bitter silence.

However, Sebastian did say that as Aaron spoke on this particular night, he sounded non-challenging. There appeared a spark of interest on Sebastian's part this time. He casually informed Sebastian that another mutual friend had died. Sebastian wasn't shocked. He had known their friend had been secretly battling with AIDS. He was also a client of Sebastian. No one else was aware of their professional relationship except the significant other. Sebastian offered his services as pro bono to those battling with AIDS. Many of his clients were without any insurance and could not readily afford the services of any counseling services.

I also knew of this guy. He was a regular on the scene. I didn't know him well, usually just the surface. In the past, Randy had told his friends that he was suffering with a form of an inoperable brain cancer. Some people actually thought he was suffering from the Black Lung Disease as he had once earlier alluded to. He had refused to admit even to himself that he really had AIDS.

Randy was an easily recognizable character and many knew of him. As he constantly was admitted into the hospitals, he had somehow kept his trips secret to the majority of all that knew him personally. Similar to Tiffany, Randy had also graced the stage as a female impersonator. His staged name was Randii Alexander.

As his stages of his illness progressed, he no longer felt attractive as a man. He now looked thin and exhausted. His skin was now extremely pale. As an over worked transformation slowly evolved each evening, he painted his hallowed cheeks and always adorned a wig that covered his balding head. Walking proved a major chore as his once gracefully structured legs were quickly overcome with painful weakness. Her determination was only stronger. Although he no longer performed on stage, he was preparing for the performance of his life: street life.

Randy still socialized at the local hustler bars. In full drag, he became a she and sat gracefully perched on one of the squeaking splintered wooden stools around the semi-circled bar. Her fingers danced nervously about her glass of beer as her rhinestone-jeweled hands sparkled under the neon lights. She would smile as one of the bought boys carefully aimed his billiard cue towards the sporadic balls that lined the billiard table. He was a blond. Scars and tattoos covered his arms and naked chest. His hair was cut close to his head. He sported the appearance of a military man. He smiled back with his forbidding eyes. He knew that Randii was a man. He didn't care. To him, Randii was trick potential.

Randii was forever known to flirt passionately with the rugged men who individually treated her as a woman she wanted to be at least for that moment. She often laughed and threw her head back with assured pride. Her smile was always genuine and sincere forever hiding the devastating truth.

Randy told us that he had been in love once and only once. The particular lover almost cost him his life. Randy and his former mate Derek had lived mockingly as man and wife for several years even while Randy was caring for his ailing mother that lived with them. Randy was extremely jealous of losing Derek to anyone else. To Randy, Derek possessed everything that Randy had ever wanted in his man. He was virile in all degree. He was an attractive man with steel gray eyes and enormous biceps. He knew just how to make Randy feel like a woman. His only flaws were his drinking and his womanizing.

Derek never considered himself to be gay. He loved the appearance of the illusion of a woman. Men had a chance with him only if they remained in full drag during sexual intercourse. Randy had threatened numerous women and drag queens about flirting with her man in the past.

Tragically, the lover was killed in a motorcycle accident only hours after one of their occasional jealous rages. Derek was in a drunken stupor with the name Jack Daniels clearly written across his breath. He cycled the rain-slicked streets looking for Randy. Randy had stormed from their house minutes after one of their infamous fights.

Derek collided head on into a tour bus filled with wide-eyed passengers. He had swerved to barely miss another vehicle on lower Broadway near the Ryman Auditorium. He died instantly as his bloodied broken body lay sprawled across the wet asphalt pavement.

Randy had returned home after struggling with himself wondering if he was indeed wrong. He was in the process of dressing in his most sensual lingerie when the phone rang. He rushed to the phone expecting the voice on the other end to be Derek. Randy wanted to apologize to his lover for his anger. Randy never got the chance to correct the wrong.

Months later, Randy had gone to Baptist Hospital for another brain scan and a biopsy of his brain tissue. He had been earlier diagnosed with Progressive Multifocal Leukoencephalopathy. Countless times Randy had

PANELS

been given false hope as he continued to experience spontaneous cases of remission. Unfortunately, there were no approved treatments for his illness. His own doctors had hoped that several of the anti-HIV drugs could aid in his defense against the virus. Randy had tried Heparin and Cytosine Arabinsoide to reduce his symptoms. He had long refused to take the Alpha interferon combined with AZT because he feared someone accidentally noticing his medications and would probably think that he had AIDS. Everyone, he felt, knew of the characteristic large pills. The risk was far too great for him to take should others find out his secret.

Complications had set in and Randy arrested during the procedure. Sebastian closed his eyes tightly and said nothing for a moment. As he paused, I reached over and touched his hand lightly.

We talked for seemingly hours although only minutes before the others arrived. Sebastian was far from being cold and filled with apathy. He had realized earlier during the first thousand deaths exactly just how many AIDS patients had not wanted to be remembered as the shallow deformed skeleton badly mangled and sometimes even unrecognizable even to their closest friends. He began speaking about Greg and Richard and his eyes began to fill. He told me that he refused to think about Seth being ill. He missed Bradley.

Sebastian appeared tense as he remembered the alluring gawking eyes of the numerous spectators that attended David's funeral. Faces he had never seen before.

He long understood why cremations were becoming so widely accepted because of the disfiguring appearance. Sebastian reached inside his heart for all of the positive memories of those who had died. If he needed to grieve, he would do so in the private moments of solitude.

As with his fashion, Sebastian remembered Randy and the various times they had spent together as friends. He carefully recalled within the depths of himself the previous conversations with Randy. Sebastian smiled as a single torn sentimental tear fell down his face.

In conversations later, while the days and the months quickly passed, Sebastian began to experience migraines with a great deal of frequency. At first, he contributed the lobe attacks to his eyestrain. Perhaps he was reading too much or possibly working too much on his personal computer terminal too long into the early mornings. Whatever caused the headaches, he knew he had to decrease whatever the activity.

He attempted to reach different perspectives on life as he continued fighting his depression. He would have his high days and would scream of unadulterated happiness. He wanted to live. He wanted to take the next flight to some far away land where he would only see the beauty that life and God had to offer. He was determined to make vital changes in his life to erase his negative outlook. He simply wanted to live life to its fullest.

Cleo and I often called Sebastian nightly. At least once a week, we would dine together. As a rule, the conversations consisted of light matters. Anything morbid was not allowed to penetrate into our fleeting moments. Each had chosen to keep our friends' memory alive in their minds. Each wanted to forget our cruel vehicles of death. But, Seth was still alive and lingering in all of our minds. Cleo fought back her words about Seth's deteriorating health. She feared pushing Sebastian further off into the deep.

His inner self remained in conflict. He was literally buried underneath the deaths and misery of others including his close friends. On his low days, his temper constantly flared. He later would credit his outbursts as being partly due to anxiety and sudden bouts with triumphant depression.

"Michal, I don't feel that there's any laughter in my life…not anymore."

"Sebastian, you just need to get out and let loose and live."

"I don't think I know how to live anymore. Everywhere I turn, no matter how positive I try to be, misery takes over. I'm a failure."

"You need a man." I laughed. "That's your problem."

"You're right…. I need a man. But instead, all I can find is a pair of britches. A true man appears to be out of my reach."

"You know what they say 'A good man is hard to find but a hard man is good to find.'"

"Not for me. I have decided to leave my desires behind." Sebastian turned to me. The most solemn look I have ever seen on his face appeared. "I have evolved into total asexuality. I become tense and rigid at the mere thought of anyone touching me. I feel that I could no longer trust my health to others."

He told me about his tortuous nights that left him often drenched with his own sweat. His dreams left him submerged in unclear fear and doubts. His nightmares called him by his birthright name. Sebastian felt alone in the world even with Cleo and I at his side. The same world that constantly changed much too fast for the troubled man.

Sebastian told me how he was beginning to feel confined to his surroundings. He soon felt imprisoned in a world that he no longer loved nor wanted to accept. He told me of an entry he made one night in his weathered leather journal:

PANELS

Incarceration

To those of us that have actually experienced life in any form of confinement, though we're all confined in a true sense, the truly imprisoned are fully aware of the bringing forth of their potentials. Rather, the actuality of their inner powers and beauty.

As in the moment of truth of each life that we first realize the depths of power, so it is, possibly that is when the moment of truth arrives. In either sense, that's when man comprehends life as it really is, without the glitter of tinsel and showcase lights. Man discards the perspective vision and takes hold of the prospective view. Firmly. In a sense, it is closely related to being resurrected from the dead and given another chance at life. Generally, the individual's views are altogether different

Through trial and error, with abundant time to contemplate the advantages and the equal disadvantages, we find it easier, once we plot our course in life, to steer a straight course. Thanks to the bitterness of confinement, whether physical or emotional. Like all bitter pills it does more help than an agreeable one.

Incarceration is designed primary for rehabilitation, when this is achieved, only the imprisoned will know.

Several days after Bradley's memorial, the continued losses were insurmountably difficult with outcome appearing undeniably dark. Above the others, I noticed Cleo visibly shaken each time I was with her. She eventually told me during lunch at Calypso Café recently of her battling with depression.

"I'm fighting with thin air. All I want to do is cry and scream. Sometimes I close my eyes at night praying the good Lord will take me before the morning."

"Cleo, sweetheart, you can not keep on living this way…You got to get some help before you really go off the deep end," I said.

"Believe you me, I am trying…I have become one of those crazy people you and Sebastian sees. I hope your drugs are better than those damn placebos I'm given." Cleo laughed.

"Have you spoken to Sebastian?"

"Yeah right, are we talking about the same guy? Sebastian is so caught up in himself right now, he sees no one else in his horizon...No, baby boy, you are my main crutch right now...Please don't ever tell Sebastian that I said that. I mean, I know he still cares but he's not..." She stopped suddenly. Her eyes wore that familiar glassy drug induced glare of emptiness.

"All these years of schooling and I'm still at a loss as to what to say to calm your fears...I really don't know what to say."

"Don't say anything...just squeeze my hand and maybe both our fears can be relieved...at least for the moment."

"A precious moment it will be."

"Michal...I really hate to bring this up...but it has really been eating at me for the longest."

"What is it?"

"I want you to be honest with me about something." She paused. Her eyes focused on me. "You already knew about Bradley didn't you?"

"What about him?"

"About him having AIDS?"

"Yeah...Sebastian also knew...I didn't say anything to you or anyone else because he made us promise."

"For Christ's sake! I'm not just anyone...I thought I was a friend...I thought I was a part of this pact."

"You are, and will always be a part of us."

"I knew already...he had told me." Cleo reached for another cold stale fry. Her voiced lowered to a whisper. "I even knew about him getting arrested for slugging that old guy."

"Well, is there anything you don't know?"

"Yeah...why did you guys leave him hanging out dry in jail?" She stirred her iced tea. "Why did you guys walk away from him?"

"We didn't walk away from him. The next day, Sebastian and I went to the Criminal Justice Center to see Bradley. At first, he didn't want to see us. We refused to go away and Sebastian became persistent with the guards warning them of possible chemical reactions from Bradley's neurotic medications. The guards knew us so they thought we were on the up and up. Although we were lying about Bradley being our client, we risked the jailers knowing the actual truth."

"Man, I know he was pissed at you two for the longest. He said he felt like you guys had betrayed him. He said you treated him like some damned mental patient."

"That would explain a lot. Bradley finally spoke with us. He was still angry.. Regardless, he was still one of us." I offered my glass as the waitress poured the tea. "Hours later, I felt somewhat closer to him for the first time since I have known him. For once, he was real, maybe even honest. Sebastian wanted to post his bail but Bradley would have none of it. He went ballistic when I asked him if Jeff knew where he was...Bradley constantly screamed that he would be all right and made us promise that we would not say anything to anyone of his whereabouts."

"That sounds like Bradley." Cleo continued eating. "But who told Jeff?"

"I haven't the foggiest idea. I just know it wasn't me! Anyway, the next day, I went alone but he was not there. He had been transferred to the jail ward at General Hospital. In order to see him, I had to lie ."

"God may forgive you that one time."

"As he lay strapped and handcuffed to the gurney, Bradley told me about his headaches that pulsated from the deep crevices of his head. He said the pain made him nauseated and light headed with anxious feelings."

"Did he ever tell you that he later thought the blows from the rangers possibly brought about the onset of vertigo?"

"No, he didn't. But it doesn't surprise me. I saw how hard he was hit."

"I suggested that he sue the bastard but he thought it would take too long. That the city would drag it out forever and a day."

"I even lied to Dr. Raffanti. I didn't tell him that Bradley was a friend. I led him to believe that I was assigned to the prisoner. Dr. Raffanti paused after looking at the chart. He took a deep breath, put his reading glasses in his left breast pocket, and went to Bradley...I stood outside the room where I heard their conversation."

"What was said? I know you're not supposed to tell me, but..."

"Does it really matter now? Anyway, Dr. Raffanti asked Bradley why was he telling people that he had AIDS. Dr. Raffanti told him that there wasn't much immunosuppresion and that there was no swelling in his lymph nodes, at least, not enough to be alarmed about...But, stress appeared to be his greatest threat."

"So, what happened next? Was he glad to hear that or what?"

"Our dear Bradley raised his voice. He told the doctor not to play him for some fool...He knew damn well what being exposed to the AIDS virus definitely meant...it meant death." I stopped long enough to sip on my watered down tea. "Doctor Raffanti kept his voice lowered and asked him if he realized that everyone HIV positive did not die. He told Bradley that he should try to educate himself about the real symptoms and take control of his real problems—Next thing I knew, the doctor was at the doorway telling Bradley that he had too many actual sick patients that needed and appreciated his care...He released Bradley the next morning to go back to jail. Then as an after thought, Dr. Raffanti turned back around and told him to take his advice and seek other professional help...He suggested my boss, Dr. Sanders."

"From the Cooperative? You better watch it or your boss is going to think all of your friends' elevators don't ever leave the first floor, especially after working with David and then Bradley." Cleo grinned.

"Well, later, Sanders told him the same thing: to stop swallowing in his drowning sea of self pity and doubt, get off his ass and live."

"Are you trying to say he didn't have AIDS?" Cleo sulked in her chair, eyes wide open.

"He had tested positive for the virus but he was not swallowing in AIDS."

"That bastard...that vain ass bastard took his life to avoid getting sick!"

"Sometimes, he and I would kick back and shoot the breeze. He really did surprise me a few times. I had always thought he was so shallow but...I found out several things about his interpretations of life. Death, he said, was indeed treacherous. The deaths of the others had scared him. He tried desperately to erase the vivid pictures of Gregory and especially David. He craved attention as a hungry vulture craved the dying prey."

"But was it really attention that he wanted or was it simply the uncontested love that he himself could not rightfully identify?"

"Cleo, my love, that is a very good question. The answer we will never know."

Hours later, while in the comfort of her home, Cleo and I sat inside the bay window sipping our glass of burgundy wine as he entered the room. She had been waiting for the moment as her smile reflected her heart. The image of renowned grace and sophistication with her slender fingers caressing the smooth glass stem constantly twirling the warm liquid around the opening in a teasing manner. She was wearing a gold brocade suit with beaded embroidered pockets and jeweled buttons. Although her matching lined slim skirt was waist less, her sleek figure was still very visually alluring

"Seth, darling, how was your day?" Cleo looked into his eyes and wistfully smiled.

"Nothing to write home about...why?" Seth became quite curious. He appeared to study the mysterious expression on the face before him. He turned and looked at me. I dropped my head. "What's up?"

"Oh, nothing really, dear...I just wanted to know how you was doing."

PANELS

Cleo smiled. "Can't a friend be concern about another friend?"

After a few more minutes of idle time consuming chit chat, Seth stood directly over her, placed his bony hands lightly on the tops of both of her hands cautiously as if he was touching fine Spanish china. He looked directly into her moist green eyes demanding for the mystery to quickly unravel. Smiling rather innocently, Cleo stared at the stem of her glass that she continued holding, took another sip and then spoke of her wishes to him.

"You, my sweets, are up to something." Seth leaned over and kissed her forehead. "So, spill it."

"Do you remember what I had wanted to do with this big old house?" Cleo became radiant. "Remember how I'd drawn out the blueprints renovating this antebellum home for individual offices on the ground floor and a small art gallery on the main level."

Cleo had wanted to invest in limited art pieces that wasn't readily available anywhere else in Nashville. She wanted to display the likes of Alex Echo, Michel Delacroix, and Asoma. Edward had suggested that the venture was a viable investment and had fully backed her financially before their separation.

Seth listened to her words carefully for any underlying signs. "Yeah, I remember...and you are telling me this because?" Seth paused. "What are you trying to say?"

"Seth, you know me all too well, don't you?" Cleo walked over to the portable bar and poured another glass of wine. She smiled discreetly towards me. Then she turned to him.

"I called you over here for a reason." Cleo took a deep sip. "I want the man of my life living with me. You no longer have to suffer those avalanching bills and that outrageous lease on that West End flat. I can help you and you can help me."

"So, Michal, are you also part of this ploy?"

"I'm just an innocent bystander." I tipped my glass to him.

"I don't know about you being totally innocent; I'm sure you have a hand in this somewhere." Seth turned back to Cleo. "I can't do that to you. I mean...I'm flattered but you can't be serious."

"I have never been as serious as I am on this." Cleo placed her hand softly against his lips, "I need you here beside me, and please don't say no."

I continued to sip my wine and smiled at the both of them. She had succeeded.

Seth didn't immediately move in with Cleo. In fact, he toyed with the concept for several weeks before the event actually materialized then only after his third bout with pneumocystis carinnii pneumonia.

I remember all too well hearing how Cleo had tried calling Seth's home for a couple of days without receiving any answers. It was common knowledge that they always spoke on the phone no less than twice a day. All of a sudden the calls stopped. Instead, it was now being answered with a recorded message of trouble on the line.

After continuing to dial his number for what she considered the thousandth time, she was beside herself with worry. Thinking perhaps she dialed the wrong number, although she knew the number by heart, she said she thumbed frantically at the pages of her Rolodex. She began to fear the worst.

"I know you think I'm probably making a big deal out of this...but something ain't right...you know that." Cleo refused to calm down.

"You're probably right, but we can't just go over there and storm down his door. By the way, how much of the bupropion are you taking?"

"Hell, Michal, I'm only taking it in small doses...and I know you think that I'm freaking out because of it. But I'm not."

"Well, two of the side effects are indeed agitation and excitement. But, believe me, I'm not making light of your fears."

"Michal, I have called the hospitals. I have called every one of you guys...and nothing...where the hell is he? Can you go with me to his apartment? I just gotta see that he's okay."

"I wish I could go but I can't get out of my next session...maybe Sebastian can go with you. I think he's available. Want me to check?"

"Yeah, and call me back as soon as you can...Now I ain't gonna wait all day."

"Give me a few seconds to get to Sebastian...Cleo, honey, I need you to relax and calm down. You won't be any good to Seth or any one else unless you chill."

"I thought about contacting Seth's family. But I wondered if that was such a great idea to unnecessarily alert his family when I really had no proof of anything. I doubt seriously if he is with any of his family. Still, I can feel my heart racing and skipping out of my body." Cleo was full of fear and concern.

Frantically, Cleo eventually was able to persuade Sebastian to go with her

PANELS

after he left work to go by Seth's West End flat. She had to be assured of his safe status.

Later, as they drove across the Victory Memorial Bridge toward the James Robinson Parkway, silence overwhelmed them. Cleo sat trembling slightly in total silence, as she nervously jingled the copy of Seth's apartment keys against her lap. Sebastian placed his hand momentarily on her perspiring clasped hands.

Cleo abruptly bolted from the parked car seconds before Sebastian killed the engine. With her keys tightly gripped, she quickly ran up the black-white marble stairs of the Jacksonian. Sebastian tried running in pursuit behind the thundering clacking sound of her high heels. Using her own key, she opened Seth's door without haste. Sebastian ran closely behind her with labored breathing.

Cleo told me afterwards how the vision of his place still haunts her. The rooms were all dark. The interior temperature made them both clammy. Clothes and numerous newspapers were scattered about the floor, spilling out into the hall. The path led to his closed bedroom door. Roaches crawled from within the cracks in the walls toward foul smelling plates of discarded molded food. The air smelled of the spoiled food and the smell of human waste.

Cleo and Sebastian stood speechless and dazed in the middle of the filth. They became mesmerized by the vile conditions. Sebastian began to fear the unknown. He told me that he noticed the unruly chaos and realized that something was definitely wrong but said nothing to Cleo to further alarm her.

Suddenly, Cleo ran quickly to the closed bedroom door. As the door opened, she screamed. Sebastian turned from the dining room and hurried to her side. Seth appeared extremely lethargic and barely breathing. Sebastian checked Seth's vital signs. His pulse was exceptionally faint. Seth didn't respond to his name being yelled out or any other stimuli. Cleo was silent. As she sobbed, her face became white with shock.

Sebastian raised Seth's limp body to an upright position. He immediately realized his friend was burning with a fever. His clothes and bedding were soaked with his liquid waste.

Sebastian picked the phone off the floor that was only inches from Seth's grasp. The phone was dead. There was neither sound nor dial tone emitting from the earpiece. Near the phone receiver was a disconnect notice from the phone company for failure to pay the previous month's bill. Sebastian banged the receiver angrily several times hard against the cradle. Disgusted,

Sebastian threw the phone against the distant wall. The phone made contact with the concrete wall and fell to the floor with a resounding ringing thud.

Sebastian immediately ordered Cleo to go into the kitchen for ice cubes and whatever towels she could find. They needed to bathe Seth's body with ice water to bring his raging temperature down. Sebastian quickly ran from the apartment.

Sebastian ran next door and banged fitfully on the door until a middle-aged black woman appeared. She yelled for him to stop before she called the police. He yelled back that he needed to use the phone to call for an ambulance for his dying friend next door.

Curiously, she opened her door enough to see his face. After seeing the urgency in his eyes, she gradually opened her door. She nervously pointed him toward the direction of her phone. Close behind his heels, with her cane slightly raised, she was full of questions about Seth. Sebastian continued to talk to the emergency operator. He prayed they were not too late for Seth.

Seth was extremely sick when he was initially found. He was close to death. Cleo, Sebastian, and some of Seth's family, and I were standing around his bed when he finally awoke. Seth had been slightly delirious due to his fever. Tubes covered his face. He received oxygen, and the IVs were fully opened. One particular flexible tube passed through his nasal passage into his lungs to obtain specimens of his lung fluid and tissue. His surroundings were quite sterile.

Seth grasped in panic. He really couldn't see anyone as clearly as he heard his or her voice. His eyes as well as his spleen had been affected by the pneumonia. Seth grimaced. He wondered how many more bouts with pneumonia he would endure before he would lose.

Due to his infections being so severe, steroids were prescribed in addition to the medication. Unfortunately, before Seth could fully digest his latest news of despair, tests results returned positive for Cytomegalovirus, a virus that was often associated with AIDS. Seth's health status was worsening.

The team of physicians overseeing his case discretely warned others about the dangers of exchanging saliva when kissing Seth directly on the mouth. Doctors admitted they were not positive about the possible transmission by actual kissing, but they suggested the family and friends take no chances. No one refused to discontinue their physical affection or place a distance between him and themselves.

I was with Seth when Dr. Raffanti warned Seth he might eventually lose some of his sight. Seth fell deeper into depression. The doctor further warned

PANELS

Seth that should he prove too sensitive to either drugs intravenously, he might possibly receive medication injected directly into his eyes.

In his lone moments, Seth felt as if he truly had leprosy. He had a catheter inserted, which proved both painful and emotionally destructive. He soon felt useless. He felt as if he was a sideshow freak for others to gawk at.

Seth's outlook was fast becoming bleak. He realized long before his various eye exams just how bad his vision was. He already experienced objects that appeared to be obstructing his field of vision. Life was also fast becoming blurred, as shadows continued to dance between his mind and reality. Seth became complacent. He wondered often if his constant chest pain was worth the trouble to live.

Four weeks after his initial admission on the hospital's eighth floor, and after much mental wrestling with reasoning against Cleo's demands, Seth was finally discharged. She still wanted him to live with her in Edgefield. Sebastian, Cleo, and I packed all of Seth's possessions and moved the items into her house. Seth's family arranged for his baby grand piano to be moved with his belongings.

The thought of the move scared Seth. He wondered just how long his relationship with Cleo would last under the rather strange arrangements. Seth also wondered how either of the two would endure the accompanying stress levels that would surely mount as his sickness increased. He realized he was dying, but honestly wondered if Cleo accepted the fact. Seth loved Cleo unconditionally and never wanted to hurt her or destroy her love for him. He worshiped her.

The street had trees in curved intertwining rows. They arched over the streets. Near their house was a public park. There were a few steps to climb to enter the park. Etched deep into the concrete steps was the shape of an upturned horseshoe. Across the imprint, on the raised platform, a green plaque rested, which read "East Park, Originally called Edgefield Park, this park was developed as a result of the Great 1916 Fire. Rededicated by Mayor Richard H. Fulton on May 14, 1983." Even the destroyed can live again.

The year was 1998. We began to laugh again. We began to trust again. We began to realize that life was indeed a gift. No longer was life to be taken for granted. Each day was actually welcomed and cherished. Above all else, we realized that if we were to survive then we must also begin to love ourselves.

Unfortunately, Cleo suffered a major blow. Her father died after suffering a massive heart attack in her Spanish homeland. The villagers were not able to respond timely to revive him. Within two months, Cleo and Theresa returned to us with her mother Helena. Seth stayed with me until she returned.

Grief is indeed a strange animal. It strikes us differently and at different times. I decided to stop by The Gallery on Russell. Everything was quite dark and quiet. The last employee had left the premises hours ago. When I found her, Cleo was alone.

Light danced mysteriously off the interior structures, causing brief shadows to give dimensional effect to the various displayed pieces of art. Underneath a mural was the familiar piano.

She was alone. I watched Cleo slowly sip on her white wine. I called out to her. She gave no response. Her eyes appeared waxed as she stared out in the openness of her life. I decided to leave her to her self-imposed solitude confinement. I left.

Days later, she did tell me that she awoke from one of her frequent mental lapses and found herself sitting behind the Steinway. She said she was startled. One of the common associations that she shared with her lover was with the ivory keys. Playing brought back too much pain to endure. She wanted to push herself away from the piano and leave. Instead, her fingers started softly caressing the ivories while careful not to disturb the serenity of her surroundings. Still holding her wine glass with her left hand, she began to massage the polished keys with the fingers of her right hand. She took a long swallow from the delicate crystal. Seconds later, she angrily flung the fragile stem in the far corner. She began playing the piano.

The notes were now echoing through the empty halls. Her voice soon penetrated the silence. Cleo's smooth articulated words became clouded with emotion.

"I stopped and slammed the cover closed. It made a loud resounding thud. All I could do then was to cup my face in my hands and cry. Michal, I didn't realize I had company."

"Was it Theresa?" I asked.

"No, it was Mama."

"Did you scare the poor soul or what?"

"She pulled my head against her breast and asked me if the pain was still tearing at me. She spoke in our native tongue."

"Did you answer her?"

"Did I ever! I said 'Is it still? Mama,' I said, 'it's never left me. It's only getting worse. It's like the ocean rushing hurriedly at me. I'm standing out in the middle of the water and the waves are coming at me. Not allowing you to catch your breath. But you still see the mountain of pain in massive waves building and coming at you. At times, I'm afraid to stay here. Watching, waiting, and even wanting the wave of death to hurry and arrive. I want it to stop taunting me. But it doesn't listen…instead, it waits, and as it waits, it tears my heart into fragmented insignificant pieces that the wind blows away.'"

Cleo said she continued to rest her head on her mother's soothing body. Cleo found comfort, as she felt her mother's heart beating against her ear. She closed her eyes briefly. Cleo paused, after having found reassurance in her mother's familiar arms. She was her mother's little scared child once again.

"I really don't know what to say," Helena said. "I'm learning myself on just how painful someone's absence can be. I remember reading your countless letters about your life here. I used to wonder just why you had invited those people into your life, but then I finally realized that they must be special people. I may not know just how exactly you may feel, but I know that you do hurt. I know how I had wished that I too had died with my Raul. If I was dead, then the hurt would die as well; it would vanish. However, is that really what your friends would want you to do? You have them still alive in your heart, right where it matters the most. No one can ever take those memories away from your heart. No one." Helena lowered her head and kissed her daughter's forehead. Tears formed in the corners of their eyes.

"Mama, how did you manage to watch the one that you had loved the most lowered into the ground? How did you manage to say bye to Papa?"

"Truthfully, I closed my eyes. I refused to believe that your father was in that casket. Instead, I imagined him somewhere behind me as usual protecting my shoulders from the abusive sun. I imagined that his massive hands were the ones that were so carefully massaging my trembling shoulders. I refused to even look upon his grave for that would mean that I had accepted his death. Do you know, several days after the burial, I still found myself holding his nightclothes against my face as I slept. I still felt his warmness and the smell of his manly body laying against my own…Later, in the night, I awoke with the cruel hand of reality shaking me. I would then find myself very alone in the dark room still clutching on his pillow…I was furious with embarrassment. Sometimes I would just cry and cry and cry. I cursed the damned darkness wishing your father to return to my arms. But I knew that this miracle would not happen. Therefore, I must make myself go on. The worst part of death appears to be the ignorance and not really knowing what is on the other side of the journey. What actually proves to be reality or myth. Your other friend that is still alive. I won't tell you to stay away from him. Your heart wouldn't allow that. If you need to, be there for him even until his end. I wouldn't want a daughter to stop loving anyone because the person was dying. Ask God for your strength to endure your pain; I have already asked him for myself."

"Mama, I worry about Seth a great deal. I don't know if I'm expecting him to hurry and die or to become sicker or whatever. Somehow, I know that I'll eventually lose him as I have the others. You may not completely understand what I'm about to say, but then again, you may wholeheartedly understand all of my emotions that I'm battling with. We all became extremely close, as our friendship flourished. I know, it makes no sense, but each instilled in me hidden qualities I didn't even know I had. Don't get me wrong, you and grandmother taught me about the duties of being a wife, but they taught me how to be a true woman without being afraid to express my emotions. I still laugh while remembering how each brought out the real woman in me, a frightened little girl. I laugh also whenever I think just how naïve I actually was when I first married Edward. Mama, Edward never loved me. Never. My gay friends actually taught me about bonding and trust. Each showed me individually how someone so different could love someone like me without much in return except my honesty. They never wanted anything from me except my sincere friendship. They taught me that a true man was only masculine when he comfortably displayed his genuine weakness without feeling threatened. I didn't give a damn about whom they slept with, as long as they were happy with themselves. I loved those guys with all of my heart. Mama, I could talk to them whenever I was feeling lonely. I literally died when the first one even mentioned that he thought he had AIDS…Mama, no one deserves AIDS. After talking with a few that lived with the virus, my breath was literally knocked from me, as some told me how their own families disowned them, left them abandoned on the heartless cold streets. Mama, this was their own blood, where is the humanity that we hear so much about? Jesus, Himself, never walked away from anyone, but those that use His name as a shield forever spur hatred for those with AIDS. Why?…but, nonetheless, I felt safe with my friends. They guarded me with their shiny armor of unconditional love forever protecting me from harm." Cleo cried. "But now, they're gone…or leaving."

"Not really. True, they are physically gone and you cannot see them. Nevertheless, you will always have them where it matters the most: deep

PANELS

inside your heart. I keep Raul there, I close my eyes, and he always appears. Love will always keep them alive." Cleo said her mother took her into her arms and kissed her tearstained cheek.

A portrait titled *Portrait of Madame M* graced the gray marbleized mantel. It was of a young woman with alluring powers. She was in full control and appeared to have captured the divine elegance of life. A pair of Italian tortures stood guard on each of the opposite sides of the massive room. An array of bright flowing cut flowers overfilled the various methodically arranged Baccarat vases. Art deco styled furnishings sparsely filled the room.

In Cleo's face, there were a hint of both a little princess and a little peasant girl. Her passive features remained intact and hidden behind her usual stoic smile. Her eyes constantly glinted sporadically about the room.

Seth was reclined in one of the huge chaise lounges, deliberately carefully choosing his words. With the numbness brought about by the combination of his medication and his grief, he feared losing his grasp with his own reality.

Cleo, on the other hand, deceptively appeared semi-captivated by the various art pieces that she had just had delivered to the studio. Several new pieces such as the Mikkio Watanabe's *Nu Couches II*, Lu Hong's *Summer Rain*, Tarkay's, Azene's, and one by Michael Eisemann. Cleo had already sold *Paris Café*, the *Red Tulips*, and *Nu Couches II*. She told us how she had admired the later work having found the piece extremely sensual and warm. They were nude bodies with souls.

Cleo realized the chances she gambled with in introducing these specific art styles to her patrons but her intuition had never failed her in the past. Cleo had a certain flair that tripled her initial investment into the gallery that later secured her place among the other established art dealers. She had made a mental note to call her customers to arrange scheduled delivery of their investments.

I have spoken with Seth in the past often about his current struggle with his health. He would always look away as if in shame. Quietly, his voice always lowered to a whisper. Seth told me how he had accepted and had even finally realized that his only certainty was one that he could not escape. Seth tried not to concern himself too intensely with his wayward sibling's death. It only threatened to wear the remaining resistance levels down. All in all, Seth still missed and loved Bradley. He will always love him. Perhaps for that very reason, each moment seemed in retrospect so uniquely memorable. His own destiny kept him here with his friends, which the fact alone failed to give him any other deep satisfaction.

In various conversations, we all appeared somewhat generally tended to be dismissive about some of our former close friends. Few of us were still present and accounted for, but where were the others who had pledged their undying friendly intercourse?

As the days drew near, I noticed that Seth's conversations appeared more and more of simple monologues. At times, his wordings were clear juxtaposed and frightfully fragmented. Dementia became his common bedfellow. Seth's memory no longer could be relied on.

Sebastian slept over often to give Cleo temporary relief. Sebastian would mention to me the details of her burning herself out as well as her growing frustration. Cleo, however, would never face defeat. Her choice was far more than a mission. We felt that Cleo was obsessed with Seth.

Patricia and Ruth occasionally stopped by the house either to assist with Seth or to take Cleo away from the house for several hours while Sebastian or one of Seth's own family members cared for Seth. Cleo was forever hesitant about leaving Seth behind.

In certain times of his delirious state, Seth would continue to ask for his brother's presence. I personally witnessed these changes. In his feeble mind, he appeared to have understood Bradley's absence as being his usual act of distancing himself from Seth out of fear. He refused to believe that it could have been out of hatred or alienation of his affectionate love. As if forgotten the actual reality, Seth worried constantly about Bradley's health.

Once, in a clear state of mind, he spoke of Cleo and Bradley's relationship. Seth had imagined Cleo's obvious disdain for Bradley had stemmed for her hatred for him deserting the others. Seth said he felt that she had indeed masked the truth as she herself often became livid as she described her vast emotional anger towards Bradley. She and Seth would argue that Bradley had tried to escape reality through his vanity.

Secretly to many of us, she admitted that she had fooled herself into believing her own fallacy of her dislike for Bradley. As she continually rode the horse of deception, Cleo secretly had known of Bradley's health status long before the others had known. When she told me the complete story, I was quite surprised at her knowledge.

"So, why do you think he chose you?" I asked.

"I stopped second guessing Bradley years ago. Too much trauma! Anyway he did. He actually confided in me after we had met for cocktails at

PANELS

Sperry's one raining evening," she replied.

"Was he drunk?"

"Are you kidding? You know he could put away his liquor. No, he was quite aware of his words to me."

"So, what did you say after he told you?" I asked.

"What could I say? I was still in shock that this man was actually talking to me about this crap. I just listened. I mean, of all the years I've known him, this is the first time he was talking straight with me without the bull…I really do think he was absolutely sincere in wanting me to know."

"Did you ever think that perhaps he was using you as a mule to tote the load to Seth?" I asked.

"Maybe, but do you know what? I was not the one to take anything like that back to Seth. Be for real, I mean, somewhere I have to draw the line," she ended.

She went on to describe the rest of their evening. During the conversation, she later reached across the table and placed her hand lightly on his trembling hands after he had disclosed barely above a whisper that a recent lover of his had died. He wasn't for certain but felt strongly that it was due to AIDS. As the thoughts circled her ransacked mind, she felt that for the first time since she had known Bradley that the hurt that actually existed within his eyes were indeed real. For the first time since she had known him, she finally felt close to him.

She felt that his words seemed sincere and frightfully honest. His pain was even real. She wondered to herself questioning his decision to tell her instead of one of the others in the circle. Why had he chosen her to open himself and allow her to penetrate his usually well-guarded fortress? Nonetheless, he had opened himself to her.

While Bradley softly cried, Cleo's own eyes started watering. Cleo realized quite soon where the conversation was heading. The all too familiar remorseful tone and the wording before the obvious was finally said. The knot inside her stomach grew and gnawed at her even as he spoke. Finally, the dreadful second arrived as he told her of his own recent diagnosis. Their hands squeezed tightly around the other. Initial silence. The knot grew larger and painful in her stomach.

Before she could ask him if he had told any of the others, he reached over and tenderly stroked a lock of her fallen hair from her face as he wiped away her tears that fell onto his fingers. Looking straight into her swelling eyes, he pleaded with her not to tell anyone especially Seth. He wanted to tell them in his own way. Choking on her own emotions, she agreed with him that it was not her place to disclose his secret to anyone. She promised to abide.

Cleo said that Bradley was extremely bitter not because his former lover had died but because he hadn't bothered to tell him that he was infected with the virus. Whether Bradley was actually experiencing psychosomatic illnesses or the real thing, he felt certain that he was slowly becoming sick. There hadn't been any actual symptoms but nonetheless he knew that he had the dreadful bug. Although he couldn't bring himself to tell others at the moment, somehow he felt he could trust her. He felt it was essentially necessary to tell someone of his predicament. Bradley knew all too well how AIDS had lived around him and his playmates. "But does anyone really have any damn hindsight?" Bradley smirkingly asked.

Cleo always remembered that night of his confession. The night that they walked hand in hand in the midst of the mild downpour of Nature's tears. The night that he had entrusted in her a truth that was so devastating that her heart was torn again but at a different place. The burden proved far too heavy indeed while it rested upon her frail shoulders. But, she had made a promise to him.

Cleo said she became angry with him because he had known of his status for well over two years but had not entrusted the others within the circle to allow them to share his fears. She later realized that even until the moment of his last breath did he make his own decisions deciding whatever fate or destiny he would have. She never really hated him. The love she had for him became devastated. Countless times, the words had almost escaped her when others came to his defense about his habits. She fought hard within the depths of her own core to keep the truth from being known. Her stoic mask appeared bitter with the realization encompassed with the deception.

Although she was caught totally off guard hearing the news of his demise, Cleo was surprisingly relieved when the actual phone call came. No longer did she have to carry the burden of his truth. She was far from being thrilled in the revelation of his death. Tears still settled in the corners of her eyes refusing to fall at Bradley's bittersweet victory. Still, Cleo finally closed her eyes. She smiled while realizing that once again, Bradley had even controlled his manner of his destiny: his death.

After placing the phone back onto the cradle, she returned to Seth's bedside. She watched him sleep peacefully. Almost for the first time in several days, there appeared neither frightful nightmares nor unruly dreams haunting his still body, just peace.

PANELS

The next morning after Bradley's death, Seth looked into Cleo's troubled face searching for answers without quite knowing the questions. Cleo tried avoiding his sunken stares. She refused to accept the chore placed uncomfortably in her hands. She prayed for strength and for the reinforcement of his family to arrive. She kept extremely quiet. We all kept silent. Who would tell Seth?

Nashville can be eminently beautiful in the fall season. Much was the case on that particular autumn day. The leaves changed. Some fell crisply onto the earth's cold hardening ground. The colors of Nature strongly resembled the ardent sun that was now setting. Mixtures of bright blues and oranges that blended as abstracting pieces across the greenish brown earth. Stillness and serenity prevailed as the brisk wind that rustled against the challenging lives. Cleo finally told Seth.

We all remembered how hard the memorial service for Bradley was for Seth. The pitiful sight of Seth's fragile body that stared endlessly as Bradley's portrait was displayed before him. Bradley's services were held at his parents' lavishly spacious Woodmont estate only a few miles from the Jewish Temple.

During one of our many chats on religion, Bradley had considered religion to be of a personal and private nature. He felt that he had not lived his life according to his Creator's words and refused to be remembered with vain senseless words at his death.

Standing erect and poised with the pain of his agonizing grief, Benjamin recited the Kaddsih for his son. There were no longer any evidence of anger in his voice. He had accepted his son's peace. All of the mirrors in the house were covered completely draped with black cloths. The spacious antiques were previously removed from the study and replaced with rough wooden crates for those in attendance to sit on.

The sealed Gothic urn rested carefully on a soft crinkled gauzed wrapped pedestal in front of his portrait. Candles burned throughout the room reflecting off the various solemn facial expressions. Together we prayed for Bradley's safe journey bidding him a fond farewell.

In less than a month, Seth was admitted to Vanderbilt Hospital. He was suffering from another bout of pneumocystis carinii pneumonia. After clearly assessing his troubled respiratory distress, the emergency medical technicians started him on oxygen hoping to correct the shortness of his breathing possibly due to the poor oxygenation of the blood in his lungs.

During the racing transport, he coded. One of the technicians immediately administered cpr until his own heart began to beat. Seth went totally limp and appeared lifeless. His coloration changed quickly from pale to a dark clammy shade. Actually a bluish discoloration of both his skin and his mucous membranes due to the excessive concentration of the reduced hemoglobin in his blood. He appeared extremely cyanotic. His body was incredibly hot as his temperature soared upwards past 104 and rising. Sweat mixed with his collecting perspiration made the body difficult to hold onto the stretcher during the tumultuous ride. His heart rapidly failed again. The medical technician constantly called out his name refusing to allow him to give up his life.

The siren whirled madly as the ambulance raced against Death. IVs were constantly being started as monitors were wired to his body to observe all vital signs. Mike Porter, medical technician for the past thirty years, had never lost a patient and was determined that Seth would not be his first casualty. With his massive strength, the compression lasted until Seth finally responded. In the process, three of Seth's ribs were cracked. Battling exhaustion, the resuscitator was started. The driver continued radioing the status of his failing health to the Vanderbilt's emergency room personnel for further instructions.

Cleo and Patricia anxiously followed closely behind the wailing ambulance. As Patricia drove, she tried to console Cleo whom was still hysterical after finding Seth's lifeless body. Cleo screamed at Seth pleading with him to live. Inside the car, she banged her head hard against the car's window while blaming herself for not being there for him. Fearing that she would either break the glass window or end up with a possible concussion, Patricia grabbed her with her free right hand and pulled her trembling body closer to her own body attempting to restrain her.

Patricia told me later how she had dreaded this very moment. She had often wished that she could cast out a wave of a magic wand forever erasing the hurt and the pain that continued to live inside Cleo's heart. Patricia pretended to be in full control when actually deep inside she herself was torn apart fearing the inevitable. She and her mate had experienced this moment too often with some of the AIDS infected babies they had kept. Through their continued friendship with Cleo, both Patricia and Ruth had tried preparing Cleo for the oncoming Hell. Can one really be ready or sufficiently prepared to accept or welcome death?

PANELS

While I was driving behind them, I noticed that the intricate loop near the Demonbreum exit had a strange quietness about the air. There were very few vehicles that were traveling in their direction. Whatever the reason, there existed an eerie feeling of something dark hovering over the land.

Seth was rushed into the emergency room as the intercom announced an incoming STAT Code Blue. All available medical personnel quickly responded as additional intravenous lines were placed in his awaiting veins. Antibiotics in large doses flowed. Steroids were injected as well as other anti-PCP medications. Crushed ice was placed around him in an attempt to desperately bring down his rising temperatures.

I watched as the EMTs collected their gear on top of their stretcher and soon left after taking one last look at their recent transport. Mike glanced stealthily at the women who had followed behind in their car. Thinking of his own family, he had wanted to go over to the women to tell them that everything would be all right, but he seriously doubted his own words. He didn't know the relationship between the people involved but he could clearly attest to their loving concern. Mike dropped his head and walked away trying to shake the earlier expression on Seth's placid face as he was pounding on his chest.

In a matter of a few minutes, others from Seth's family had joined them in the emergency waiting room. Eloise and Benjamin were both physically escorted to their neighboring seats by some of their remaining children. Eloise held Cleo's hands as Cleo described through her tears having found Seth unconscious and burning with a fever. Cleo cried as she further went into vague details of the ordeal. When she started blaming herself, Eloise grabbed her and held her against her breast. She rocked Cleo in her arms. Eloise was crying softly until Sarah wiped her mother's tears away. Speechless, we hurdled around each other and waited. Tears fell from my eyes. I was scared for Seth.

Everyone had expected the moment to occur although no one was really ready to fully accept the obvious outcome. Benjamin closed his heavy-laden eyes. He silently prayed for his dying son. He had already yielded one son to death just a matter of days earlier, and now death was asking for another child. When will it ever end, he questioned the silence. Maybe it was for the best that Seth no longer had to suffer his hell on this earth. But why always death?

Sebastian arrived only moments before Seth's attending physician started walking towards the family. I ran to him to brief him.

Cleo was the first to see the grim, broken expressionless face. She knew then that Seth had left her. Immediately and abruptly, there was silence among those gathered. Benjamin reached over to his wife and tightly held her hands. He squeezed her hands ever so gently and compassionately. Eloise braced herself fearing for the news of his demise. Her heart raced to a thundering halt as he started to speak.

"I don't have to tell any of you just how sick he is…He is still in a great deal of discomfort and pain…He is extremely weak at this point…We are doing all that we can, but regretfully it is only a matter of time…" Finally, the stranger cloaked in white said. "I'm assuming that you are aware that he has on file with this hospital a request for a DNR? Unless the family has strong reservation regarding his last request, I feel obligated to respect his decision…At this point, we feel that the left side of his brain is dead…He is currently being stabilized using a respirator…If you would like to see him, I must first warn you that his appearance may frighten you initially…He is very weak…I'm sorry…" Dr. Matt Neilsen finished.

Extremely exhausted, Dr. Neilsen leaned against the sterile wall. He wiped the perspiration that had formed around his face. He closed his tired eyes momentarily as he wished to change the entire scenario. Instead, he waited for their decision to discontinue the life supporting machines.

No one would publicly consciously contest Seth's choice. What quality of life did he now possess? Would death not be an actual viable alternative to his current hell? Would their silence prove any less in their love for him? Looking for an answer in Eloise's crushed face, Benjamin instructed the tired physician to allow the will to stand. Cleo carefully stood and approached the physician. She asked if she could please see Seth before it was too late. Although he was somewhat hesitant, after looking at the family for some type of reassurance, he finally allowed Cleo the chance to say good-bye to her friend.

Suddenly, she stopped outside the examining room where Seth was laying. Dr. Neilsen turned and faced Cleo. He wanted to be sure that she did want to see her friend in his failing condition. Would it not be better to simply remember Seth as he once looked instead of living with this vision forever embroiled on her mind? Cleo looked straight into his eyes with a very stern stare. She refused to relent.

Sebastian and I ran behind her. The appearance of the room gave us a sudden brake. Around his bed were arrays of countless monitors with numerous snaking tubing injected into various orifices of the disfigured mangled thin body. Fighting back the tears, Cleo held his unrestrained hand delicately inside hers.

His eyes were so black and empty as they stared aimlessly into space. Cleo prayed to all of her saints for their assistance. She refused to allow him his freedom. She remembered the two of them laughing once at the mere thought of Seth being chained to a tree near the graveyard of the Saint Haji Sher. Although they had joked about the myth, each had wanted the saint to rescue his soul from dying as many believed the Pakistan tradition that dated back to AD 750. She wondered now how many days it would take the saint to give her back her best friend. She leaned over the railing and kissed his hallowed cheek as she softly caressed his thinning hair. Suddenly, Cleo felt a response within the hand that she held. His hand tightened around her finger. Did she imagine this or was there really tightness?…The monitors no longer beeped.

Cleo lost all control and emotionally ran outside screaming. Her tears streamed down her distorted face. Sebastian quickly ran behind her until he finally caught her in the parking circle outside the emergency entrance. Cleo began to hit him as she tried to get away from him. He, along with myself, were finally able to restrain her. Cleo continued struggling wanting to be free. Sebastian held her tight until she eventually calmed down. She cried as she told us that she wanted to run far away from everything that reminded her of Seth.

"I just lost my very best friend…I loved him…God only knows just how much I really loved him…I can't accept that he is gone from me…My heart is hurting real bad. If I could have died in his place, I surely would have…There is nothing that you can possibly say that will ease any of my pain…No one has ever loved me the way he had…..Why, Oh my God, why take him from me?" Cleo collapsed in our arms.

Later, as Sebastian, Cleo, and I were resting on the curb near the hospital's entrance, the life flight helicopter whirled away from the neighboring rooftop. The turning of the blades drowned much of the noise around us. Nothing could drown our sorrow.

Cleo laid her head across Sebastian's lap. Sebastian stroked her soft hair as she stared aimlessly into another space and time. Both their eyes were still swollen from crying. I tried to say something but I could not. I just sat there.

"Why did he have to leave me? Was I not there for him?"

"I don't even know what to say without sounding so damn patronizing…or having a mouthful of nothingness except some damn tired clichés…I really don't know if he is really better off where he is now, I can only hope that he is…Hell, maybe he's up there playing and singing duets with Richard, who knows," Sebastian retorted

"Hell, maybe he's kicking Bradley's ass, what do you think?" Cleo briefly raised her head from his lap and asked with a weak smile.

Holidays invaded the atmosphere. Although the last death had been several months before the winter, I still was not in the festive mood. In fact, none of us was the least cheerful. The transitions of our friends continued to haunt us individually.

Over the course of the change in our lives, I began to share much time with Sebastian. I tried to mask my need for him by citing work related issues although I knew it was because I really needed him. In my mind, he was the remaining patriarch. It was his shoulders that I leaned onto for strength.

On the week before Christmas, all were not asleep, as the fable would say, as the vast lights inside his windows decorated the night. Rain fell hard against the cold earth. There were no carolers singing the seasonal melodies outside the candle-adorned windows. Although there were indeed holiday decorations dressing his lonely confinement, the spirit of the season simply surpassed his domain.

One night after work, Sebastian and I went for drinks at a few pubs on Ellingston Place. Our conversation appeared quite above surface for the first hour. Nothing major was presented on either part. We laughed and joked about others around us as well as ourselves. But I began to notice that he wasn't the same person I had always known. I felt as if I was talking to a stranger. I was puzzled.

While consuming his third rum and coke, he slowly began to open my eyes. Sometimes, knowledge can be worse than ignorance.

"If you ever tell Cleo or anyone, then I will swear that you are a damn liar," Sebastian said.

"What, pray tell are you talking about? Tell who what?" I asked.

"Promise me that you won't talk until I'm ready to tell the others," he said.

"Omigod, please tell me it's not what I think…I can't take it…I really can't take it anymore…Please Sebastian."

"Maybe I misjudged you. I just thought I could get this off my shoulders…"

"Sebastian, I'm sorry…but I…you just caught me off guard." I closed my eyes. I wished this moment would erase itself from my mind. "What can I do?

PANELS

"God only knows…just be there for Cleo…and me," he asked.

"When did you find out?" I asked.

" Today…That was why I missed the staffing…I was too busy crying my eyes out and cursing God for allowing it to happen…You see, I have been having these God awful headaches that won't go away. I decided to bite the bullet and had the battery of tests done," he said.

"I'm really bummed out…somehow I guess I just thought you was invincible and immortal. You have always been there for me. I can not possibly fathom not having you set the pace…What can I do?" I asked.

"Nothing, I guess except maybe ask the good God in Heaven to forgive me for cursing him." He nervously laughed.

That conversation between he and I took place what seems ages ago. Over time, I finally was able to put that night in the back of my mind. It never existed unless I wanted it to. The mere thought of the subject remained asleep until tonight. I had called him about tonight's event.

Sebastian complained to me tonight that his headaches were beginning to blind his sensations with the unbearable pain. He constantly remained nauseated. I did notice that he appeared to have lost weight but I said nothing.

We were still understaffed at the agency, which resulted in many sleepless nights for both of us.

I was still talking to Sebastian when his other line beeped. Cleo called to ask him if he was ready for their festive evening. Her voice was very giddy and gay, anticipating the planned events of the night.

Dulled by the penetrating surges going to his brain, Sebastian barely listened to any of her words. He told me that Cleo had to repeat herself several times.

Sebastian usually never shared his concerns over his health with anyone. Sebastian confided in me that he merely discounted his fears as silly notions. He need not worry. He was neither yet ready nor prepared to see God's eyes.

Hours later, I watched as a dazzling Sebastian escorted a glamorous Cleo through the crowded Hyatt Grand Ball Room to our table. I noticed with glee several heads turned as Cleo walked past their tables. Dangerously beautiful with her ever-commanding piercing mint green eyes, her petite charming figure accentuated the color of gold. Her sensual form was captive in gold silk with a bead-covered bodice, as more golden sequins slinked down in slim lines to her ankle-length hemline.

She wore her hair in a French twist with mess headdress of beige pearl-like baubles attached. Her back was encased with a beaded strap that formed an X at her exposed back. To warm her soft skin, a gold silk stole caressed her shoulders. Sebastian proudly stood close to her side, while he wore his black tuxedo with the matching gold vest.

During the lavish dinner, I felt that Sebastian appeared distant. He appeared so predisposed others soon found it difficult to involve him in any of the circulating conversations. True to her nature, Cleo made polite amends for his attitude.

As I leaned over to speak with him, Sebastian looked startled. He said his vision was blurred, as his eyes traveled around the candlelit room. The candlelight made the faces distort and run together. He whispered that he wanted to run from those strangers in the room. But, he couldn't move. He said his head whirled with pain.

Suddenly, music began to play from somewhere. The music became louder and louder, as movement appeared around him. I watched him grab his ears as if they were hurting. I gave him a shrug at his arm to stand. He opened his eyes while Cleo whispered softly into his ear that she wanted to dance.

As they slow danced, Cleo held him tight. Cleo told me how she had noticed his rather sluggish movement, as they swayed to the music. She was surprised at his awkwardness with his feet almost dragging the floor. Twice she stopped briefly to look into his eyes but never said anything. She simply held him closer. She closed her eyes and prayed for the dance to last forever.

Moments later, Sebastian made a faint uttering noise. He collapsed in her frail arms. Startled, Cleo screamed out his name. There was no response from him. Several people including myself hurried to their side. We carefully carried him away from the dance floor area and away from the growing audience. I saw tears run down Cleo's face. Reassuring strangers comforted her. Cleo wiped her eyes dry, attempting to mask her fear, as she walked over to where we were.

Someone checked his vital signs. Cleo stared up into my eyes. I saw her mumble something. She told me later that it was a silent prayer.

Patricia Sedler stepped forward with her husband, Daniel, to drive him to the hospital. Without speaking a word, Daniel quickly grabbed Sebastian around his waist and hoisted him onto his massive shoulders. Patricia and Cleo hurriedly followed behind. Once again, I followed enroute to the hospital. This time I was cursing and very fearful of the night.

The almost barren streets were wet and slick with a mixture of salt, rain, and ice. Frozen slush covered the roads. Still, the brisk cold wind whistled throughout the car. Cleo felt the heat that rose from Sebastian's body. He continued to tremble violently. He lapsed into another seizure. He remained unresponsive to her touches. She wiped the mounting moisture from his forehead. She cradled him closer to her breast.

Sebastian was rushed inside the emergency room. A nurse immediately detained Cleo and I at the admission desk. The nurse wanted to know about his medical history. Frantically, Cleo started crying. She was overwhelmed with the questioning. She couldn't remember anything other than his age.

All she had known was the fact he was constantly complaining of severe headaches and was under a great deal of stress. She blacked out momentarily. Faces appeared queerly distorted and warped. Each seemed to blend into the others, creating a kaleidoscopic view, before splitting apart. We moved to the waiting area where Daniel was already seated. I placed my arm around her trembling body. Cleo laid her head on my shoulder. Her body shook with silent tears.

"Are you the people who brought Sebastian Michals in?" The doctor said.

Cleo opened her eyes fully to take in the vision of the young man in the hospital blues. She wasn't listening to his words. Instead she noticed the innocent charm that was accentuated by the sparkling eyes of a cherub. His voice was non-threatening and slightly reassuring. Cleo repositioned herself in an upright angle, trying to focus entirely on the friendly intruder's dialogue.

A caravan of names and faces ran through her head twirling fast. She asked me about calling Sebastian's new friend Scott but she didn't know just how much Scott knew of Sebastian's health. I looked directly and asked her what could we say since we really didn't know anything specifically ourselves.

I was quickly snapped into reality when the doctor explained that Sebastian would have to undergo several extensive tests within the next few hours. He would not say anything specific. Unfortunately, because none of us were Sebastian's relatives, he could not divulge any pertinent information. However, the doctor did say that Sebastian had been stabilized, and they started fluids into his system intravenously.

"Sebastian was bathed in crushed ice to decrease his fever." The doctor tenderly caressed Cleo's trembling hands, as he told us that hopefully our friend would pull out of it soon.

"When could I see him?" Cleo said. He suggested she might want to wait until later, after he had been admitted into the hospital. Cleo became furious. She stood in angry defiance demanding to see Sebastian immediately.

"I'm sorry, but that may not be wise, especially the way your emotional level is right now. His appearance may alarm you," the doctor said.

"May alarm me? How dare you try to patronize me! Who the hell are you to keep me from seeing my friend. I don't want to leave here without seeing him. What have you done to him? Why doesn't he want to see me? Where is he?" Cleo wanted quick answers.

"Look, I understand your concern for your friend. Perhaps even some of the frustration that you may be experiencing. Maybe you can see him tomorrow. Definitely not tonight."

The physician left as quietly as he had entered, without raising his voice to meet Cleo's of anger. Cleo sat fuming. She appeared confused and laded with doubt. Cleo toyed with the idea of simply bursting through the doors to where he was. Out of the corner of her eye, she noticed two burly security guards stationed near the double doors. She wondered if she should wait until the next morning.

Patricia assured her she could return the next morning and perhaps his status would have improved enough for her to see him. Her soft compassionate eyes told Cleo she somehow understood. Reluctantly, Cleo quietly rose from her chair and left with them.

Early the next morning, Scott, Cleo, Duchess, and I stood quietly over Sebastian's bed, as he began to stir. He tried to regain consciousness. Cleo held his hand against her face, as she softly stroked his face. As he appeared to utter faint words, Cleo leaned closer to hear. A tear fell from her face onto Sebastian, as the Duchess turned and left the room. Sebastian was still very weak, but obviously wanted to tell us something. Cleo strained to hear every word from his parched lips. She replaced her anger with anxiety and reverence.

"Will you ever forgive me? I never wanted you to see me like this. Like the others. I'm sorry. I'm really sorry," Sebastian said in his faint whisper.

"Just get your ass up from that damn bed, then we can fight. Hell, it's no fun beating the crap out of you right now since you can't fight back." Cleo laughed.

"Sebastian, you really look like shit, " Scott said. "What the hell do you mean to try to upstage me, anyway? I'm the one that's supposed to be laying there not you. And if you don't fight and get your ass better, then I've already decided how to dress you for your funeral. Imagine yourself going away making a queen's fashion statement. You'll be wearing a pink tutu with matching slippers. You remember that purple wig I wore one Halloween?

PANELS

Well sister, guess who will have it perched on his head?" Scott prodded Sebastian's feet with his cane and smiled.

"You're really touched in the mind. Both of you. I may have to take a rain check on the fight for now. What day is it anyway?"

"You mean you didn't hear good old Santa scaling your windows? Merry Christmas, darling." Cleo smiled, as she wiped a strand of his hair from his eyes. She had been crying earlier, and the swollen wet eyes and the occasional hint of a sniffle were still evident. "So, where's my gift? I've been a good girl."

"Oh, God, No. Why are you both here on Christmas? Where's your family? Why aren't you both home celebrating with your family?"

"We were out slumming and we thought about coming by to see just how many piles of coal the old fart brought you," Cleo said, as she sat on the bed.

"Seriously...why aren't you guys at home with your own families?" Sebastian stirred in bed.

"Look, asshole, you're a part of our family or have you forgotten that. Anyway, I will not leave here until I know that you are okay. So, quit your bitching, and get well. I can bitch too, you know. I've had the best teachers."

"How well I remember. Seriously, why are you guys here? Haven't you seen enough misery and death from within the circle? Are you both to be my keeper? Why put yourselves through my hell?" Sebastian stared angrily into Cleo's eyes.

"There's nothing worse than a bastard drowning in his own piss of self pity," Scott said. "How dare you expect us to walk away from you! I hope to God you are okay. I hope to God that you'll never see the shit I have to deal with just to see another day. Have you ever heard of loyalty? If I wasn't so damn tired, I'd beat the living hell out of you with this goddamned cane." Scott started shaking the cane at him.

"Look, don't give us this shit. We are here because we do give a damn about you. Obviously, you don't give a damn about yourself. Instead of fighting whatever the fuck is affecting you, you prefer to lay here in your own self-pity. God damn it, do you think that you're the only one hurting? Do you think that everybody is simply going to run away from you just because you refused to accept us? Fuck you and the unreal horse that you're trying to ride. I care about you, and yes, I even love you but I will no longer sit back and watch you destroy yourself or destroy the love from those around you."

Cleo whirled around and found herself looking at Dr. Sanders' bewildered face. Angrily fighting back her tears, she assisted Seth in standing and stormed past the psychiatrist. "Please, talk some sense in that damn fool's head."

As time passed, Sebastian finally matured enough to allow himself to engage in conversations with us, the Duchess, and with the psychiatrist on a daily basis. Although he had known of the specialist on a professional basis, he was slightly embarrassed to disclose his deepest fears. Eventually, Sebastian allowed some of his barriers to crumble.

After he was discharged from the hospital, Sebastian participated in an HIV support group held at Comprehensive Care Clinic that was facilitated by Dr. Sanders, where others similar to him were dealing with the impact of living with the virus. For years, Sebastian had facilitated similar groups for others. Now, the tables had turned, making him an unwilling participant.

After each counseling session, Sebastian disclosed to me that he was not a pessimist but was actually a sentimentalist. With the start of his world dissipating into the countless deaths starting with his first friend Gregory, he simply wanted to hold onto the memories. Sebastian purposely balked at the possibilities of accepting new alliances, because he feared becoming too close to someone only to have them eventually leave him. Sebastian's rather dogmatic doctrine was simple. He felt that if reciprocating expectations didn't exist between them, then they couldn't let him down. Sebastian had always been the strong one who forever continued smiling on the outside to mask his own hurt and fear. He had always been there for others but felt remarkably guilty for reaching out for their help.

In his past, his life came to a halt simply when others needed him. Sebastian never considered himself worth troubling any of the individuals within the circle with any of his problems. His barriers remained unsheltered because of all of the pain that he had tolerated.

Sebastian greatly removed himself from reality. He appeared to no longer feel a part of anyone's life, with the exception of Duchess, Cleo, and myself. He refused to cloud his limited life with illusions of love being around him. He realized his limitations. Sebastian knew all too well that even the most seasoned person that dealt firsthand with AIDS eventually became tired.

When Sebastian finally left Vanderbilt Hospital accompanied by Cleo and me, he left in a cloud of misery and ignorance. He admitted feeling the

PANELS

ignorance and doubt because he didn't know his eventual fate. He would have to wait for all of the test results to arrive. Although he felt as if he had all of the answers, Sebastian still would have to experience the wait.

Sebastian continued attending a support group at the Comprehensive Care Clinic. Initially, he felt ill at ease with being on the other side of therapy. His position had turned participator instead of the facilitator. Believe me, this is not a comfortable change.

He told me how he would initially sit on a session quietly. He said he could never simply relax and disclose his feelings to those strangers. He wanted desperately to be in control.

During this process, he first met Scott. Although he said he vaguely remembered Scott when he first arrived to the group, Sebastian said Scott took extra effort to always sit near Sebastian and would prompt him for his responses. Sebastian said he was annoyed by this guy but was also somewhat intrigued. He went further to say that Scott had been positive for twelve years. Over a period of time, Sebastian finally opened up to him.

"Believe me, I do understand not wanting to get close to anyone after losing your friends. I know all too well of the Hell and the prospect of starting over with different people. Tell me, if you refuse to open the door, when no one can come inside and hurt you, are you any safer?" Scott asked.

"I don't know...I really don't know. Unlike you, I don't have all the answers. I'm just starting out," Sebastian said.

"Not necessarily true. However, if you leave that door closed, you simply stop living altogether...I, too, have lost those that I have loved very much. My lover left me after fifteen years...It took me years to stop talking in the plural. I had to say I instead of we or tell others to come and see me instead of us...I had to relearn life in the singular sense...Friends have left me...Friends that were closer to me than my own family had been...But, I close my eyes, cry a few tears, and then open my eyes to see another day. The sun still rises regardless of the pain...I'm not saying that it is easy to go on, because it is not. But you have to try, if not for yourself, but for the others that have passed on...Cry, scream to the top of your lungs, kick some ass, do whatever it takes to survive...Don't ever keep it all bottled inside," Scott responded.

Somehow, listening to Sebastian tell me of their conversation, I really felt if Scott had actually gotten to him. Scott's words appeared to have lifted his spirit. I just knew that Sebastian was climbing out of his gully.

I was standing at my office window staring into the open nothingness. The trees were no longer naked but clothed in green. The coolness of the brisk air had been replaced with the fluttering of birds in flight. Hours turn to days turning to months. Seasons change bringing renewed possibility of life. I noticed that the grass was no longer brownish in color. I began to drink in the beauty of the serenity when I heard the knock on the door behind me. I was quite annoyed at anyone intruding on my daydream.

"Spring has arrived without much fanfare. But that is what I like about the uncertainty of life. The sun continues to rise and set," Liz Tomlin announced as she stood beside me.

"There is much beauty in God's growth cycle," I returned. My words seemed strange even to me. Why did I feel the need to respond to her invasion?

"Any day now, the sound of children's laughter and the patter of their playful feet will take hold of the silence."

"Then, we return to our hellish nightmare called reality."

"My, aren't we quite the positive ones today!"

"Whatever!"

"Ooh, I do believe someone got out of the bed on the wrong side this morning!"

She teased back in a baby like voice. She stood less than an arm length away from me. I closed my eyes. Maybe if I wished hard enough, she would disappear.

I gradually turned to glance at Liz. Liz Tomlin, the girl from somewhere in Minnesota, who just graduated from college. She stood there with her glistening blond hair dangling over her eyes. She had that irritating bubbling personality that always appeared cheerful and unadulterated. I looked at her and wondered just how long she would remain so positive when the entire world around her becomes an emotional basket case.

Initially, my first impression of Liz was of distrust. She appeared too eager and way too friendly. I got the impression that she was interviewing to be everyone's best friend—but not mine. I refused to allow her to cross my threshold as Sebastian had allowed. Although I really couldn't place my finger on anything specifically, there was something about her that scared me. I was not going to open myself to her and disclose anything. I began to wonder what was her hidden agenda and if she was attempting to climb the career ladder by stepping on the weak. I have learned from past experiences how associates can win your trust only to try to destroy you later. Anyway, no one is that genuinely nice especially to strangers without any forms of reciprocation.

Liz persevered until my boundaries eventually crumbled. Perhaps Sebastian had been right in saying that he did not see her as a threat but an ally. After her initial arrival, Sebastian and I had spoken as to her sincere merits. I began to digress to our previous conversation concerning Liz.

"Michal, You know me, you know that I don't trust anyone easily. It has to be earned not given...but I think that Liz is okay," Sebastian said.

"So, you trust her enough to tell her everything?"

"Be for real, as long as I have known you, do you think you know everything about me? You're fooling yourself if you do think it."

"Oh, so you admit to have secrets even from us...from me?"

"My dear Michal, you never tell anyone everything. Always keep them guessing."

Until this moment, my own life appeared to have been on hold. Frozen in the sense of point in time. For whatever reason, my struggles didn't matter that much compared against my friends' lives. Don't get me wrong. I actually love my friends. It was just that all our conversations as of late always depressed me. The fun that once existed in our circle had vanished without a trace. I began to miss the laughter and the joking. Now, in their places existed a void only to be filled with tears and despair—my tears and despair.

Often, I was able to leave them momentarily and pamper myself. I began to wonder if I was actually trying to leave their misery or was I trying in a feeble attempt to avoid my own. However, fate had other plans for me.

"Hey Michal, do you have plans for next weekend?" Liz touched my shoulder.

"It depends on who is asking."

"In other words, a big no! Good, because I want you to help me facilitate a support group during a weekend retreat."

"I don't really think I would be the best choice for a retreat."

"Oh, Michal. Stop being so modest...Anyway, I could learn a great deal from you. You know, my approach in confronting and transferring the clients' aggression away from me so that I stop personalizing non-essential issues. You even said so yourself that I still was quite green..."

"Since when did you stop to listen to my critique?"

"Hey, you'd be surprised as to what I listen to." She smiled. "Anyway, think about a weekend getaway to the mountains. The early morning dew freshening your face as the sun begins to rise. Nothing to listen to except the crackling of the trees as the wind blows through…Better yet, no pagers going off."

"Well…Just that thought alone may be worth the trip."

"Good! You give it some thought and I will come back in thirty minutes for your answer…just kidding, maybe I can ask you on Monday." Liz laughed as she left. I was still annoyed with Liz's abrupt invasion when Sebastian walked by the open door. I yelled out his name and motioned for him.

"Hey guy, I'm jealous…I just heard that you might be going to camp next weekend."

"Yeah right, I haven't told her that I would go. How dare she take those liberties."

"Calm down, rover…No need to show your teeth…Anyway, I think you should go. You know, just to get away from everything. It's not like you will miss anything here. I would go if I didn't have clinic rounds."

"But, one question, why should I go?"

"Why not, what do you have to lose?"

"Why did she choose me? What is she after? I mean, this sounds like a set up and with you helping her. So, what's in it for you?"

"Man, you should hear yourself talk. Can we say major paranoid! You're beginning to sound like some of our clients…what's the big deal? Do you think you can't handle it? What gives?" Sebastian buffed. "Hell, take it as a compliment from someone that actually appreciates your approach and style. It really doesn't have to be anymore than that."

"Do you know if she asked anyone else?"

"Yeah, she did. But, no one else was free. Anyway, you can use this time for your annual regs. Hell, you get three days credit for what…one to four hours of session…so, you actually get off lucky and now you won't have to desperately run around searching for other volunteer sessions to meet your requirements unlike myself."

"I guess you're right."

"Of course I'm right…just because she may want to have her way with you in the woods means nothing."

"You don't honestly think she wants me, do you?"

"Yeah right, be for real, she's not that green. She's been working here long enough to know your flavor of Kool-Aid"

"I just don't know. I don't think I'm ready for my weekend to be swallowed by someone else's issues."

"So, instead you are staying here and listening to our little circle moan and groan. Man, suit yourself…personally I think you would regret not going." He walked to the door. "You're an adult; I'm sure you will make the right choice for yourself."

After considerable thought later that night, I decided to take Liz at her offer. Listening to her describe the remote mountainous setting far away from my world sounded quite attractive so I agreed to participate as one of many facilitators in a weekend retreat at Camp Hill Mont.

On Monday morning, I was ready and willing to assist. I was standing in the middle of the break room floor waiting to get coffee when she walked in. As I reached for the coffee pot, I felt this rush of air breeze by me.

"Good morning, Michal!" Liz greeted. "So, what did you decide?"

"I assume that you are referring to the retreat?" I asked. My eyes still cocked with my partially closed lids. I hated Mondays.

"Well, of course! What else?" She chuckled as she poured the coffee into my mug.

"What retreat? What are you guys talking about?" another female voice rang out from behind me. Before I could respond, Liz ecstatically jumped to the chance.

"Oh, Michal and I are co-facilitating a few sessions at a retreat that's being held at Camp Hill Mont this weekend…Rachel, girl…no more four walls to restrain us, just the openness of the open sky!"

"Man, that sounds like a blast! So, Michal…what is the theme?" Rachel asked.

"I'm not really sure…I think it's just general mental wellness," I stuttered back. I felt foolish not knowing what I had volunteered for.

"Oh, Michal…forgive me, I thought I told you that the topic was AIDS…the theme is simple— 'Let Go and Let God.'"

My stomach began to knot tightly. My heart began to race. The theme was simple, "Let Go and Let God." The words repeated over and over in my mind that the concentration was on AIDS. Up until now, I was able to swallow anything about AIDS in small quantities and always avoided anything major. Now, I'm being asked to live in it for an entire weekend. But it was too late for me to back out. So, I closed my eyes and prayed for deliverance as Liz beamed that damn smile.

The days leading up to the weekend appeared to have been the longest God forsaken days of my life. Somehow, I opened my eyes and found myself at the camp.

PHIL MICHAL THOMAS

I watched as several people arrived at the rather remote campsite. Numerous cars filled with luggage and eager faces. The glorious sun was beating across the tree-lined horizon. For whatever reason, I began to wonder if angels ever slept. The sky was a calming blue with scattered clouds. The rustic cabins edged the rows of carefully manicured graveled lanes. With much apprehension, I parked and walked towards the main building to check in. As my feet sunk into the gravel while I walked, I was very much full of fear.

Even with numerous people present in this spacious surrounding, I still felt very much alone. I so wished that my friends could have been present. But, that was not to be.

Each step that I took towards the main house to register, each step I took to the full realization of the real life around me.

"Hello, everyone, on behalf of Wonderful News, I would like to personally welcome you to Camp Hill Mont; this weekend we promise you only what you allow yourself to take away from this time."

I turned slowly around to face the speaker. With a deep sigh, I realized it was another associate. Robb was one person that I personally was not too fond of but one that Liz obviously had accepted. I had previously battled with him on countless issues. I hated him; I really detest his mere presence. I wanted to retreat to my car and leave his miserable ass standing there. However, my anger made me stay. I decided that if anyone left, he would be the one. So I stayed.

"Hopefully, it will include a more positive outlook in what already may appear quite dismal. This is your weekend. I look forward to meeting each and every one of you over the course of this time spent. Once again, welcome and thank you for coming to Camp Hill Mont."

While standing in an apparent self-imposed fog trying to ignore Robb, Liz approached me. Liz was wearing a faded tie-dyed denim dress with her bangs parted on the side. Without much fanfare of my current status, she told me that she thought this might help me deal with silent needs. I acted as if I didn't hear her. What silent needs was she referring to?

She touched me on my shoulders and called out my name again. She was smiling. Without much to say, she hurried me off to my quarters before I could hear anymore that was being said to the multitude.

From a distance, I noticed people scampering about the grounds armed with their sleeping bags and luggage scattering down the gravel drive to their designated cabins. I noticed some of the faces were smiling and engaged in conversation while several appeared distant and even afraid.

During the weekend, we participated in various exercises of personal and spiritual healings. Music played a significant role in relaxation. There were no anger nor dogmatic teachings applied, simply love and acceptance. This was the first time I had actually heard a religious organization actually speak of loving one.

At one session, I felt a rather strange revelation of my possible purpose for being there. One half of the group sat in an inner circle while the other half stood directly behind us in a human chain. The music was of Celine Dion, a young Canadian singer whose words professed of being our angel that would always be there for us, a promise to never leave us no matter what the outcome proved. No mountain was ever too high to climb as long as we had faith.

In the extreme center was a small clay figurine of a circle of people with a candle burning. As the music played, the outer circle would gently lean over and whisper comforting words into our ears and in a slow methodical dance would move to the next person. I was a bit uncomfortable at first having someone so close to me but I soon relaxed and closed my eyes and listened.

The lyrics began to take shape in my mind. I have heard this song numerous times over the radio but never actually listened to the words. The possibility of having someone take away my burdens, even if just for a few moments, gave me reassurance. The moment appeared to encompass most of my fears, and as I glanced around the circle, it may have possibly took hold of others as I noticed tears being wiped away. As the music ended, we took our turn as the outer link as they took our seats. Now, it was my turn to reciprocate and give comforting words to others.

I stood over my person and literally froze. I didn't know what to say. I searched over and over in my head for the right words but nothing formed from my lips. As I leaned over, I mumbled something about "He loves you regardless." The young woman reached up and grasped my hands resting on her shoulders and thanked me. I stumbled onto the next person. This time, I was the one crying.

By the time we had finished, I felt somewhat polished and prepared. I no longer felt like the bumbling fool but someone that recognized my own limitations. I soon realized that none of my book learning meant anything if there existed a void in my heart. I felt that my words were previously worthless without meaning.

The outcome for me arrived in numerous channels. From the very first death that took away a link from our circle and continued to the present, I was angry. Beforehand, I had felt unclean and unloved. There was no way that anyone including God could love me. I felt alone, desolate, depressed, and unworthy.

Although I attended as a staff, I left feeling that I was not alone. One surprising gift awarded to me came from a participant during another session that I co-facilitated with Liz. Listening to others speak of their lives sparked an embarrassing awakening for me. One particular moment caught me off guard. I could no longer distance myself emotionally and I simply lost my composure and began to disclose my own fearful distrust. However, although I considered this to be quite earth shattering, no one else appeared offended. In fact, a stranger looked directly in my eyes and thanked me for bringing his own life into a clearer perspective.

"Thank you for being honest with us and to yourself. It always angered me to talk to therapists about my issues and you people always maintained that uncaring apathetic stone face. I never really felt that they were listening to me. That perhaps you guys are all trained to stop caring for fear it would weaken you and make you not very effective. Thank you for being real. Man, this shit is not easy to deal with, no matter who you are."

I didn't know how to respond. Liz reached over and clenched my hand and gave me that familiar reassuring smile. "You did well; be proud."

Amidst the beauty of God's work with the surrounding kaleidoscopic summer colors, I was taught that I was still loved by God unconditionally. It was the first time that I shared tears with others around me while realizing our worth. Can you ever imagine the simple touch of someone as they whisper that they love you and that God loves you?

That weekend at Camp Hill Mont, the God of compassion was indeed shown to us through loving angelic faces. I'm no longer grieving my past, present, nor my future. Somehow, I felt that I gained some insight on the mounting deaths of my friends and as if completing some form of a figurative makeover. My previously hated foe Robb and I actually stole away and conversed with much comfort. I began to see him in a totally different light.

"So, what are you taking away from this weekend?"

"Believe it or not, somewhat a sense of peace," I said.

"Yeah, I can relate…I know that we don't know each other too well although we often work side by side at the agency and I'm not blind to see that I'm probably not one of your favorite people…So, be honest with me for a second…Were you a bit put off when you first saw me here when you arrived?"

PANELS

"Yeah, I was, at first. But not any longer."

"Would you have come if you knew I was coming."

"Probably not."

"Well, truth hurts...but I will get over it...always remember to never ask for the truth if you don't want to hear it...anyway, I am glad that you came."

"If the truth be known, I'm glad that I came...things are not always as they appear. Life doesn't have to be some mystified struggle which I think I sometimes create for myself."

"Michal, my dear man, if I may be so brave as to suggest this to you but one key to life is to be open with yourself. Realize and accept the simplest things in life...the certitude of the simplest pieces of our life offers us that security that we so desire."

"Robb, I think I know what you mean...but even in the simplest things in life, there is a struggle. I have developed more phobias than I can have ever imagined."

"Michal, you can overcome your fears...all you have to do is to confront them head on...you confronted me, didn't you." He laughed.

As I drove home on Sunday, mental images of the recent days captivated my thoughts. Perhaps I really did misjudge people. I really didn't open my heart to others. At least not fully, I will take baby steps. Surprisingly, I now felt somewhat strengthened. I wasn't as scared anymore.

The faces, no longer strangers, taught me that it was okay to let go and let God into my life. Through these now familiar voices, I felt that God still loved me.

Fall was resplendent in Nashville this particular year of the Dragon. The dry golden leaves made crackling rustled sounds. The cold wind swept harshly underneath between the branches and the solid earth. Although earlier forecasts of cloud burst, the sun defiantly and brilliantly coveted the earth with its incandescent rays. Laughter and in camera conversations filled the surroundings. Nature's process for coloration was as magnificent as ever which was evident by the inciting ineffable changes of the trees with their leaves coloring before each fell from their hosts.

The sky was void of any dissipating clouds. Various breeds of four legged animals walked strikingly close to their masters. Their leashes only restricted their total freedom of abandoning flight.

I was leaving building when I noticed her as she stood inside the foyer while glancing at her reflection in the mirrored lobby. Her porcelain features appeared weathered and a bit frayed. The innocence that she once possessed had been impregnated with soiled misery. Her youth juxtaposed with experiences too mature for her naïve choices. Could she ever stop the present madness and relive her life in a more satisfying manner? I wondered silently to myself as her steps took her gradually in his direction.

Would he now welcome her or would he become outraged at her mere presence that clearly violated his domain? Why was he so bitter towards her, I wondered with slight fear?

Having braced herself, she walked past the other distraught appearing visitors clutching their various floral gifts and nervous smiles, and summoned the elevator with an assured gesture.

Cleo had a true mission. One that would try to captivate Sebastian's life into her domain. In reflections years later, she admitted this fact to me as she described to me how a date with she and Sebastian for lunch.

Her face gleamed as she gave me her details of the event. Seconds quickly changed into decades as she stood on the moving platform. Her stomach knowingly turned with various mixed emotions as fear emitted forward. Thoughts tempted her to simply walk away from the impending hell without ever looking back, thus forever voiding the friendship.

I knew that the sensation that burned inside Cleo's heart was fast becoming unsettling and bothersome. I realized this after a recent argument between us regarding Sebastian.

"Have you ever heard about being careful at what battle you choose?"

"Michal, I'm not that naïve…I may not have a degree in psychology but I'm clearly aware that I have become an enabler within our relationship. But do you know what? I don't care. I have resigned myself in accepting the fact but I will never accept turning away from Sebastian."

"I'm just worried about your own welfare and the child."

"Don't worry about us. We are doing just fine." Her voice turned cold. "You can choose what battles you fight…if Sebastian is not one of them, that's up to you…I don't walk away from my friends!"

Sebastian was dressed in his French ribbed cream colored cotton pullover with the silhouette blue fitting knit cotton pants underneath his single breasted sleek vent-less rice-weave sport coat. He was also smiling as she walked into his office. He briefly told me how he had been expecting her with alarming anticipation. They had planned on having a quiet lunch together to quietly celebrate his birthday. Sebastian seriously made her promise to

PANELS

disregard any lavish thoughts; her presence was all that he needed.

Sebastian beamed brilliantly as he left his office arms interlocking with Cleo radiantly close to his side. Cleo remarked just how dapper Sebastian was looking which embarrassed him slightly. He had always felt genuinely flattered by her kind words. Both friends were in their own private world. Nothing else mattered.

I knew that Cleo and Sebastian had become closer as the years drew and the deaths mounted around us. It has been almost two years since Seth's death. Our lives were slowly building back up from the drudges and the hell that we had to endure. In our personal solitude, tears were allowed to flow freely for our deserted circle of friends.

Although our numbers had greatly decreased, we shared a great deal of our individual lives together. We shared our limited joys and our laughter. We also displayed our affirming bitterness and anger towards life. At separate times, one even allowed the other to ventilate our heartfelt frustrations while using the others in our circle as a passive venting board. Although their anger surfaced, their ideal love appeared to have always prevailed to soothe the wrong. Alienation was not to be in our rules for living nor was it ever contemplated.

By now, Cleo's art gallery was flourishing. Her clientele increased drastically, which gave her the necessary means to hire additional staff. Her promotional literature described "The Gallery on Russell" as being the visual arts anchor within the district of the historic Edgefield. Occupying over 4,000 square feet of combined gallery space, which included the renovated first and second floors. Cleo had the third floor renovated as her personal living space. Several other pieces were on loan from various numerous artists who had attempted extremely radical interpretations. In her role to further publicizing the nefarious effect that AIDS has on society, her gallery was joined with other galleries playing hosts during a benefit to raise money collectively through awareness of the world of art.

Even today, as one entered the gallery's foyer, attention is immediately directed to a mural with certain undeniable likeness of each face within the fallen circle. Cleo had commissioned Tony Teek to create their effigy and to preserve their individual personas to constantly serve as a reminder of their strong willed past. Cleo told me how she always paused to glance at their smiles and to say a brief prayer under her breath. At times, she caught herself actually talking to the images as if they were actually standing before her in the flesh. She laughed and she cried often while still missing her men. At each of the anniversaries of her deceased comrades, Cleo made a sizable monetary contribution on behalf of the individuals to Nashville CARES or to the Meals on Wheels.

Sebastian continued to work long incredible hours still due to the staff shortages. Relief was constantly promised although nothing ever materialized. He had used the increased workload as a crutch to avoid his troubled empty life. Sebastian's only source of relief came indirectly from our insistent arguments for social ventures. He had very little if any contact with his family other than the occasional dinners with the Duchess. It appeared that Sebastian had refused to allow anyone else to penetrate his massive thick barriers—It would also appear that he distanced himself to avoid any further heartache.

Living in his shell, Sebastian grew uncommonly silent over the last few months. He overcompensated for his losses through his self-mounting counseling duties. The actions, I felt, appeared as his defense mechanism in protecting his weakening vulnerability. Sebastian stayed bitter towards life. He always expected only the worst that life had to offer. Beside his employment, we became his surrogate lovers.

Cleo still beamed as she went into details, even the minute ones, about the picnic. As Cleo drove, she appeared full of girlish charm and giggles. Sebastian was visibly relaxed and even appeared slightly himself and even somewhat elated with her presence. Their in camera world ostracized all others from the depths of their endless boundaries. Both were familiar with each other without any fear of any rejection.

Relinquishing total control from his hands to hers, Sebastian allowed Cleo to dominate the moment. Rarely had he ever had the chance to fully relax under someone else's powers. The controlling factor decreased gradually to non-existence, which finally appeared to reduce his stress levels. Their sincere unquestionable bond was the foundation for their trust levels. Sebastian compared these intimate moments with the time spent in the fetal position, deep inside the mother's womb; unconsciously wanting that what is familiar.

"Not that I really give a flying damn, but just where are we going?" Sebastian asked as he finally raised his head from the slouched position.

"Honey, I know you all too well. I know that the only way I can truly have you all to myself is to get the hell out of Dodge. But don't worry; I'm not going to kidnap your trifling ass. Why bother, no one would pay the ransom."

"With my luck, lately, you would probably have to pay someone to take me back." He sheepishly grinned.

"And I would certainly pay a King's bounty," she laughed as she playfully pinched his cheek lightly. "Actually, I think I will keep you just for your adorable cheeks."

"You mean to tell me that you actually took the time away from your precious gallery for me! Oh! Don't I feel privileged? But what is going to be the price that I must one day pay for this loving being thrown from my soul mate?"

"Believe me, you don't have enough money to compensate for my terrific services. No, baby, there's no red light stuff here. So, sit back and give me your total destiny."

"Where's my god child? Why didn't you bring her?"

"Theresa is over at Justin's...I wanted this to be just the two of us."

There was a small cove off the beaten paths near Percy Priest Lake near the Seven Points entrance. As the civil engineer designed lake circles the numerous bends, there were several areas available for the amorous few. For those predisposed with other matters of solace, hidden alcoves were readily available. Located within the midst of one of the bends was a twelve-foot wooden pier.

Cleo further described the water being extremely calming as the rippling circles formed and gradually dissipated into the masses. She watched an elderly fisherman stir from his silent corner while casting his bait of worms into the rushing rising waters. Cleo parked close to the pier. Mesmerized by the milieu scenario, both sat still. They stared endlessly into the watery surroundings in total silence. Sebastian's disposition turned lively. He smiled wickedly. He had been here countless times before. We all had been to this place a time or two.

"Isn't life so damn full of contradiction? Isn't it ironic how something so beautiful in creation and form can be so cruel in death?" Sebastian whispered softly breaking the silence. "You know, I constantly think about death—my death. I don't know whether or not if it is partly my own selfish continued grieving process or if I'm just too scared to live anymore. What gloomy words, right?"

"Well, I can't really say that it sounds very uplifting especially with today being your birthday. Each to his own, I guess. Actually I have wondered about my own mortality. The other day, we received a flawless, and I mean a flawless, painting by Teppei Sasakura titled *Arcos de la Frontera*...Sebastian, it was a painting of various buildings high in the air in the clouds. I sort of envisioned heaven looking very much like the structures in the piece. Hell, I even thought that I saw Seth waving from one of the windows. Tiffany was doing one of her drag numbers in another window…Of course, Richard was reading and our Bradley was cruising the clouds below. God, how I do miss those guys. So, you had better think twice about leaving me. Enough of this, burgeon the miserable sentiments," Cleo nervously laughed.

"I don't know if I believe in Heaven. This time on earth is definitely the Hell that we all have always been forewarned about. I'm waiting for the storm to at least subside momentarily. There is days that I hate going to work to listen only to other's trivial misery. No one ever seems happy anymore. Always some form of some dysfunctional conflicts surfacing daily. What is it all worth?" Sebastian rested his head against the car's headrest. He stared across the water. His outlook was being enhanced not with self-pity but with tortuous reality.

Shifting gears in the directions of the planned outing, Cleo grabbed the white wicker basket from the back seat and walked towards the floating pier as Sebastian hurriedly walked behind her.

While on the pier, after spreading me blankets across the splintered dock, Sebastian soon became slightly nauseated. He quickly passed the sensation off as being due to the floating movement of the removable dock. Facing each other as their bodies rested against the covered railings, Cleo spread their elaborate prepared menu across the blankets. Sebastian uncorked the chilled bottle of white wine. Their past remained quiet, as their future appeared ignored while their current status experienced needed intimate joy.

As he lay on his back facing the cloudless sky, she stroked his hair softly while she prayed for this moment to extend. She leaned forward and kissed him on his lips.

In later days, while drinking coffee at Fido with Cleo, I listened to Cleo describe in detail her picnic with Sebastian; I strangely remembered a song being played in the distance. It was Kathy Mattea singing of angels being sent from above. Through her gentle voice, I began to visualize Cleo's scenario. I lightly reached across the table and pushed away a fallen hair from Cleo's eyes. I wonder if angels ever sleep?

The year was 1999. Research in AIDS brought the virus into a different realm. AIDS wasn't yet cured but rather the horizon appeared to have hope. No longer as dismal AIDS could be maintained with the proper regiment followed. The rate of infection among homosexuals was on the decline. AIDS no longer meant immediate death.

Within four years of Seth's death, Sebastian was admitted back into the hospital. His health faltered to the point his counseling duties were seriously affected. He would become angry for no apparent reason. Sebastian became uncommonly late for his sessions and case conferences. His usual patience with his clients decreased. Sebastian would leave in the middle of management meetings and his sessions. He blamed others for his crucial errors on his consultation reports. He badgered everyone he came around including me.

After the administration found him no longer able to perform his required duties, he was asked to take a medical leave of absence until his health improved. He laughed at me while saying how polite his supervisor was for not firing him outright. He knew there would be no return for him. As he left his office on his last day, few people would look him in his eyes. He had been loved so well that no one wanted to say the final good-bye. I purposely stayed home that day. I could not face him, especially not at that moment. I was frightened but didn't know why.

During my course of writing our memoirs, I was informally introduced to Sebastian's grandmother. Although she was quite cooperative with my efforts, it was several months later before she would talk about him freely. Before that moment, I remembered that first day that I saw her outside his hospital room.

As the Duchess neared the sterile corridor outside his room, her sojourn gradually became very emotional for her. Tears that quickly filled the crevices of her swollen eyes were visible, as she stood waiting momentarily outside his door. Her aged hands, wrinkled with despair, were cold and clammy, as they reached hesitatingly to open the portal. Ironically, across the hall, someone was playing an old African-American spiritual.

She told me later that in her younger years, an older African-American woman named Ella, who once ironed for their family, used to sing those very same words, as she went about her duties of starching each of the white cotton dress shirts for Mr. Michals.

The Duchess remembered, although vaguely, how that same woman appeared to have found some relief in singing something about one day there would be peace in the valley.

The significance of the lyrics hadn't struck any chords related to her rather fortunate life until now. Uncommonly for her, she stole back to her past. She stopped to that moment the small seventeen-month-old infant was laid in her anxious awaiting arms. She said how even at that early age, Sebastian's eyes gleamed up at her. He had captured her heart.

Although the penetrating gospel song wasn't being played very loud, she heard enough of the words to realize she knew so well of that particular song with the somewhat familiar honey-laced singing of Mahalia Jackson. Mahalia was at that moment filling the sterile white silent halls. Anger, fear, and slight hope were among the various feelings she said she personally felt at that second. Anger dominated the others, because it was her grandchild that was in such a regressive present stage. Her fear prevented her from having the slightest inkling of thinking of his future.

In our lengthy conversations, I soon learned that with the Duchess's age, time had certainly brought much wisdom and grace. Her character was never to dwell on the past. Duchess had long accepted the fact no one could alter nor change history, but she could certainly indulge in her present environment. Duchess easily could be considered characteristically overpowering and equally determined. She was a big-boned woman with clear traces of her German Dutch ancestry. It was definitely the power other provoking character that appropriated her graceful statuesque form.

Duchess vivaciously advocated the rights for racial minorities as well as heavily supported the women suffrage movement. She always spoke her mind without fearful remorse. Duchess, similar to her grandson, was doggedly determined in her committed stances no matter how rewarding the end would prove. She was left with a rather sizable substantial inheritance, which she parlayed to her advantage. Her controlling investments in the community and in certain politicians made the Duchess a force to reckon with. Unfortunately, she did not possess the power to cure her ailing child.

It appeared that immediately after Sebastian's first birthday, Zachary coerced a drunken Julie to sign away any and all custodial parental rights to Sebastian.

Zachary's sincere intent was to place Sebastian in an orphanage. However, during one of Julie's raging fits of drunken anger, she called his parents and told Duchess of their son's hidden agenda for their only grandchild. Horrified and bitterly outraged at his actions, Duchess immediately called one of her judicial associates and obtained an injunction, which abruptly stopped his treacherous deception. Duchess proceeded to file for petition with the courts for the guardianship of Sebastian. With her established movement within the judicial circles of friends, she was literally no contest for either wanton parent.

Even to this day, she said that bitterness still existed between her and her son. Her bitterness stemmed mainly because he had always refused to accept his son. He regarded Sebastian as a separating force between his parents and himself.

I watched as the Duchess slowly entered the room in complete control. Her staunch shoulders imposed impressions of weathered strength. The grave figure that rested on the bed could not move her, she decided. Nothing could damper her mission. She simply displayed no weakened emotion, even as she brushed his thinning hair from his skeletal eyes. Initially, she collected her leaking emotional thoughts and donned her most gay but stoic mask.

Sebastian asked me if I would bring his Victorian rocker from his grandmother's home. He said he wanted something familiar in his sterile room. I took this opportunity for another interview. In this one, the Duchess paused momentarily as she remembered that dreadful day Cleo had driven Sebastian to her home.

"At first, I hate to say, I didn't recognize the frail stranger that stood on my porch, even after I had extended my hand to greet the sulked person. I almost fell back against the door when I heard him say in a raspy voice the name Duchess."

"When was the last time you saw him before that day?"

"Oh dear, it must have been some time ago. I mean, we spoke regularly by phone. I knew he was tired and working a lot. But I had no idea he was sick."

The weather was slightly warm with faint touches of the wind scarcely blowing.

Sebastian stood before his grandmother cloaked in an oversized sweater, while Cleo stood directly behind physically supporting his every step. As he spoke, Duchess subsequently caught sight of his profile. Without thinking, she raised her hands in utter despair. She was clearly shocked by the figure in front of her. He nervously smiled and greeted her with a trembling raspy voiced "It's me, Sebastian."

She quickly pulled him into her arms. They embraced tightly. She felt her stomach churn from horror, as she felt how thin he really was.

Although Duchess had been ignorant to the threat of toxoplasmosis in her grandson's life, she searched throughout her medical journals for answers to his unknown plight. She constantly called the Center for Disease Control in

Atlanta to explain to her in laymen's terms.

The Duchess was formally informed of his homosexual lifestyle the same moment she was told of his diagnosis. "The gayness was no real surprise to me...I always known but said nothing. Nonetheless, Sebastian was still my grandchild, and the fact he was gay had no bearing on my heartfelt love for him. In my heart, I knew and long accepted his hidden identity. Until that moment he disclosed his sexuality, I had only known a part of him. Now, I was able to love the whole person that he was."

As her interest in his health status increased, the actualizing woman grew in self-awareness with a firm identity. She ultimately became keenly receptive to what was factual and worthwhile, giving notice to that which was dishonest or that which was superfluous. She kept vigil around the last stages of her child's life.

While Sebastian was still at Vanderbilt, I befriended a nurse that appeared to clearly understand and accept our friendship with Sebastian. From the moment any of us stepped off the elevator, she was there with a reassuring smile. The smile belonged to Belinda Bames.. This angel in white often told us about his previous nights of unrest. One night in the middle of the early hours before dawn, Sebastian suddenly frantically rose up in his bed. His bed was covered with profuse sweat and blood. It was still dark, as his bed appeared to glow with the whiteness of the starched linen. It was assumed that a nightmare possibly caused him to stir, which caused him to fling completely free from the portable IV monitor. The monitor interrupted the pregnant silence with its electronic whaling siren. He couldn't see around him, which probably terrified him even more.

Sebastian told me the next morning about his night. He said he immediately felt strong massive pressure on his body. Someone was trying to make him lie flat, as other extensions of human flesh grabbed at his flailing arms. The bright lights blurred his already limited vision. He tried clutching his painfully cramped stomach, but he couldn't move his body. He was restrained to his bed. Sebastian cried out hysterically, as the IV lines were injected back into his body near the broken veins. He blacked out.

The lesions duplicated themselves. His battle chest of medications had been discontinued or quickly changed due to him falling in dangerous toxicity levels with his liver failing. His "helper" lymphocytes were rapidly being destroyed.

PANELS

Sebastian appeared to be resting after he just returned from having an additional series of MRI brain scans. He experienced headaches with much frequency that appeared to accompany his seizure disorders. His usual well-mannered disposition drastically evolved into Dr. Jekyll and Mr. Hyde characters without warning. He experienced repeated episodes of abrupt awakening from his drug-induced sleep, with vague but intense anxiety. He often sat in bed with frightened expressions with either emotional or psychological signs of anxiety and confusion.

Although he wasn't too fond of the idea initially, the Duchess persuaded Dr. Sanders to take care of Sebastian's emotional needs. She once had served on the women's auxiliary for the hospital and still knew her strengths. Sebastian was her only weakness.

Dr. Sanders termed his behaviors as being "pavor nocturmus." Sebastian also experienced episodic behaviors, such as the incident where he threw his food tray angrily at us. At times, he saw objects around him that others didn't see. Paranoia set in, as he contemplated others were trying to kill him, especially those dressed in white.

Dr. Raffanti ordered additional testing of CAT and MRI brain scans attempting to determine the growth and the actual locations of the brain abscesses. Another physician on the team, Dr. Lisa Brumble, contemplated another brain biopsy that further diagnosed toxo, although the presumptive diagnosis of toxo had already been determined.

Sebastian could no longer visually recognize the figures that lurked over his bed. He felt the breathing shadow of the Duchess, while fighting back the rising tears, called his name softly. She delicately stroked his face. Sebastian appeared to relax with ease. He smiled toward her movement. Duchess refused to look at the various life-supporting equipment around his bed nor acknowledge the numerous IV tracts that ended in his arms. She also refused to see her Sebastian as being so helpless and lifeless.

Duchess told me how she imagined Sebastian as being that forever-stubborn little boy that always refused to freely admit his mortal errors in life. In her mind, he transformed back into that same spoiled rambunctious nuisance she realized she molded. Sebastian was definitely a fighter and would eventually conquer whatever was affecting him fatally.

The latest additions to his list of infections were pneumocystis carinii pneumonia, dementia, and pneumothorax. His days were equally good as they were bad.

Dr. Raffanti ordered a set daily routine attempting to reduce further unnecessary stress until he could go home. Sebastian developed pneumothorax after several traumatic events, which included bronchoscope and intubation with positive and expiatory pressure. His lungs finally collapsed, as the aerosol pentamidine prophylactic therapy appeared to no longer prove effective.

By now, Sebastian already experienced randomly four bouts of pep. He would live to experience further cases of pneumothorax. Cultured organisms included staphylococcus aureus, and Aspergillus niger. He appeared not fully aware since his last partial seizure left him apparent wakefulness with grossly diminished response to any outside stimuli. Still, Sebastian continued fighting. A fact alone the Duchess knew in her heart.

I began to notice his father now standing for hours outside the actual nursing station. I got the impression that he refused to go look at his son closer. Perhaps, he felt ashamed and yet guilt ridden. Maybe he sincerely believed his earlier resistance that alienated his own blood had somehow driven Sebastian to his own unfortunate lifestyle.

Perhaps he should have spent more quality time with his son instead of allowing his obviously ineffective parents to nurture the manly side of Sebastian. Whatever made him that way had nothing to do with his father. Zachary told his mother that he knew he was normal and found it difficult to accept what he considered his son's abnormalities.

I decided to take a chance and talk with him. He was Sebastian's father, after all, right? Our introduction was quite cold. Nonetheless, he did agree to speak with me but only for a few minutes.

Zachary concluded to me whatever defects Sebastian possessed were definitely due to his mother's drunken stupor crazed history. Perhaps Julie was drinking booze while she was still pregnant, he wondered. Looking over his own family, he shook his head. No one on his side of the family ever possessed any of the lower qualities that would have conceived the notion of homosexuality. Introverted focusing on the perverted thoughts of two men entangled sexually sickened his very manly soul. He became emotionally nauseated. I winced as he mentioned a thought if perhaps Sebastian ever once looked at him in that same manner.

Later, I watched as his mother Julie and Zachary passed each other in the tight antiseptic halls as total removed strangers. Neither acknowledged the other's presence. Each appeared to blame the other for the reason their son was dying. They stared bitterly with expressionless glances. Finally, after he muttered something of vile contempt in her direction, Zachary left the hospital. Why should he remain? Hadn't the destruction taken its toll? In his weakened moments, Zachary promised me that one day he would return and stand by his son's bed. Maybe he would even forgive Sebastian for his wayward life.

Relinquishing Immortality

In one of my courses on spirituality, I became aware that for mankind, a significant rule of life was to accept and not question. Another rule, which was incomprehensibly, indecipherably clear, denoted neither possible deals nor bartering being allowed. Perhaps the printed words were now reality for all of us.

For whatever reason, I felt compelled to stay by his side. I would steal away from my workstation and return to his bed late at night. Often we said nothing. Often I sat in a corner and watched him sleep.

The light raised shadows around Sebastian, seated in a wooden rocker facing the open window. His trembling bony limbs desperately clutched the sides of the chair. His head whirled heavily with dizziness encompassed with vague but familiar feelings.

Across from him, on the floor, a designer mallard print comforter had fallen heavily from his unmade bed. He watched, as if in total awe, the material descended downward, as if he was fascinatingly disturbed by its quickness. He related his very existence with the fact his life also changed rapidly, which included the onset of impregnated desolation. Nonetheless, he appeared still somewhat troubled by the insignificance of the fallen linen.

On the bedside table was the makeshift altar of sorts. The materialistic collection of memories included a sculpture of a pair of silver mallards in boundless unrestricted flight. He stole curious glances at the objects while wincing a quick smile halfhearted, as if the structures gave a fragmented kind of reflection into his past life.

His face appeared somewhat darkened distraught and shadowed with the complications of beard stubble of days growth. His once-massive frame transformed was now imprisoned in the fragile figure with his starched bedclothes hanging as loose sails that rested on the calm seas. It was as if his soul was waiting.

Once considered very distinguished and darkly attractive, his skin now clung tightly to his bones. His eyes were incredibly dark and hollow, complete with emptiness within the deep massive circles that reflected simple destructive but reasonably reflective doubt. His eyes jaundiced with tormented sorrow. He appeared deceptively as an elderly man covered in swollen raised liver spots. The markings further accentuated his graven features. His persona was drastically aging, as seconds developed into years. In actual reality, he was just thirty-four.

It had been close to three weeks since Sebastian was readmitted to this same room on the eighth floor. He told me once that he felt as if he was to live there for the remainder of whatever life he still had to endure. Countless times, he wanted to run from that room, that floor, that hospital, from himself. He didn't want to bear this cruel cross after all, especially not alone. Please, he prayed, direct the Angel of Death to him. He wanted me to say words to console but I really knew of none. I actually felt defeated and not worthy of my own degree in divinity. I hated myself to realize that I knew Sebastian was involved in a hopeless battle. His unworthy opponent was quite witty and powerful.

Sebastian could no longer defend himself. His strength was fast succumbing to the painful endurance of the suffering already inflicted. The fight had been decided but who would be triumphantly happy? He was beyond finding solace in the arms of pity. He blamed no one for his lack of indiscretion. His bitterness was newfound; he was ready to depart life and all it held for him. I hated myself for not only knowing this but thinking it as well. Where was my own faith?

No one else was in the room with us. The attending nurse just left him after attempting to give Sebastian his evening medications that he refused once again. There was simply no angry verbalization between either party that time. There was only silence, as the rain fell quickly upon the earth. A tear also fell down his face, as he continued to stare outside in oblivious concentration. Car horns and sirens broke the code of silence below but not with him. He was ready. He was still afraid but ready. Once again, Sebastian was in his frightfully familiar room on the AIDS floor.

Although there were several doctors assigned to his team, two doctors in particular continued to stand out in Sebastian's mind. One reason was extremely obvious: his pain had not prevented him from falling in love with Dr. Sanders. Sebastian had known Dr. Sanders wasn't much older than he was which Sebastian appreciated. With his boyish charm and his wicked smile. Dr. Sanders' heart was certainly filled with sincere gold. Sebastian gradually grew very fond of Dr. Sanders, who spent hours talking to him from the beginning.

PANELS

Sebastian once told me that when he first learned of his fatal predicament, he confided to the psychiatrist that he had already decided on the perfect technique to end it all.

"Dr. Sanders, I know that you probably don't agree with my choice, but I can no longer live the rest of my days like this—Days that have sadly become so damn desolate and insignificant to me…I don't want to live by these measures put upon me—With whatever strength that I may have still left, I'm prepared to take care to end my hell," Sebastian whispered in his faint coarse voice.

"It's a sign of vanity. Suicide was the best way to get back at life and shows control of one's actions to the fullness. An act in grand fashion," Dr. Sanders, not at all surprised, calmly responded.

"Then consider me a grand queen—But better than that, imagine yourself in my place…then tell me that I'm wrong."

"Is this a way to a mean?" Dr. Sanders asked while ignoring his suggestion.

"Is there any other way to deal with life that has no certain future except death?"

Dr. Sanders possibly did take Sebastian's decision extremely serious. He tried

looking deeply into Sebastian's soul imagining his own personal hell and torrid fears.

Painfully, he realized the man before him had long lost his will to fight. How could he argue with Sebastian while knowing full well there was no cure on the distant horizon? Who was being rational and who was persistent in maintaining partial truth?

Sebastian was always the caregiver with the firmest shoulders for others to cry on. He was the Rock of Gibraltar. He hid his feelings of true mortality. Perhaps Dr. Sanders realized the fight was indeed over, but he refused to accept the obvious defeat.

The other physician Sebastian favored was Dr. Stefhan Raffanti. Dr. Raffanti went far beyond the realm of the call of doctrine in order to heal the sick and ailing. He was conditioned to only accept prolonging life without fail.

I recall how Sebastian fondly remembered Dr. Raffanti seeking to find an ailing destitute soul dying from AIDS stricken anger. Sebastian knew all too well how Dr. Raffanti climbed through a second floor stairwell window and crawled through the stench of human filth and the jagged pieces of the broken glass from the window. He was searching for one of Sebastian's clients to administer to his failing health.

Without pity, aglow with only heartfelt warmth. Dr. Raffanti tracked down his prey for the sake of sustaining life. Although the incident was rarely ever discussed, no one had ever forgotten the deed of the unselfish internist.

Before he became a mere statistic, Sebastian previously counseled with numerous patients of Dr. Raffanti. He already established a close working relationship with the physician with respect. Even Dr. Raffanti could not shield the mask of disbelief when he eventually realized who Sebastian really was during his initial admission. Dr. Raffanti's facial expression became chalky white with horror from the realization of the identity in the examining room.

Having counseled numerous terminal ill patients assigned to them, I had the opportunity to get to know both physicians quite well. Dr. Sanders and the graying Dr. Raffanti long stopped paying their last respects to the dead. Both painstakingly cringed each time they turned the sterile sober white corners seeing new or familiar faces arriving on that floor. So many times their individual thoughts took them away from this morbid atmosphere. Unfortunately, they only escaped briefly.

Collectively, on the immediate horizon, they waited with others for the ultimate cure for AIDS. All had observed enough of the damned control groups and individual subjects. No more, they cried.

From our various conversations, I knew that Dr. Sanders was beyond the juxtaposed confusion and pain for his own clients and friends, as well as the world around him. He lost numerous friends that he couldn't even help even with his medical knowledge. Since leaving the fast-paced life of New York's Sloan Kettering Hospital, Dr. Sanders aged. His life appeared to have inherited a renewed vague life-saving campaign.

He was fueled by his bitter hopelessness and ignorance. He feared for his own past life surfacing and threatening his immortality. Certainly, he saw himself clearly through Sebastian's eyes.

Once while eating my lunch in the break room, I overheard the following conversation between the two men:

"Hundreds of years from now, someone will be standing before a large class of eager beaver medical students dissecting our decades as being the period of years of unnecessary mortal defeat. Laughing their fool heads off at how we watched ourselves die without knowing we had the answer within our midst," Dr. Raffanti barked, as he poured the thick settled percolated coffee with the loose caked coffee grinds into his weathered, stained mug. As he collapsed into the massive wooden Danish chair, a copy of the *Proceedings of the National Academy of Sciences* was thrown across the cracked, aged Formica table in front of him. Dr. Sanders stood nearby waiting for Dr. Raffanti to read completely the yellow highlighted article. Mechanically, movements void of any emotions available. Dr. Raffanti quickly studied the carefully chosen passages. His face changed to crimson.

"I actually fool myself into believing that I'm actually doing something to ease the troubled minds of those with AIDS. I try to even fool myself into honestly believing what comes out of my own mouth...This hell just tears my flesh as easily as a jagger of glass would have. One of our sainted benevolent leaders himself...who incidentally found a way to conquer polio...now warns us that our efforts to prevent the spread of AIDS through immunization is senseless."

Dr. Sanders leaned against the nursing station threshold, as people continued to walk past him oblivious to his disheartening words. His ageless voice seemed cold with a broken spirit. His eyes fixated to form a glassy stare, as he continued with his desperate soliloquy.

"What really bothers me is not necessarily his suggestions for searching for a cure of a different ailment, but the fact that there are others out there with powers to be who may disregard AIDS the same uncaring way that Sabin had...Hell, instead of us running from the nefarious virus...why can't we try to find the son of a bitch...God only knows what other virus may also evolve into this same stage."

"How much longer can this epidemic go on? How many more needless deaths do we have to witness? Are we to become goddamned robots masking our own fears as we look into their dreadful eyes while we stumble with asinine excuses simply because we don't know what the hell's happening to us?" Dr. Raffanti released..

Dr. Sanders caught Dr. Raffanti's eyes. Dr. Raffanti's face expressed a bitter solace. The reality of living up to their individual aspiration and dreams frightened them into anger. In total reflective silence, Dr. Raffanti reached over and squeezed Dr. Sanders' shoulder for assurance, as he walked away to begin his morning rounds.

Malice shadows danced around Sebastian. He was in his wooden Victorian rocker when I arrived. He faced the open window. I called his name out so that I wouldn't startle him. He didn't turn but nodded. The vintage rocker had been with him throughout his entire life. In his past, he told me that his grandmother would rock him seemingly for hours. She cradled him close inside her arms, as she read poetry or recited her own created simple stories of her past. Now, he imagined that he still felt her arms tightening around him, as they encircled his frail body, trying to keep harm away from him. He found serenity within his wooden splintered host.

As I continued my watch, I soon realized just how his body had drastically changed. I closed my eyes shortly while hoping that when I opened them again, I would see the old Sebastian. Instead, my hope vanished as reality took hold.

Sebastian now wore a wool cap to protect his bare head from the sharp wind. His hair loss was a result of the numerous radiation procedures used to reduce the swelling of his massive tumors. His once thick mane of black hair that I loved was now lost along with his innocent youth. He closed his eyes frequently. He told me how he tried to imagine himself young again, and not dying. He felt somewhat safe seated within the enormous rocker, as he had once while still in the Duchess' motherly clutches. He was assured no harm would ever come his way while she held him.

During one of her visits, his mother shared a conversation with me that she had with Sebastian during this period. Amidst her own pain, she said she felt vindicated and comforted in knowing that Sebastian did not hate her.

On one of the last times he ever spoke with his mother, there appeared a great deal of contention. Sebastian's solitude faded quickly. Julie's voice penetrated his stillness. He displayed no emotional reactions. Instead, he turned back to the window and possibly to his private thoughts.

"So, what are you thinking about?" she asked.

"I'm contemplating whether or not to simply close my eyes and never open them again at least not until the very end."

"Why on earth would you want to give up so easily on life?"

"In case you haven't noticed, life gave up on me. I'm just being the ever-polite loser and bow out gracefully. Why shouldn't I give up? Isn't that just what you and my father did with me? Didn't you both simply turn and walk away just when I needed you both the most? It must not be too hard to call it quits!"

"So, you're still very bitter about what I did in the past? Is this how we are to leave with whatever bitterness between ourselves? Drowning in a sea of hate because of a mistake on my part? Ending the last moments with sharp

PANELS

jagged words of hatred?"

"Whose' hatred?" Sebastian said. "Certainly not mine. I've long accepted your rejection as well as my father's. I realized years ago that I was never quite the son that either of you had wanted...So...Why did you ever come back?"

"Honey, it wasn't until last week that I even found out about your condition. Your grandmother called me. I would've been here sooner, but I had to get my act together to be strong for you or rather strong for my own self. I can't bear the thought of losing you again. I don't know if you're listening to a word that I'm trying to say, but believe me, if I could take your place in all of the misery, I definitely would."

"Bravo! How damned wonderfully honorable of you to even suggest replacing me in this hell. Don't bother. Isn't it a tad too late to start playing the ever-concerned loving mother role? What a superb act. I can already hear the heavenly nominations for your Oscar. In a rather short matter of time, I will no longer exist in either of your lives. Only a mere memory. A bad one at that. You're wanting to trade places with me is quite a twist. Maybe you'll be well remembered and rewarded one day for the sincere thought."

"I really don't know what I expected from you by me coming here. I can't change anything about the past. I believed foolishly in giving a person a second chance. But it is obviously clear that you still hold against me the foolish things that I did when you were a baby, placing you with your grandmother. I can never justify what or why I did what I did at that time but at that time I really thought I was doing the right thing for you." She stopped, regained her composure. "I know that you can't forgive me, and I don't forgive myself, " Julie stopped. Tears mounting. "Somehow, though, I had hoped that we could still be friends. I've never called upon you for anything. Even now I don't want anything from you except for your love. Maybe one day in your past, whenever you made a mistake that had involved others beside yourself, maybe you remembered that no one, not even yourself, was ever perfect. I hope that you're listening and remembering that I do love you. Go ahead and scream, yell, do something to let me know that you've heard me. What else can I possibly say?"

"Momma, I'm sorry...I've never totally blamed you for deserting me. Time will heal even the weakest of hearts. Momma, I knew the real score. Believe it or not, I actually understood. What I mostly hated and despised about my life was that I've never been able to tell anyone directly just how much I love them. It's never been very easy for me...For whatever it is worth,

I forgive you, and I even love you regardless." He paused. "Do you forgive me?"

Sebastian turned and faced his mother. He looked into her face for the first time, wanting to reassure her. Julie leaned forward and kissed him on his forehead. Tears formed and fell from both of their eyes. Sebastian reached out his bony hands to wipe away her tears. His arms would not reach her. The intravenous tubing restricted it. His failing strength was passing quickly. Julie rose to leave. Sebastian returned to the open window. I passed his mother as she left the room. She grabbed my hand and squeezed it.

Slowly, Sebastian tried to return to his bed. His body was numb with pain. I tried to help him but he pushed me away. A nurse had previously administered a continual flow of morphine for his discomfort. The medication, together with any movement from time spent in his rocker, made him faintly nauseated. Although his bed was only inches from him, his movement took great effort. Still, I tried to help but he still pushed me away.

"Why are you here?"

"What do you mean?"

"Why are you here? Is it to watch me shrivel up and die?"

"Sebastian, I'm here because I want to be here. I want to be with you." I paused. I really didn't know what to say. "Do you not want me here?"

"What good am I? I can't do a damn thing. I can barely talk without gasping for air."

"I'm here because we are friends and I don't walk away from a friend no matter what."

"Michal, that's what I like about you. You are so full of crap that I actually believe you." Sebastian attempted to smile. "Just promise me that you won't remember me like this."

"Sebastian, my life is full of memories of you and this is only a small part."

"Good." Sebastian tried to get out of the chair and almost fell to the floor.

A familiar nurse, sporting shoulder-length red hair, rushed to his side. I watched as she gently pivoted him around. He held onto her thin waist until he felt the bed underneath him. Gingerly, she reached for his feet to position him on the bed.

Belinda Barnes was more than just a nurse to us. As it turned out, besides coming into our life as a nurse, she attended the very same church where Richard's memorial was held. She appeared to understand the struggle. Often while he slept, she and I conversed quietly. Although a total stranger, her piercing eyes looked in my very soul and comforted me. This road of travel was all too familiar to her. However, I don't think she ever gave up hope.

Sebastian had grown to love the nurse whom he considered his angel of mercy. Her mannerism reflected sincerity without fail. He had also remembered her previously taking care of Richard before he died. Sebastian told me he also remembered she was there during Richard's memorial. He even remembered her very swollen but dry eyes. Now it was him that she helped.

She reached over his balding head to reposition his pillows. She kissed his forehead, as he lay extremely exhausted. He smiled his weak smile. Her eyes silently acknowledged.

Looking into her eyes, Sebastian notified Belinda he wasn't looking to create any new marathon records of being admitted into hospitals. He didn't need their sugar-coated expensive remedies. Belinda listened attentively. She routinely checked the needles to assure the continuing path of the intravenous fluids that flowed into his partially collapsed veins.

I was staring out the window when the Duchess came in and stood next to his bed. I started to leave but she beckoned me to stay.

"Guess what, Duchess. I'm scared. I'm actually scared of what's happening to me," Sebastian said.

"You mean that you're actually scared of something? Am I in the correct room? Where's my Sebastian who's too stubborn to fear anything?"

"What do you think death is really like? I mean, I know that you really don't know about dying firsthand, but maybe you may have heard something about the other side. Perhaps I should have listened more closely to those sermons when I was younger. What do you think?"

"Life itself may have taught me a great deal, but unfortunately death never gave me anything except a broken heart. I can only wish to believe what your grandfather always believed about death. He would say that whenever someone starts their final transition into the other world of darkness and light, that there was someone waiting for them at the end of the tunnel. Supposedly, that person or spirit was actually someone that the dying person had known and had loved very much while both were still alive on this earth. God uses loved ones to welcome individuals into heaven to begin their serenity."

"So the light at the end of the tunnel is actually Grandpa and the rest of my friends?"

"If they're the people that you loved the most, perhaps they're the ones waiting at the other end for you."

"They're the ones that have already died. I do love them but you're here with me. Above all others, you're the one that I'll always love more than life itself. Don't you ever forget my love and respect for you."

"Don't you ever forget my love for you, " she said. "Oh, God, if I could just take your place, I would. This isn't fair for me to have to say good-bye so soon in your life. I'm sorry for crying,.Damn it, it hurts seeing you this way. I feel so guilty, at times, wanting you to suffer no more. I feel guilty whenever I realize that your own faith and hope to endure this hell are much stronger than mine. I feel guilty that I cursed God for allowing this to happen to my child. Whenever your battle finally ends, then I must find strength to accept the defeat, but not until that moment." Duchess paused. She took a deep breath.

"I never meant to drag you into my hell. I never meant for you to see me like this. I'm sorry for all of the pain I've ever caused you and Grandfather. Having you here with me right now gives me assurance that everything will be all right eventually." Both cried softly.

As delicately as if holding angel hair in her hands without the slightest ruffling, she rocked her child close to her heart. She lowered him ever so gently, kissed his face, and left the room. Sebastian no longer avoided the truth falsely replacing the fiction with reality.

Later that night, I sat and stared at him as he slept. My own thoughts betrayed me. I may have had a stoic expression plastered across my face, but inside I was emotionally torn. I screamed on the inside. My heart raced with fear. I wanted to run from this room but I also wanted to stay and fight that damn virus that was taking another one of my friends.

As the cold barren rain fell quickly upon the earth, it shattered the silence. The rain danced wildly on his windowpane. A song filled the air from his small portable radio on his nightstand. A woman was softly singing a ballad of the pain that hurt leaving her with a broken heart and feeling scorned. As she said the word "best friend," I thought I noticed that Sebastian appeared to have smiled.

I watched as Belinda offered Sebastian his evening medications. He politely refused everything except the morphine. There were no angry verbalizations just agreeable silences. No pep speeches on any of the significance of receiving the pills—just silence.

He closed his eyes. Before the morphine could fully take effect, Sebastian winced at his unbearable pain.

I imagined someone had reached for him at that moment. Perhaps he now saw them, but still could not make out their identities. Maybe he felt another

PANELS

touch, one he was somehow strangely familiar with. A smile formed on his face. Sebastian tried desperately to gasp for his breath. Maybe Sebastian felt he was ready.

A firm smile formed on his face, as his breathing slowly ceased. Tears fell from my eyes. I walked over to where he was lying. I kissed him softly on his lips. I whispered to him to have a beautiful journey home.

The Duchess once again was holding onto her dear grandson. She held onto the beveled crystal urn that briefly housed his remains. Methodically, Cleo stood very close to the shore at the Duchess's side. We watched, as the frail aged woman carefully knelt closer to the water.

With tears absent from both faces, the Duchess opened the urn, exposing his ashes. As she gingerly poured some of his ashes onto the miniature wooden Viking ship draped with tiny red ribbons, some of the embers were caught in the strong untamed wind across the cold stillness of Percy Priest Lake near the cliffs.

Cleo ignited the starboard of the ship, using one of burning candles present during the memorial. With a swift steady push from the Duchess' hand, the tiny vessel floated away toward the center of the water, where the flames overwhelmed the wooden pieces. His ashes dissipated into a bluish green hue. Cleo and I took the remainder of his ashes and buried the ashes underneath a newly planted Dogwood tree at Radnor Lake, as he requested.

Regardless of what happens in one's life, no matter how cruel or kind it seems at that moment, life around you continues to carry on. Time was definitely essential in healing. I would give anything to have my life as it once was. Staying optimistic can really be trying especially if most of your loved ones have left you. Each day becomes a challenge but one that I cherish because it gives me hopes to fight, not just for myself but also for the others.

Days quickly evolved into months and then years. Cleo and I continued being there for each other but not as often. She did tell me that at night, as Theresa slept, Cleo found herself often alone downstairs in the gallery facing the mural. The memories of the past years continued to haunt her. The numerous candles that illuminated the darkened corners failed to illuminate her darkened heart.

In remembering her fallen friends, she reflected with pride over each one.

She missed their presence. She still longed for the day she would recapture their smiles. I couldn't agree any more.

One recent night, she called me was right after she had found the lost letter. Cleo had been crying. She told me that she had read his letter over and over. Sebastian had written the letter after their last conflict. The letter was not delivered until after his death.

Sebastian wrote following words:

My Dearest Cleo,

My concepts of life have all but turned dim, as fate itself appeared deemed to totally separate us. Yet, my love, I do take great courage for the memory of you that still remains intact, now and forever, to console this rather desolate aching heart of mine. In my every thought, you dominate. In my every breath, it is your precious name that I declare, and the very beat of my heart echoes the word of "I love you," endless to you, my darling Cleo, because I do love you as only love itself knows why or even how. My heart went out to you many times. One of my fondest memories was that one summer picnic from whence the most tender and the most affectionate feelings of love, pure love, have ever radiated.

From which I derive my own limited strength, my joy, and yes, even my life. For you see, before you and the others in the circle, my life was null and void. Although I smiled, danced, and even held my life at surfaced ease, it was only a simulated farce. For within, I was already dead. But alas, Cleo, you brought life to the dead, you gave me insurmountable joy to my lonely heart, and above all else, you inflamed a heart, my heart, where there wasn't a spark.

Unfortunately, I never took the time to actually tell you just how much I do love you. Yes, I have every reason to be proud of you, because you have loved us individually in return in such a way that only love could love. My friend, always remember that you had earlier realized that we all must not fight someone because they have AIDS but to fight for what that person actually symbolizes which is indeed the mortal soul of mankind. Omni a Vincit Amor Ad finem.

My sincerest love,
Sebastian

It was nearly a year after Sebastian's death that Cleo closed her art gallery. While advocating for the rights of those living with AIDS, she became aware

PANELS

of the need for housing. With her investment from the gallery, she opened her home as an AIDS hospice. She named the hospice "Circle of Friends." No one was ever turned away.

Almost ten years past before I saw Cleo again. I had moved away from Nashville and far away from my past or so I thought. I purposely stopped all contacts including with Cleo. Or at least I thought it was possible to do.

I found myself living in Savannah, Georgia. I had entered into a partnership with a local mental health agency. The life was slower and humid but full of Southern relic charm and hospitality. I felt safe within the weeping willowed streets. I could live my life free from harm that was until I learned of my own diagnosis. Then, I wanted to go back to my past. I wanted to go home.

I decided to attend a symposium on AIDS in Nashville especially after reading a familiar name as one of the presenters. Cleo was one of the speakers.

She looked somewhat weathered but still quite the graceful woman I have always known. At first, I wondered if she still remembered me. She did! She caught my eye and smiled in return.

As Cleo spoke, she stood ever so proud. She mentioned that she rejoiced in thinking her best friends were still there beside her. Believing that, she smiled. Tears formed in both our eyes. Someone from the audience asked why she cared to speak on behalf of those living with AIDS. Cleo rose defiantly from her chair. She stated with firm convictions that although it may have helped her to deal with her own loss, others who were still ignorant to the cause needed to hear the truth. "When I first arrived in this country, I read a story of how a few people made a difference in their lives because of a promise to their dying leader. He was very wise. He long realized that the mere differences that existed between the individuals would forever separate them. How could anyone avail himself to total knowledge if he refused to open his eyes fully?

"One night as the young men slept, the frail elderly leader secretly wrapped an enormous crate. He quickly sealed the package and gave strict instructions that the package could not be opened until they reached the mainland. The crate was designed in such a way that all of the youth had to assist in handling and transporting. The weight could never be shifted.

Each youth had to promise him they would abide by his words. I don't remember the exact reason that these men were lost deep in the forest in whatever inhabitant land that they were in. What I do remember vividly was how they struggled through countless conflicts and strives, not only with the foreign soil but also with each other. Through their tears and sweat, they managed to survive.

Months later, as they emerged joyously from within the thickness of the dense forest, the crate was finally opened. To the amazement of each individual, the contents appeared to have been nothing more than dirt and mortar. Inside the box was another letter from the leader explaining the purpose. The purpose was simple. Together they would survive, alone they would perish."

As tears formed in the corner of her eyes while stealing a glance at her healthy teenage daughter, she concluded. "There's still too much turning away from reality."

I really missed Cleo. I missed hearing her sweet laughter. I missed the closeness we once shared. I missed everyone.

Up until this moment, the last time we were together was when some of the panels of the AIDS quilt came to Nashville. Even now, every time I hear a song of Kathy Mattea, I still close my eyes. I can still see the ground blanketed with panels. I can still hear the baby voice of Theresa asking me about her uncles. The selected panels circled the entire Parthenon and people walked around, exploring the displays of affection. The pain is still real as it was then.

It was great seeing her again especially since it wasn't for someone's memorial service. Walking down the aisle to a seat, I saw the Duchess in the audience. She saw me and beckoned me to the empty seat beside her. She remembered me and even asked how the manuscript was coming along.

There's never a day that I don't miss Cleo tremendously. I still think of our circle. I think mostly of the good times that we shared. I miss our laughter and our joy. But, I now find myself alone. I constantly think of the past and how I have become quite bitter. Actually, I am angry. But at whom was my anger directed?

Much to my surprise, when the panel discussion ended, Cleo ran over to where I stood. We kissed and embraced. It felt wonderful holding her again after all this time. Theresa stood nearby smiling that customary cherubic smile. I reached out and squeezed her extended hand.

"My, you have really grown into a beautiful young woman." I twirled her around. "Let me look at you." Her body was void of the flatness of her youth. She now sported height and curvature.

PANELS

"Uncle Mike, you have always been so sweet. I have really missed you. I ask Mama all the time if she ever hears from you. How have you been?"

"Yeah, Michal, how have you been? I haven't heard from you in ages. I was afraid you had dropped off the end of the earth." Cleo continued holding onto me. "It's so good seeing you…Listen, I'm gonna have to go and collect my evaluations and meet with the council briefly. Why don't you come over to the house tomorrow for lunch?"

"I would be honored. What do I need to bring?"

"Not a thing, just yourself." Cleo turned to leave. "Oh God, it's so good seeing you! See ya soon."

The next day, the hours appeared to crawl as slow as aged earthworms in the rain. I dressed and redressed several times trying to find the right choice. I wanted something to hide my sulkiness and thin frame. I wanted to hide the new me.

I arrived a few minutes before noon. The weather was untraditionally warm. In the mist of fall, there was a premature of new growth. The red, three-floored home still appeared as the way I had left it several years earlier. The only differences were the fresh coat of black paint on the wrought iron gate and the name on a signpost. Seeing the words "Circle of Friends" emblazoned on the massive double doors made me stop to rethink my past.

I took a deep breath and then knocked on the door's windowpane. There was a quick sound of clacking across the hardwood floors and the door opened.

"Yes…may I help you?" A young man asked.

"I'm here to see Mrs. Castleman."

"You must be Mr. Cameron! Please follow me; she has been expecting you." The doorman with the boyish charm ushered me in. "She's waiting for you on the veranda."

I followed him through the now unfamiliar house. The mural was still hanging with what appeared fresh cut flowers on a pedestal. The room where was once the gallery now supported various couches and small intimate tables. I walked past people coupled in conversations. There were soft sounds of laughter in areas. Amidst the folksy furnishings were the presence of IV strung bags.

"I knew you wouldn't stand me up." Cleo winked as she sipped on her glass of iced tea.

"Believe me, that was the last thing on my mind. You look great!" I leaned over and kissed her.

"You don't look so bad yourself...I hope you brought your appetite." Cleo stood. "Let me look at you. For Christ's sake, you haven't changed much after all these years."

"Maybe a little...gained a pound, lost three pounds. You know the routine. I still cry at Julia Roberts' movies."

"Always the romantic...speaking of which, is there anyone in the horizon?"

"Yeah...myself. For the first time in my life, I have started to love all my flaws and myself. I have even forgiven myself."

"Good for you. You deserve it." Cleo appeared to be examining me closely. "After all these years, you are still quite attractive."

"Not bad, considering, right?"

"Well, since you brought it up. How are you doing?"

"I have my good and bad days. My count stays 500 to 600. So, I guess I'm just peachy keen." I smeared jam across my bagel.

"So you are taking care of yourself?"

"Yeah...in fact, I have developed a plan to live."

"Good for you!" Cleo poured more wine. "Is it something we can incorporate here? We can use a little cheer and hope around here."

"Perhaps...I simply started to forgive myself and stopped hating myself because I contracted the virus. I stopped looking at the advent of a new day as being a day of misery and began seeing it for its newness and as a gift."

"If I could just bottle your emotions and serve it to those living here, I would probably have lengthened many of their lives. How did you come to this thought?"

"Realizing that I can still love myself." I paused. A shadow of a thin soul cloaked underneath a blanket slowly walked past our window. Each step appeared excruciatingly labored and painful but determined. It sat down on a glider on the far end of the porch. "Cleo, doesn't it bother you to see this day in and day out?"

"What? Oh, you mean the guests? Not really. After the first couple of years, you tend to get used to it." Cleo smiled. "For many, I'm the closest thing to their families that they have."

"But, why do you do it? What possibly could you get out of living your life as some death caretaker?"

"Michal, I love you and I love you dearly...but don't you ever say anything like that again to me. I do it because I want to...I do it because I know they don't have any other options but the streets...I do it because none of you guys ever allowed me the chance to show you that I cared for you. There is never a day that doesn't go by that I don't remember our little circle. Michal, it hurt like hell losing the others but somehow I felt that you wouldn't push me away…but you did."

"Cleo, I never meant to push you away. I just didn't want to…"

"Want to what? Damn it, Michal, I'm your sister. We were a family. Family doesn't turn away from their own regardless of who they are."

"You're right. I'm sorry that I didn't stay around. I'm sorry that I pushed you away." I grabbed her hand and gently squeezed it. "I'm back if you will have me."

"In my heart, you never left me. Only in my eyes."

There we were, just the two of us. We are the last two links of the circle. Over the next few hours, we became as one again. We laughed and we cried. I glanced at the forgotten scrap book she had maintained. A pictorial history of how it once was with all of us. We both fought back the mounting tears.

"Michal, I have a confession to make…promise me you won't think ill of me. Okay?"

"You…our sainted sister has a confession to make?" I laughed.

"Yeah, I do…But, don't get me wrong…I'm not asking for any repentance because it was something that I don't ever regret doing."

"You gotta be kidding! You are so squeaky clean and pure that you make the Pope look like a deviant."

"I cheated on Edward while I was still married to him."

"No offense, but who could rightly blame you. You weren't getting it from home. We all knew he didn't love you…So, was it someone that we knew?"

"Yeah, someone we all knew." Cleo paused as she pushed her tea aside and poured white wine in a clean glass. For the first time, I noticed she was shaking. Her eyes no longer made contact with mine. "Would you like some?"

"As close as you and Seth were, I'm sure he knew. Did he blame you? Did he say that you would go straight to hell for adultery? He did know, didn't he?"

"Oh yeah, he knew…He knew everything. In fact, it almost cost me his friendship. That was the only thing I did regret about the whole thing. Possibly losing his love."

"Naw, you didn't have to worry about that. He worshiped the ground you walked on. No matter what you did, he always loved you…So, who was this mysterious guy that almost tore you and Seth apart?"

"Seth." Cleo locked her eyes deep into mine.

"Seth who?" My eyes turned into disbelief.

"The one and only…"

"Talking about missing the boat on this one. I'll be damned." I started laughing. "I'm sorry, I'm not laughing at you but…you just blew me away. Cleo, honey, I have always known that there was something about you two but I could never pin point it. You go, girl!"

"I'm glad you found it so comical…It has bothered me for years."

"Being unfaithful to Eddie boy?"

"Naw, I got over that years ago…"

"Then what got to you?"

"Allowing one intimate night with someone that I loved as a friend come between he and I."

"Cleo, what you and Seth had through the years was special. One night of passionate rolling in the hay wouldn't erase that fact. We all knew that he loved you and that you loved him. Who knows what would have happened if he had lived."

"You know, I would have done anything for him. I would have done anything for all of you guys."

"So, when did this take place?"

"Remember when we used to get together at his father's studio…One night, there were only he and I. It all started quite innocently. He was playing the piano while I stood behind him softly massaging his shoulders. For whatever reason, I leaned over and I kissed him…He kissed me back…moments later, we were lying on a pallet across the floor. I began unbuttoning his shirt and caressing his chest. He rolled me over and began making love to me…He was so gentle and ever so passionate." Cleo's eyes glistened. "Afterwards, we never acknowledged that night. It was as if it never happened."

"I can't think of a better person to experience what true love is all about."

"Thank you for being who you are and forever my friend."

"Always, until the end and then some."

"You got a few more minutes?"

"Yeah, why?"

"Come on, I want to give you the twenty-five cent tour." Before I could refuse, Cleo was standing and pulling me towards her.

We strolled through the homely structure arm in arm. Being so close to her, I smelled the familiar fragrance of Chanel perfume, her trademark. Her

PANELS

hair was still very black although there were sporadic strands of gray interspersed. Cleo was still the beautiful woman I had always known and loved.

"Do you notice anything about the different rooms?"

"No, should I?"

"Stand back…look over the thresholds."

"Omigod! This really is a tribute." I was quite surprised.

"Call it obsessive behavior…call it whatever you may. Somehow it gives me a feeling that they are here with me." Cleo paused. "Each room not only have their names engraved but also each room is decorated with something that reminds me of their personality."

"Lord, I can only imagine what you did with Bradley or David's rooms."

"Well, I did have to scale down their madness just a tad. I didn't want anyone freaking out thinking they were taking some bad trip on their meds." Cleo laughed.

" I'm surprised that you didn't just put up mirrors all over the room…including the ceilings."

"Surely you are not suggesting that either of the two of them had the slightest problem with being vain? I mean, I thought everyone had a room full of nothing but rhinestones and mirrors."

"Don't forget the drag music and the strobe light with the disco ball."

"Last, but certainly not the least…this is Seth's room." The laughter appeared to have left her very soul. She became as sedated as the room was.

The room had a soothing tone of color, not too much of a bore nor too drastic. Earth tone linen covered the three single beds and matching side chairs near the stained glass windows. Vintage black and white photographs of musicians from the past graced the walls. Current residents' personal items were scattered on the adjoining nightstands of each bed.

"When I come in this particular room…my eyes always swell. Sometimes, when this room is empty, I come here and just stare out the window…sometimes I can feel his presence in this room."

"Wasn't this the last room he stayed in before he died?"

"Yeah, the very one…the room he began to lose his mind."

"How I remember that all too well. Seth began to experience bouts of dementia. He forgot who anyone was."

"Michal, I think that was one of the hardest times of my life seeing someone I love so much lose their mind. Some days he would just look at me and stare as if to ask who the hell was I. I would kiss him every night before he went to sleep. He would only stare."

"I remember a few nights he would become angry and wanted to go home."

"I hated those times…I hated holding onto him trying to tell him he was already at home. He cursed me and told me that I was lying…then he would look straight into my eyes and ask me why was I treating him like he had done something wrong. He would always ask why was I punishing him." Cleo wiped her eyes. "I loved him but he hated me."

"Cleo, Seth never stopped loving you. That damned disease that took over his body was talking, not Seth."

"Michal, I know that. I truly do. But there were times when I doubted if I could be there for him. I went to hell and back trying to understand what was going on with him…I know what you are going to say…I know that you and Sebastian tried to talk me out of letting Seth stay here with me…But do you know what, I don't regret a single day that I shared with Seth."

"Cleo, you should be proud to realize that you gave him as well as the rest of us our dignity. You were certainly there when we were not there for ourselves. And girl, we love you for it!"

"I was just thinking…you are staying at that hotel wasting money…why don't you move in here. You know I have plenty of room."

"There you go again…Cleo, while I do appreciate your old big generous heart, I think it wouldn't be a good idea."

"And why not?" Cleo's voice turned cool. "Why wouldn't it be a good idea? It's not like we don't know each other. I need you…the others have left me."

"What about Theresa? Have you thought about her feelings?"

"What's bugging you, man? Ooh, I'm so not dealing with you…Theresa has no problem with you living here, you know that." Cleo paused. "Look, I'm not trying to crowd you, I just thought…"

"I promise that I will give it some thought, okay!" I placed my finger against her lips. I kissed her cheek and left.

The next day, I attended a support group where someone spoke about a gathering of African-American gay men living with HIV and AIDS. My interest peeked so I waited afterwards to speak privately with Wayne Jenkin, a dreadlock angel with a soft distinctive Bronx brogue that had that certain smile of innocence across his cherubic face. The name of his organization was "Brothers Untied."

Through "Brothers Untied," I was able to find hope in my despair. I was able to meet other black gay men living with this disease. I began to see my life in different perspectives. Wayne's sincerity and his mission were essential in my growth. With my new "bros" I no longer felt ashamed of neither my gayness nor my illness.

Over numerous cover dish dinners of fried chicken, spare ribs, collard greens, ham hocks, hot water cornbread, etc, I rediscovered my blackness with pride. Wayne and the others helped me to fight my illness through knowledge and emotional support.

Another sparkle in my life appeared to be that I attended that very same place where we had so many of our friends' memorials: Edgehill Church. The place had a new meaning for me. It has definitely started to fill a void. I felt accepted and even felt that my faith had been renewed. I felt as if I belonged to something again.

I invited Cleo and Theresa to join me one Sunday in October. At this particular service, the congregation celebrated what they referred to as "All Saints Day." The dead were remembered and a bell was rung for each of them as their names were called out. In front of the congregation, attached to the highest window, was a structure shaped in the figure of a dove. It was made of small crystals.

While standing in a human circle as we held hands, we recited "presente" after each name. As I called out our friends' names, I felt a reassuring squeeze from Cleo.

Moments later, I listened as a petite beautiful woman named Connye sang. Her startling delivery of "Sometimes I Feel Like a Motherless Child" touched me. I shuddered in remembering my own life. I so wanted to feel my own mother's arms around me. I didn't want to wait until it was too late. I desired her love now.

Connye's eyes were closed as her voice dominated and filled the entire room. Each note was clearly defined and passionate. Chills covered my body as she sang that song like no one else I had ever heard before.

Instead of wanting to run away from my hell, I wanted to stay and confront it. Perhaps this was my vehicle to return to my own faltering faith and make amends with myself and to my God.

I have learned that I was not unworthy of His love. Although one day, I may have AIDS, I am still accepted as a child of God unconditionally. Somehow, I think I may know exactly how the prodigal son felt upon his return home. I am no longer afraid of death. "Thou preparest a table for me in the presence of my enemies...and I shall dwell in the house of the Lord forever."

Considering my possible limited options that life had dealt me, I now know what I must do to win the battle but on my own terms. As my dear friend Sebastian had once stated: *Omni a Vincit Amor Ad finem!*

Did you ever see the classic film *The Children's Hour*? One particular scene that continued to strike me was the very last scene. The scene was the burial of her friend. The way she turned, with her head held high, and walked away without saying a word to anyone. The only emotions were dignity and grace. Without appearing too dramatic, I always wished that I could be as svelte and demure as Audrey Hepburn when she walked away from her past.

It has been six months since his death. He simply went to sleep—a peaceful rest. His head was nestled on my lap. As the last breath left him, he surrendered. I leaned forward and kissed his forehead. I wished him farewell as he began his journey.

At this very moment, I find myself gazing into the nothingness of an autumn day. I'm sitting alone on the aged glider while staring into the clear dark sky. I'm numb and my tear ducts were dry. Only the sound of the screeching metal of the glider reminded me where I was. Near me, the loose pages of his manuscript nestled inside a sturdy box, rest. I have just finished reading our story.

The pages relived the many years I shared with them. I was no longer saddened at the loss. Instead, I felt proud of my friendships. I did not regret anything I did with them. That was the type of love we had shared: honest but life saving.

It's amazing how accurate or inaccurate someone's perception of others may prove. Having read both Michal and Sebastian's depictions of myself, I doubt if I was as adolescent as either had described. Sure, the lifestyles of my closest friends were not anything that I was raised around but I certainly didn't freak out over their differences either. Each had taught me something about loving and accepting myself. With them, I felt like a real woman. With them, I was Cinderella and they were my fairy god brothers, no pun intended. With Edward, I felt as if I was only his little child. I was merely an inanimate object to be seen but never heard.

It was time to finish the last chapter of Michal's manuscript...It was time to give our lives closure. I don't aspire to write as well as either Sebastian or Michal had written but I do owe them the very best that I can do. As I struggle to find the right words, a song played on the radio. I closed my eyes and listened as someone asks to be my hero that will kiss away the pain and will stay with me forever. I imagine myself dancing with my friends. Twirling and twirling and twirling, in and out of each other's arms. Laughter filled the stoic air. Then, suddenly, the song ended and I'm left alone. Again.

"Mama, I brought you a sweater…It's getting a bit nippy out here, don't you think?" Theresa was standing directly in front of me. "Don't you think it's getting pretty dark out here to be reading?"

"Thank you…I guess I just lost track of time." I wrapped the sweater around me. "What are you doing here? I thought you and Brett were going to dinner."

"We are…I just wanted to make sure you were okay before we left." Theresa hugged me. "You're sure you don't want to go with us?"

"Lord no! There's nothing worse than a third wheel especially when two people are engaged and still play google eyes with each other." I smiled. "I will be fine here. So, you both go and have fun."

"Mrs. Castleman, it won't be a bother to have you join us. It would be a pleasure to have your company." Brett offered his hand.

"No, really. I have things I must finish here before it gets too late. Now, shoo! Neither one of you is too big for me to put across my lap and spank." I waved them away. For a brief moment, I glanced at them. How lovely they looked together. She leaned over, brushed my hair from my eyes, and kissed me on my cheek.

" I miss my uncles too!" Theresa pointed at the pages on my lap. Without waiting for a response, she grabbed Brett's hand and walked away. I watched them leave arm in arm. The love they shared appeared so untarnished and blemish-free. I clutched the box tight and whispered to my friends that they need not worry about Theresa because she had found someone that really loved her. Our little angel will be okay.

Michal's last days were beautiful. He and I often spoke about his final journey. I have never known of anyone that didn't fear death nor welcomed it as freely as he had. At first, I found the conversations quite morbid and wished for something else to talk about. But he was determined to stay on task. Over time, I began to wince less and hear more of the macabre thoughts. Perhaps it made me feel uncomfortable because I was made to address my own mortal needs. Perhaps it made me realize that I wasn't as immortal as I had once believed. For once, I realized that I too would die one day.

One morning after leaving Mass, I stopped and browsed around in St. Ann's Bookstore near the Cathedral. There it was! Sparkling in the dull light of the day was the perfect gift. Without the slightest hesitation, I purchased a St. Christopher medallion for Michal. Perhaps St. Christopher could protect Michal on his journey.

Michal had long accepted and forgiven himself. There was never any bitterness or hatred only love. Although his own family had disowned him because of him being gay, he still loved them, especially his father. Each day proved a gift, one that he cherished to the fullest.

One warm night, Michal and I were swinging on the weathered glider. All of the others had gone to bed or retired to themselves. So we were all alone. The flickering fire from the citron candles cast shadows around us. It had been a long tiring day for both of us but neither wanted to be alone at that moment. At least, not from each other. So we did what came perfectly natural to us; we talked.

" You never cease to amaze me."

"What am I guilty of doing now?" I caught his eyes.

"You continue to live here amidst all this sickness and death…You are a regular Mother Theresa, you know that!" He patted my knee.

"I guess that's a compliment. Thanks! " I moved closer to him. "I just do what comes natural to me."

"But caring for the dying…doesn't that get to you knowing that not a one of your guests will ever leave here. That they are here on a one way ticket." He turned his eyes away from mine.

"At least, when they go, they will go knowing someone cared."

"Cleo, I can see it in your eyes the sincerity with a tempting taste of hope in you. But I wonder if you are giving yourself the same care and love you give others. I wonder about the pain that lives deep down inside you that you try to hide. "

I felt a tinge of resentment. I stopped the glider and reached up and touched his face. "People always take the small things for granted. No one ever stops to really look at the clouds in their strange formations or even listen to the chirping birds."

"We become too busy with all the unnecessary garbage in life to take time."

"Cleo, why is that so? Why do we wait until it's too late to see God or his beauty?"

"Because we move away from God. Our lives become so bogged down with bull that we walk away from all that's good. Sometimes we use God as a weapon against others."

"Perhaps you're right…perhaps we do that…you know, I used to believe that I was evil. I believed that God had turned and walked clear out of my life because of who and what I was. At least that was what others had me to believe."

"That's because they didn't take the time to get to know the real you, only a part of you."

"Yeah, I know. My own flesh and blood speaks of me as if I have already died. After all these years apart and our struggle to bond again, my father still doesn't want to hear anything about me. Did I ever tell you why he divorced my Mom?" Michal paused. "Since I had failed him by not being able to pass on the glorious family name, he wanted another woman to give him another boy. Maybe this one would come without defects. It would serve that bastard right if my little half brother turned out queer as well." Michal paused. "But it really doesn't matter anymore…does it?"

"I guess not."

"One day I may start to love my family again, even with all their faults…Right now, it's a bit too painful."

"Michal, my dear, that's what love is." I patted his arm.

"I guess you are right…but do you know how it feels to love the only family you have that encompass no reciprocated love. To be hated merely because of your birthright!" The veins were raised in his neck. "I never wanted anything from them except for their love…the lowest cut was when they tried to turn my grandmother against me. I felt so damned worthless. I could not do a thing but hope and pray that she didn't listen to their lies. I would have never done anything against her. Lord only knows just how much I loved her."

"Never feel the need to defend yourself. You certainly did nothing wrong." I looked him stern into his eyes. "Only you and the Lord knows what you did, and that's all that really matters."

"I can only hope he may have forgotten some of what I did." Michal smiled his mischievous smile.

"It could have been worse…at least you are not Bradley nor David." Michal walked over to the edge of the balcony. There was a slight glimmer of the moonlight peaking through the scampering clouds. He stood and stared. I walked behind him and watched him stare into space.

"Carlin and I used to go to some of the remotest places and just star seek. I mean, we would let our minds travel far from here simply admiring the constellations…Nothing else mattered to us, nothing."

"So, what happened between you two? I thought he was good for you."

"He was…in fact he was too good for me. All my life I wanted someone to love the real me without any of my adornments. I am just plain simple old boring me. Beyond that, he was extremely honest and loving, you know husband material. When I was with him, I felt empowered. I wasn't afraid to explore my spirituality."

"So…what happened?" I was becoming quite perplexed. "Why are you guys not together anymore?"

"I just couldn't do it to him. I refused to drag him into my hell. Surely you haven't forgotten that this isn't a glamorized death…So, I consciously pushed him away."

"But he wanted to be there for you."

"Honey, Carlin was scared…he was scared that he would one day see me as one of those living corpses…Don't get me wrong, he never said it but I knew he didn't want that picture forever engraved in his life…Truthfully, he left me."

"Oh, I'm sorry. I didn't know."

"No, you didn't…you also don't know how I wish that I would never hear anyone tell me that they loved me. It only lasts for a fleeting moment…almost like a climax where you quickly leave once you're off…For all of my life, I have been searching for that one person to just love me and all my flaws. Trying to find that love has cost me my life."

"Are you afraid to be with anyone?"

"I'm here with you aren't I." Michal attempted to smile.

"You know what I mean…are you afraid of being intimate with a partner?" I turned to him. He didn't look me in the eye, merely stared into the wind.

"That, my dear, died when I found out that I was positive." He had tears in his eyes as he turned and faced me. "Now, there is no hope for finding love of any kind. My search in this life was all in vain."

"But…" I began to protest as he placed his finger to his lips."There are no but's." He stood and walked to the edge of the porch. "What a beautiful clear night. The stars are ever so distinctive. Rivers belong where they can ramble,

PANELS

eagles belong where they can fly…I got to be where my spirit can run free…gotta find my corner of the sky." Michal broke out in singing slightly under his breath. He stopped and turned back to face me. Even with the weak dying fluttering of the candles, I saw an expression of peaceful closure on his face. "One day, I will find my corner."

"You know something, Michal? I just know you will." I stared at Michal. I wanted to see his face in the candlelight. I wanted to see his smile like old times. This time, the smile was different. "You amaze me at how positive you are in face of whatever."

"Oh, don't be fooled. I haven't always been this cool about it." Michal raised his head and looked straight into my eyes.

"I don't follow you…"

"Let's just say…I haven't always been in love with God. In fact, for quite awhile, I resented the almighty. Yessirybob! I loathed everything about the great oz. I cursed the rising sun and the raised moon. I was pissed at the cards dealt me."

"But…you kept it all inside of you. I never knew how you felt about being sick."

"Hell, I could handle being sick. It was realizing that I am indeed dying. It's not like I thought I was any better than the others but…somehow…maybe I thought I would have been given a reprieve by the almighty. But obviously that wasn't in the plans."

"Michal…I don't have any of the answers nor do I know what to say. I will not lie to you and say that it does not piss me off knowing that I will someday lose you like the others. I go to Mass, light candles, and pray that I will not be alone. Maybe, He's not listening to me either."

"It's getting late. Thanks for listening to my drivel and being my friend." Michal kissed me on my forehead. "I'm going to bed. I will see you in the morning. I do love you."

"Sweet dreams." I leaned over and blew the fire out. "I love you."

The pieces of fabric were already cut and ready to be placed onto a larger swatch of material. I had searched at length for the vibrant colors to use. Each color had to be radiant. Michal had left me almost three months ago. Although I knew he was gone, I was in no hurry to complete this task…the last thing I could do for him. But still I sat motionless.

Each time I attempted to thread the needle, my eyes clouded with tears.

PHIL MICHAL THOMAS

My hands shook, not with grief, but anger. Yet, pride replaced my anger. I am proud to tell everyone about my friends. Each individual helped me become the person I am today. No longer a weak-willed, pitiful soul, but a woman with convictions.

"Mama, I want to help you." Theresa sat beside me. She began to smooth the wrinkles out of the fabric "Have you thought how you want it decorated?"

"Yeah…I have…but then, no, I haven't. It has to be something really him. Something that yells 'Michal!'" I reached over and pressed her shoulder tightly against mine. The sparkle in this young woman's eyes takes away my pain. She lives. She fought HIV and won. I know her uncles gave her that strength.

"You know, Mama, I was looking at one of the old scrapbooks. I came across this picture of you, Uncle Seth, and Uncle Michal. It looks like one from your college days!"

"Omigod! I had forgotten all about this one. It was taken on the opening night of Pippin, the first musical we did at Vanderbilt. Michal played the role of Pippin…Oh God, just look at him…He's smiling in all his glory." I kissed her cheek. "This is it!"

Several days later, Theresa, Brett, and I carefully spread the panel across the living room floor. Before we shipped this panel to Atlanta to be with the Quilt, I had to make sure everything was perfect. Tears filled my eyes. Not tears of sadness, but tears of joy. The joy one felt while seeing a dear friend honored. I stood back for a full inspection of the design.

Theresa and Brett had the photograph of Michal, Seth, and me enlarged and placed in the center of the panel. Michal's smile was still gleaming! Above our photograph were images of eagles soaring, children playing, nightingales singing, and rivers rambling. Near the top of the panel were the words:

Michal Anthony Cameron,
September 1959-June 2002.
Searching for his corner of the sky.